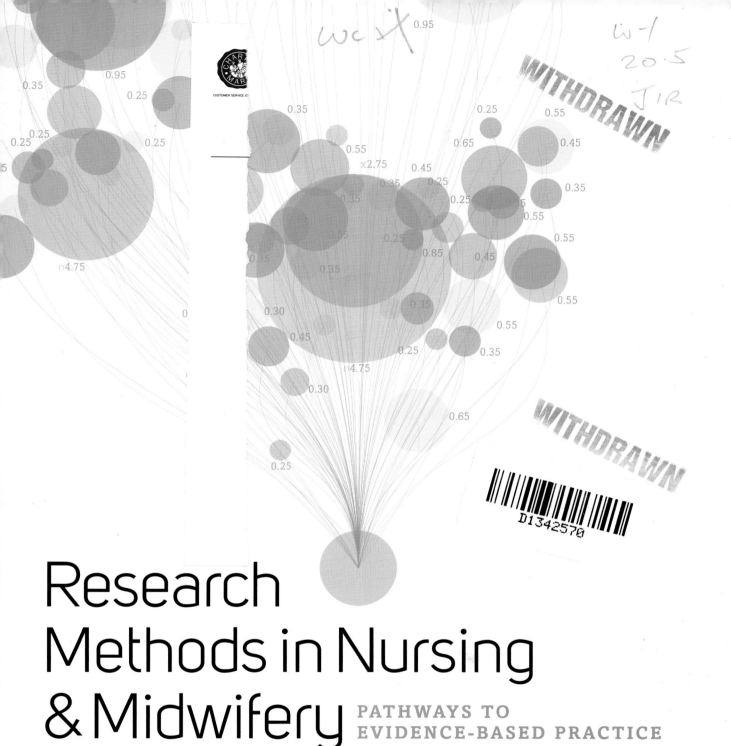

Research Methods in Nursing & Midwifery

PATHWAYS TO EVIDENCE-BASED PRACTICE

edited by

SANSNEE JIROJWONG ▸ MAREE JOHNSON ▸ ANTHONY WELCH

OXFORD
UNIVERSITY PRESS

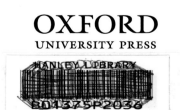

OXFORD
UNIVERSITY PRESS

Oxford University Press is a department of the University of Oxford.
It furthers the University's objective of excellence in research,
scholarship, and education by publishing worldwide. Oxford is a registered
trademark of Oxford University Press in the UK and in certain other
countries.

Published in Australia by
Oxford University Press
253 Normanby Road, South Melbourne, Victoria 3205, Australia

National Library of Australia Cataloguing-in-Publication data

Author: Jirojwong, Sansnee.

Title: Research methods in nursing and midwifery : pathways to evidence-based
practice / Sansnee Jirojwong ; Maree Johnson ; Anthony Welch.

ISBN: 9780195568189 (pbk.)

Notes: Includes index.

Subjects: Nursing–Research. Midwifery–Research.

Other Authors/Contributors: Johnson, Maree. Welch, Anthony J.

Dewey Number: 610.73072

Text design by Cannon Typesetting
Typeset by Polar Design Pty Ltd
Edited by Venetia Somerset
Proofread by Anne Mulvaney
Indexed by Russell Brooks
Printed by Sheck Wah Tong Printing Press Ltd

For Bob and the Jirojwong family, in particular Po' Pravat.
SANSNEE JIROJWONG

I would like to dedicate my contributions to this book to my parents and family,
without whom such an achievement would not have been possible.
ANTHONY WELCH

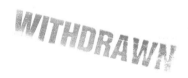

Contents

Part 2: Making Sense of Research Methods   107

List of Figures

List of Tables

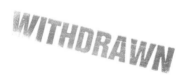

List of Abbreviations

ABS	Australian Bureau of Statistics
ACHA	Australian Community Health Association
ADHD	Attention deficit hyperactivity disorder
AHPA	Allied Health Professions Australia
AIDS	Acquired immune deficiency syndrome
AIHW	Australian Institute of Health and Welfare
ALP	Australian Labor Party
APA	American Psychological Association
ARC	Australian Research Council
ATSIC	Aboriginal and Torres Strait Islander Commission
CALD	Culturally and linguistically diverse
CAM	Complementary and alternative medicine
CAT	Critical appraisal tool
CATI	Computer assisted telephone interviewing
CCFR	Centre for Child and Family Research
CI	Confidence interval
CINAHL	Cumulative index to nursing and allied health literature
CNC	Clinical nurse consultant
DRG	Diagnostic related groups
EBM	Evidence-based medicine
EBMid	Evidence-based midwifery
EBN	Evidence-based nursing
EBP	Evidence-based practice
ED	Emergency department
EMS	Extended midwifery services
GD	Gestational diabetes
GP	General practitioner
HAPI	Health and psychosocial instruments (database)

HGP	Human Genome Project
HIV	Human immunodeficiency virus
HRECs	Human research ethics committees
IQR	Inter-quartile range
JBI	Joanna Briggs Institute
MAStARI	Meta-analysis of statistics assessment and review instrument
NFER	National Foundation for Educational Research
NHMRC	National Health and Medical Research Council
NICU	Neonatal intensive care unit
OR	Odds ratio
PLS	Plain language statement
QARI	Qualitative assessment and review instrument
QUAL	Qualitative
QUAN	Quantitative
RA	Research assistant
RCT	Randomised controlled trial
RN/M	Registered nurse/midwife
RR	Relative risk
SD	Standard deviation
VAS	Visual analogue scale
WHO	World Health Organization
WMD	Weighted mean difference

About the Editors

Sansnee Jirojwong (PhD) is a Senior Lecturer at the School of Nursing and Midwifery, University of Western Sydney. Sansnee has taught nursing and midwifery students at undergraduate and postgraduate levels. She has undertaken research projects in Thailand, Brunei Darussalam and Queensland, Australia. Sansnee's research projects have focused on the health of disadvantaged groups such as migrants and rural people. Migrant behaviours while they are in a host country or returning to their home country have been explored. She has been involved in a number of projects in Queensland rural communities and has worked closely with local health practitioners. She has also worked with local communities and disadvantaged groups to increase the accessibility of health and social services to migrants. The most recent project has used the participatory communication concept as a framework to develop health education resources for Vietnamese-born pregnant women who have gestational diabetes. Sansnee's research articles are published in international refereed journals and conference proceedings. With Professor Pranee Liamputtong, Sansnee has recently co-edited a textbook published by Oxford University Press, *Population Health, Communities and Health Promotion: Assessment, Planning, Implementation and Evaluation*.

Maree Johnson (PhD) is a Clinical Professor at the School of Nursing and Midwifery, University of Western Sydney. Maree is a nurse and epidemiologist with 27 years experience of research in the university and health sectors. In addition, she is a visiting Professor to the School of Nursing, Midwifery and Health Systems, University College Dublin. As Director of the Centre for Applied Nursing Research (a joint facility of the University of Western Sydney and Sydney South West Area Health Service and Joanna Briggs NSW Collaborating Centre for Evidence-based Health Care) she has assisted academics and clinicians to successfully complete research projects, including at Honours, Masters and PhD level. Her expertise includes the use of complex sampling procedures from population sampling frames, conducting population-based surveys, instrument design and testing, advanced quantitative research designs and analysis procedures, and grounded theory and ethnographic studies in qualitative research. Other aspects of her current role include undertaking systematic reviews and developing clinical guidelines for health professionals. Professor Johnson has published in national and international refereed journals in nursing and health, as well as books, monographs and commissioned government reports. Professor Johnson has taught undergraduate research units in the Australian Capital Territory, New South Wales and Victoria and has a contemporary understanding of the textbook requirements of undergraduate and postgraduate research students.

Anthony Welch (PhD) is a Senior Lecturer at the School of Nursing, Queensland University of Technology. Prior to his current appointment Anthony was Associate Professor, Mental Health Nursing at Royal Melbourne Institute of Technology University. Anthony has held a number of positions in nursing in both the private and public sectors of the health care industry (Australia, New Zealand, Hong Kong and Singapore). Anthony has been Director of both undergraduate and postgraduate programs at a number of universities. Anthony's research projects have involved the use of both qualitative and mixed-methods of enquiry. The focus of his research has been on mental health concerns, particularly in relation to men's health, transcultural issues and humanbecoming. Anthony is a recognised senior international Parse scholar and researcher within the Humanbecoming School of Thought.

About the Contributors

Petra Gertraud Buettner (MSc, PhD) is an Associate Professor at James Cook University, Queensland. Petra studied Mathematics and Physics at the Friedrich-Alexander University of Erlangen/Nuernberg, Germany. She completed her PhD on measurements of consistency and conformity with the Technical University and the Free University of Berlin, Germany, in 1994. Petra moved permanently to Australia in 1995 and has been working at the School of Public Health, Tropical Medicine and Rehabilitation Sciences, James Cook University, since then. She has more than 20 years experience in lecturing undergraduate medical, nursing and allied health students as well as postgraduate Master of Public Health students in research methodology, epidemiology and biostatistics. Her main research interests are quantitative methods in epidemiology, design and analysis of epidemiological studies and clinical trials, and cancer epidemiology, especially skin cancer epidemiology. She has co-authored more than 100 original research publications in peer-reviewed journals as well as several book chapters.

Monika Buhrer-Skinner (RN, MPH&TM, PhD cand) completed her education as a registered nurse in 1985 in Germany and as a certified registered nurse anaesthetist (CRNA) in 1988 in Switzerland where she subsequently worked in several roles as a CRNA including aero-medical retrieval and clinical education for more than 10 years. In 1996 she completed a Bachelor of Nursing Science (Post-Registration) and in 1998 a Master in Public Health and Tropical Medicine at James Cook University, Australia. Monika started working in clinical and research nursing roles in sexual and reproductive health in Australia in 2000. In 2003 she joined James Cook University and has been a lecturer teaching quantitative research methodology to undergraduate and postgraduate health science students. Her main research interests are in the area of sexually transmissible infections, especially *Chlamydia trachomatis* infection, which is also the topic of her doctoral project.

Sungwon Chang (PhD) has extensive experience in quantitative data analysis, mainly in the areas of large data set management and collection. She also has advanced knowledge and skills in sampling, psychometric testing procedures and multivariate analysis including structural equation modelling. Sungwon has used her biostatistics expertise in a number of collaborative research projects within health services and clinical research. She currently teaches in research methods and biostatistics to undergraduate and postgraduate students at University of Western Sydney, School of Biomedical and Health Sciences. Her areas of research interest include exploring a range of measures in clinical trials including composite endpoints.

Keri Chater (PhD) completed her nursing at the Alfred Hospital in 1980. In 1984, she completed her Bachelor of Arts from La Trobe University and then continued her study and completed Master of Nursing at Royal Melbourne Institute of Technology (RMIT) University and a doctoral degree from La Trobe University. Until recently she was employed at RMIT University as a lecturer in nursing. Her areas of specialty are aged care nursing and nursing ethics. She has extensive experience in aged care research as well as being a member of the University Ethics Committee. Currently she is employed at Westgate Aged Care facility where she is the Clinical Coordinator. She is an active researcher and the coordinator of the facility ethics committee.

Ritin Fernandez (PhD) is a Senior Lecturer at the School of Nursing and Midwifery at University of Western Sydney. Before this appointment she was the Manager of the South Western Sydney Centre for Applied Nursing Research (CANR), held from May 1999. Ritin is also the Deputy Director of the NSW Centre for Evidence Based Health Care, which is the NSW Collaborative Centre of the Joanna Briggs Institute. Ritin has over 20 years of clinical experience, mainly in coronary care and intensive care nursing. She is actively involved in secondary prevention research related to heart disease management and is a strong advocate of the use of technology in this area. Along with other projects, Ritin is the principal investigator in the DHARMA Project, which aims to develop effective interventions for heart disease reduction and maintenance among Asian Indian people living in Australia. Her teaching and research interests have focused on chronic disease management, cardiovascular disease, evidence-based practice, randomised controlled trials and diagnostic studies. Ritin completed her first research project in 2000 and since then has been awarded research grants of more than $800 000. She has published 47 peer-reviewed journal articles and over 70 peer-reviewed conference presentations. Ritin is currently co-supervising five research higher degree students and is an active peer reviewer for several national and international journals.

Rhonda Griffiths AM (PhD) is Head, School of Nursing, University of Western Sydney. She is also the Director of the NSW Centre for Evidence Based Health Care. Professor Griffiths completed her first research project in 1988 and since then has been awarded research grants of more than $3 million. She has published more than 120 peer-reviewed journal articles and book chapters and over 100 peer-reviewed conference presentations and 40 invited papers. She has extensive experience in research translation, having been a member of a team that has published 10 systematic reviews. She also has completed research utilisation projects with clinicians in a tertiary referral hospital. She is currently a chief investigator of an NHMRC-funded project to develop evidence-based guidelines for the management of type 2 diabetes mellitus.

Cecily Hengstberger-Sims (RN, PhD) is an Associate Professor at the School of Nursing and Midwifery, University of Western Sydney. Cecily has extensive experience in the development and implementation of units of study relating to nursing research. She was the Foundation Director of the Graduate Nurse and Research Practice Unit (now the Centre for Applied Nursing Research), a conjoint appointment between a local Area Health Service and the University of Western Sydney. Cecily has successfully supervised a number of Honours and research higher degree students. She retains an active interest in evidence-based practice and nursing research and her current research interests include effective team communication, transition to new graduate practice, innovative teaching and learning strategies in nursing research.

Jackie Lea (MN) is a registered nurse, lecturer and clinical coordinator in the School of Health at the University of New England. Jackie's career has focused on patient care within medical and surgical settings and the clinical education of student nurses. Jackie has extensive clinical nursing experience within rural and metropolitan health care facilities and she has provided clinical education to undergraduate nursing students from the University of New England, University of New South Wales and Curtin University, Western Australia. Jackie teaches clinical nursing practice and patient care to students in the external and internal undergraduate and postgraduate nursing courses. Her research interests include new graduate nurses, rural nursing practice and recruitment and retention issues in nursing. She has presented papers at numerous national and international conferences and workshops, and has published in a number of nursing refereed journals.

Janice Lewis (MBus, DBA) is the Program Leader for Health Policy and Management courses in the School of Public Health, Curtin University, Western Australia where she teaches health services management and qualitative research methodology at postgraduate level. Her main areas of interests are health policy and qualitative research methods. She developed a doctoral subject in qualitative research that has a strong mixed methods component. She has also developed a research methodologies unit for Open Universities Australia, which combines both qualitative and quantitative methodologies. She has presented papers on mixed methods at international conferences.

Pranee Liamputtong (PhD) is a Professor at the School of Public Health, La Trobe University, Australia. Pranee has particular interests in issues related to cultural and social influences on childbearing, childrearing and women's reproductive and sexual health. She has published several books and a large number of papers in these areas. Pranee is a qualitative researcher and she has also written several textbooks on research methods, both traditional and innovative qualitative research methods including *Qualitative Research Methods* (Oxford University Press, 2009), *Researching the Vulnerable: A Guide to Sensitive Research Methods* (Sage, 2007), *Knowing Differently: Arts-Based and Collaborative Research Methods* (Nova Science Publishers, 2008), *Research Methods in Health: Foundations for Evidence-Based Practice* (Oxford University Press, 2010), and *Performing Qualitative Cross-Cultural Research* (Cambridge University Press, 2010).

Phillip Maude (PhD) is an Associate Professor at Royal Melbourne Institute of Technology University. Phil is the Director of Research Programs and a coordinator of mental health/addictions programs at RMIT University. Phil has more than 16 years experience in nursing education and is a fellow of the ACMHN and a member of both the RCNA and DANA. Phil's research interests include historical work, practice development and cognitive behavioural interventions for violence, self-harming and addictions. As such he has supervised PhD students who use diverse research methods and has an interest in engaging students in the use of research evidence to improve clinical practice. He holds a PhD, Master of Nursing (Research), Postgraduate Diploma (Primary Health Care), Bachelor of Health Science, a Diploma of Mental Health Nursing and Certificate in Addictions.

Reinhold Muller (MSc, PhD) is an Associate Professor at James Cook University, Queensland. Reinhold is the Principal Epidemiologist/Biostatistician of the School of Public Health, Tropical Medicine, and Rehabilitation Sciences at James Cook University, a position he has held since 1995. He holds a PhD in epidemiology, an Honours degree in statistics and a Masters degree in informatics. Over the last 20 years, Reinhold has been conducting, analysing and publishing as principal investigator a wide variety of quantitative epidemiological studies covering diverse areas such as infectious diseases, occupational health, nursing, rehabilitation and cardiology. His experience comprises two decades of teaching quantitative research methodology (epidemiology, biostatistics, research design, statistical software) at undergraduate, postgraduate and doctorate levels. He has also been consulting and collaborating with various government departments, non-governmental organisations and diverse industry bodies. Reinhold's publication list encompasses more than 200 articles in international peer-reviewed scientific journals and three textbooks on evidence-based quantitative research methodology.

Penny Paliadelis (PhD) is a registered nurse and senior lecturer at the University of New England and the Nursing Course Coordinator and Deputy Head of School of Health. Penny's clinical expertise is in critical care and paediatric nursing. Penny teaches undergraduate and postgraduate nursing courses and supervises higher degree research students. Her research interests include the broad area of rural nursing practices as well as the organisational culture of health care systems, particularly in relation to the roles of nurses in managerial and leadership positions. Penny has published a textbook, book chapters and journal articles and has presented her work at numerous national and international conferences.

Glenda Parmenter (PhD) is a registered nurse and lecturer at the School of Health, University of New England (UNE). Her clinical background focused on aged care nursing and community-based palliative care and she teaches these topics in both the undergraduate and postgraduate nursing courses at UNE. Her research interests concern the social lives of rural nursing home residents and the experience and professional development of nurses working in rural areas. She has published a book chapter and journal articles on these topics and presented her work at national and international conferences.

Karen Pepper (PhD) is a lecturer in the Discipline of Behavioural and Social Sciences in Health at the Faculty of Health Sciences, University of Sydney. She teaches units of study on research methodology and data analysis for the health sciences, as well as units of study on behavioural sciences. Her research interests include investigating the relationship between psychological factors and health, with an emphasis on the application of statistical analysis to health and psychological research.

Jamie Ranse (MCritCareNurs) has a nursing background in emergency and intensive care. At different times his career has focused on aspects of clinical, education and research. Jamie is actively involved in research within the pre-hospital and critical care environment and has a number of peer-reviewed publications relating to pre-ambulance, pre-hospital care and resuscitation experience. He has presented his work at various national and international conferences. Jamie is an editorial board member for the *Australasian Emergency Nursing Journal* and an invited reviewer of manuscripts submitted to a number of Australian and international journals relating to primary health care and critical care nursing.

Jan Taylor (PhD) is a midwife and a senior lecturer in the Faculty of Health, University of Canberra. She has been involved in teaching research to nursing and midwifery students for the past 10 years as well as supervising higher degree research students. Jan is particularly interested in quantitative research methods and her research and clinical interests revolve around women's experiences following birth. She has presented her research at numerous national and international conferences.

Jane Warland (PhD) is a registered nurse, registered midwife and lecturer in nursing and midwifery at the University of South Australia. Jane teaches in the undergraduate nursing and midwifery program and also supervises research students. Jane's research interests include population health (epidemiology and health promotion), mental health (maternal and child mental health) and maternal health (midwifery). She is also active in conducting project work in the area of teaching and learning. Jane has conducted research projects using qualitative, quantitative and mixed methods. She has published a textbook, book chapters and journal articles and has presented her research at numerous national and international conferences.

Lisa Whitehead (PhD) is a senior lecturer and Deputy Director at the Centre for Postgraduate Nursing Studies, University of Otago, Christchurch, New Zealand. Lisa convenes postgraduate research methods papers and manages a research program focusing on long-term health condition management. The program includes research studies on symptom management, with a focus on the assessment and management of fatigue, improving patient and family experiences of long-term conditions and the role of internet interventions in managing long-term conditions.

Acknowledgments

This book could not have been completed without the support of many people. The University of Western Sydney—School of Nursing and Midwifery provide support through their library and office resources. Students who studied research subjects have made comments on their learning experiences and their reflections. Useful information has been used to frame our book concept and revise the overall pedagogy of the book. Their ideas and opinions are valuable to us as they represent the majority of the readers of this book.

The first author would like to acknowledge Sally Schukking, Karen Mannix and Isragul Flemming for their help with administrative aspects. Dr Sharon Hillege and Heidi Creed made valuable suggestions on many figures in Chapter 6. Professor Robert MacLennan, an experienced researcher and epidemiologist, has provided critical comments as the book has been progressing through time. Sansnee is grateful for his support.

Anthony Welch would like to acknowledge his companion and friend Stephen Gellion for his continuing support and encouragement over the years as he has ventured down the path of his professional pursuits and personal aspirations. To his sisters and brothers who have been an ongoing source of pride and love. A special thanks to his beautiful Old English Sheepdog Pierre who, on many occasions corralled him in his office and maintained the watch to prevent any disruptions or distractions throughout the process of working with Sansnee and Maree on this book.

We also would like to thank Debra James at Oxford University Press for her patience and understanding of our situations as university academics, researchers and laypersons. Her collegiality is much appreciated by all of us. We value the important contributions by all contributors, who have been so marvellous in responding to our emails, requests and explanations. They have shared their research experiences in their individual chapters.

The authors and publisher are grateful to the copyright holders for granting permission to use the various figures, examples (or modifications of) and data in this book. Every effort has been made to trace the original source of the material reproduced in this book. Where the attempt has been unsuccessful, the authors and publisher would be pleased to hear from the copyright holder concerned to rectify any omission.

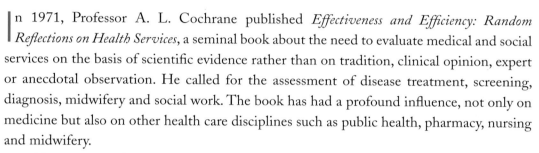

Introduction

Sansnee Jirojwong and Anthony Welch

In 1971, Professor A. L. Cochrane published *Effectiveness and Efficiency: Random Reflections on Health Services*, a seminal book about the need to evaluate medical and social services on the basis of scientific evidence rather than on tradition, clinical opinion, expert or anecdotal observation. He called for the assessment of disease treatment, screening, diagnosis, midwifery and social work. The book has had a profound influence, not only on medicine but also on other health care disciplines such as public health, pharmacy, nursing and midwifery.

About antenatal care, he wrote:

> This service is basically a multiple screening procedure, which, by some curious chance, has escaped the critical assessment to which most screening procedures have been subjected in the last few years and there seems no reason why the same approach that has proved so useful elsewhere should not be used here.

He went on to say, 'Much more doubtful is the therapeutic use of iron and vitamins… My general impression is that the emotive atmosphere should be removed and the subject treated like any other medical activity' (p. 66).

Over the past 40 years, especialy since the 1990s, evidence-based practice has been adopted world-wide as an important principle in health care. Despite Cochrane's achievement, much still needs to be evaluated.

Over more than seven decades, the professions of nursing and midwifery have made considerable advances in the development of discipline-specific knowledge and clinical expertise. Such advances can be attributed to the application of new information to clinical practice. This has led to quality improvement in all areas of nursing and midwifery professional practice. The generation of new knowledge has not occurred in isolation but as a result of applying a systematic and rigorous approach to the search for answers to issues arising in everyday professional practice. Research is the process of questioning and searching for answers to a problem or issue of concern.

Within contemporary nursing and midwifery practice there are few clinicians, educators and students who fail to perceive that learning about research is relevant to their practice. They acknowledge the benefits of research but still see it as something 'out there' to be accessed if needed but not viewed as part of professional practice.

We read the results of research published in the press or listen to discussions about research findings on the radio. They can also appear as a short message flashing on internet websites. Health care consumers who are searching for information from these media to improve their health may use these findings. As health care professionals, we need to be able to read and decide whether the results are credible, whether they are to be used by health care consumers or not. This means we need to understand the concept of research process and research methodology.

Evidence-based practice depends on a careful recording of evidence, such as is widely carried out in health care. For example, What is the evidence for deciding to have flu vaccination? can be asked when you suggest to a patient to increase their immunity against flu. Evidence is also based on the synthesis of research results. People who take on the task of generating or creating the evidence need to be able to identify and differentiate the evidence from 'good' projects from that resulting from 'not so good' projects.

Different kinds of knowledge can be generated by different pathways. Researchers can generate knowledge by conducting research and collecting data from participants in the field or in clinical areas. They can have data retrieved from records kept by hospitals, long-term care settings or community health organisations. Knowledge can be also generated by analysing and synthesising the results of a number of research studies. This research textbook is written in order to demonstrate that research is a process and there is a pathway that readers and researchers can follow.

Many health issues are complex. Clinicians often ask why such issues are occurring. There may be so many questions to ask about a particular health issue that it will be difficult for clinicians to answer all of them at once. Many questions may be answered by the findings of quantitative research; let us think, for example, about a warm sponging and rest as ways to reduce body temperature. Many others can be answered by qualitative research; let us think about having elders included as important persons who can link health care workers and Indigenous patients in some communities so the care can be increasingly accepted or adopted by the patients.

We use schematic pathways in order to identify the solutions of health issues. Health issues and research questions can be raised and then answered quantitatively or qualitatively. Some can be answered by using both approaches in what is called mixed methods research. After the research question has been asked, a certain pathway will guide the researcher on what research design will be used, how data or information can be collected and what methods can be used to analyse the data so that the questions can be answered.

In this book we use a schematic pathway that readers can use when analysing research publications or planning a research project. We hope that students, clinicians and researchers can understand why certain aspects of research are used by researchers in a given context or environment. The pathways will also help researchers to stand back and ask themselves whether all research steps follow a coherent sequence. The strong and weak points of a project can be identified from analysing the research pathway.

This book has been written for undergraduate nursing and midwifery students who study research or an evidence-based practice subject. It is of particular interest to lecturers who teach research, evidence-based practice and evidence-based nursing. The book provides information on research principles, systematic reviews for evidence-based practice, and emerging issues of practice development using evidence-based practice as a guide.

The overall approach of the book comprises principles used in conducting a research study and systematic review for evidence-based practice, beginning with major principles of research such as the research process, specific research methods, population, sampling, data collection and data analysis.

The emphasis throughout is on evidence-based practice. Generally, evidence-based practice is now required in all health care settings. It is taught as a single subject or combined with traditional research subjects. The connection between research and evolving practice has been increasingly recognised in major health care institutions. Undergraduate students are required to know about research to be able, for example, to understand the steps in making a systematic review of published research and clinical guidelines. The book discusses the application of these concepts to various health care settings and conditions.

As far as possible, each chapter is self-sufficient and can be understood without having to read the whole book, but maximum utility can be gained by reading the chapters in sequence. Case studies in different settings are used as examples when discussing the content of each chapter. Selected health and illness conditions are used as examples or case studies.

Although many nursing research and evidence-based nursing textbooks have focused on research methodology and evidence-based nursing, little is available on systematic reviews, and there is not much work clearly demonstrating a link between research and nursing/midwifery practices. Some books have used Australian examples and some have in-depth information useful for postgraduate students. This book covers general principles of conducting a research project, a systematic review for evidence-based nursing, and its application to practice development. References and additional resources are provided in context and enable readers to explore the material in greater depth. We suggest internet sources as resource materials at the end of each chapter, under the heading Weblinks.

In each chapter, the following features are individually presented: chapter objectives, key terms, concepts relevant to the chapter and various exercises in critical thinking, practice and problem solving; answers are given for self-assessment. The reader will find the boxes that highlight cases or specific points a useful reading tool. When possible, examples or case studies are based on clinical settings throughout Australia.

The book is divided into three parts. Part 1 presents issues to be considered before undertaking a research project. Part 2 discusses principles, processes, steps and issues relating to the conduct of a research project. Part 3 discusses various components of the dissemination of research findings. The application of the important aspects of evidence-based practice is emphasised throughout.

The first chapter outlines the importance of systematic research in generating knowledge, and the relevance of this to nursing and midwifery. The general purposes of conducting research in health care disciplines in developed countries are set out and research development in nursing and midwifery at a global and national level are analysed. The principles adhered to in conducting research include paradigms and methods for nursing and midwifery research and the use of inductive and deductive approaches. A general overview is given of the implication and application of research to evidence-based nursing and midwifery.

It is widely known that research is a systematic process whereby a series of related activities are developed or planned and then enacted, and the outcome of the process is presented to the scientific community for scrutiny and ultimate acceptance as new knowledge. In Chapter 2 on the research process, the authors introduce the reader to the key components of the research process: selecting a topic; refining the research question; literature review with a focus on synthesis and argument development; developing aims or objectives, hypotheses, questions; exploring research methods and examining analysis procedures; setting up timeframes; and finally, budgeting and potentially grant-seeking for projects. These components are presented within a research proposal structure and are elaborated in the other chapters.

Chapter 3 outlines the legal and ethical considerations in research, starting with the history of bioethics and research. All research undertaken has to adhere to a strict set of legal and ethical guidelines and nursing research is no different. Ethical comportment in research had its genesis in the Nuremberg Trials after the Second World War and was formalised in America in 1974 under the National Research Act. This act set the standards for conducting bioethical research and delineated concepts such as autonomy, beneficence and justice. Australia followed with a national Australian Human Ethics Committee; hospitals, universities and government departments have human research ethics committees that guide the conduct of research and approve research applications.

This chapter addresses the legal and ethical issues nurses encounter when conducting research. The principles associated with ethics, such as autonomy, rights, confidentiality, beneficence and non-maleficence, are described. A section deals with vulnerable populations, in particular research with/on Indigenous groups. The final section suggests how the legal and ethical principles outlined above can be applied to the actual process of putting together a research proposal.

It will become difficult, or even impossible, for researchers in nursing to avoid carrying out research regarding vulnerable and marginalised populations within the 'moral discourse' of the postmodern world, because it is likely that these population groups will be confronted with more and more problems in their private and public lives as well as in their health and well-being. In Chapter 4, salient issues for the conduct of research among vulnerable groups of people have been brought together. The task of undertaking research with such groups presents researchers with unique research opportunities, and yet dilemmas.

Chapter 5 discusses qualitative enquiry and qualitative research designs. A brief account of the evolution of qualitative methods and the rise of the human sciences is presented to provide a context for the various qualitative approaches to research. Particular attention is given to a discussion of the ontological and epistemological underpinnings of qualitative research designs and methods, and their potential to contribute to advancing existing knowledge of nursing and midwifery practice. The place of qualitative research in evidence-based practice is discussed in light of contemporary nursing and midwifery practice and the social imperative to demonstrate outcome effectiveness. The use of case studies and critical thinking exercises gives the reader opportunities to engage in critical reflection on the significance of qualitative research in contributing to the generation of new knowledge that informs nursing and midwifery practice.

Quantitative research designs are presented in Chapter 6. A number of quantitative designs can be applied in nursing and midwifery research. Setting a research question determines what type of research design will be used. This chapter provides information on major types of quantitative research including both experimental and non-experimental research designs. Other quantitative research designs widely used in epidemiological studies are discussed. In addition, other types of quantitative research such as program evaluation and audits in practice development are explained.

Mixed methods research is discussed in Chapter 7. This is a class of research where the researcher mixes or combines qualitative and quantitative research techniques, methods, approaches, concepts or language into a single study. Although this type of research has a long history, it is only recently that mixed methods approaches have been a focus of mainstream research. Mixed methods research is not without its debates and controversies. As an emerging discipline there are still a number of methodological challenges to be resolved. It is, however, a rapidly growing area of research enquiry. The chapter describes the main positions regarding mixed methods—whether or not it is appropriate or indeed possible to combine qualitative and qualitative methods. The incompatibility thesis is debated. The purpose of mixing methods—the classification of purposes of corroboration, elaboration, complementarity and contradiction used to structure the discussion—are presented. The strengths and weaknesses of mixed methods research and the challenges for the researcher are explored.

Chapter 8 discusses various important aspects of research populations and sampling. The principles that underpin normal populations and the central limit theorem are outlined and graphic presentations emphasise these principles. The importance of sampling frames, types of sampling frames, and examples of how to access and use them are defined. The chapter deals with quantitative sampling methods such as random selection, systematic sampling, cluster sampling, purposive and convenience sampling, and quota sampling. Sampling methods used in qualitative studies, such as theoretical sampling, snowball sampling and convenience sampling, are also explored. Finally, the authors explore some important aspects of recruitment and managing bias in sampling.

Chapter 9 introduces the reader to the procedures and processes involved in qualitative data collection. A range of data collection methods and tools, for example individual and focus-group interviews, participant observation and videotaping, are discussed in terms of their usefulness for eliciting research data. The issue of ensuring rigour, a criterion of qualitative enquiry, is examined from several points of view. Particular attention is given to the achievement of rigour and trustworthiness in the philosophical and methodological tenets underpinning a study design. The chapter examines the use of triangulation as a way of strengthening a study by combining different approaches. The process and means of data collection in relation to evidence-based nursing and midwifery practice are discussed.

Quantitative data collection methods are presented in Chapter 10. The methods used to collect data are a crucial element in determining the quality of research. The emphasis in this chapter is on practical information to support the selection of a method to match the research purposes and to maximise the quality of the findings. Commonly used approaches such as surveys, interviews and observational methods are outlined and their advantages and disadvantages are discussed. The use of tools, checklists and rating scales to collect data are detailed using examples from nursing and midwifery research. Measurement is an essential component of quantitative data collection and the principles underlying measuring concepts are described.

Technological advances have expanded the options for generating and collecting data and the problems and challenges of using computer programs and the internet to design and collect survey data are outlined. Particular methodological issues such as sample bias, response rates, and privacy and confidentiality are discussed, along with strategies designed to minimise the disadvantages. The usefulness of internet sources such as SurveyMonkey for creating and managing surveys is considered.

Chapter 11 gives readers an overview of qualitative data analysis before focusing on the processes of analysis related to three key methodologies: grounded theory, ethnography and phenomenology. Various topics presented in this chapter include general considerations when conducting qualitative data analysis, the qualitative data analysis process, matters to be considered to ensure rigour in data analysis, and data management and organisation. The use of software to facilitate organisation and management is briefly described.

Chapter 12 presents concepts and examples of quantitative data analysis. A solid understanding of statistical methods is vital to evidence-based research in all scientific areas that use quantitative studies. This chapter provides an overview of the main concepts of statistical analysis, focusing on practical applications and the correct interpretation of results.

Basic principles of the description and presentation of quantitative data are introduced. The underlying theory and implications of statistical hypothesis testing are outlined and the main bivariate statistical tests are presented. Basic steps to prepare quantitative data for multivariate analysis are discussed. An overview of the most common multivariate techniques used in medical and allied health research is presented together with some basic guidelines.

A critical review of research is presented in Chapter 13. This chapter introduces the concept of critique and gives guidelines for the critical appraisal of published literature. A health professional's ability to critically read and understand research publications is essential to any practice development activity, when considering a reason for changing practice or when implementing evidence-based care. The chapter guides readers through a series of steps to assist them to develop a sound approach to critical appraisal of literature. Critique methods for qualitative and quantitative articles are presented using case study examples.

Chapter 14 presents the steps in making a systematic review of research, which is important in the development of quality nursing care. It outlines the principles used when formulating clinical questions, and identifying, searching and critically appraising the relevant literature. Findings, including meta-analysis for quantitative data and meta-synthesis for qualitative data, are summarised. The use and availability of computer software programs and tools for undertaking critical appraisals as well as conducting systematic reviews are detailed. The chapter discusses the role of collaborative groups such as the Cochrane Collaboration and the Joanna Briggs Institute in developing and promoting evidence-based health care.

Methods used to disseminate research and its results are discussed in Chapter 15. In order for nursing and midwifery practice to reflect an evidence base, research findings need to be disseminated. Dissemination of research can take the form of theses, books, reports, scholarly journal articles, conference papers, posters and media releases. In other words, research is meaningless unless an account of the study and the findings adds to the body of knowledge and is shared with others. Becoming a published author is also a positive achievement and is vital for career development for many senior or specialised nursing positions. Thus the aim of Chapter 15 is to demystify the process of writing for publication and presenting conference papers and reports. Many nurses and midwives find this part of the research process daunting, so the chapter focuses on understanding how and where to disseminate research and describes ways of sharing research knowledge and outcomes locally, nationally and internationally. Approaches are outlined that will assist in maximising opportunities to publish or present research findings, by choosing the right journal or conference. Case study examples of Australian conference papers and journal articles are used to demonstrate the process of turning research outcomes into publications, reports, media releases and conference papers.

Guided Tour

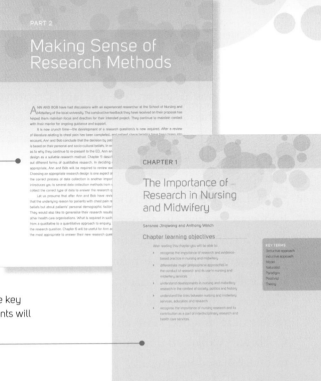

Part openers introduce and follow the characters of Ann and Bob as they embark on a research project, drawing out the main issues dicussed in the following chapters

Chapter openers introduce the key terms and objectives that students will explore throughout the chapter

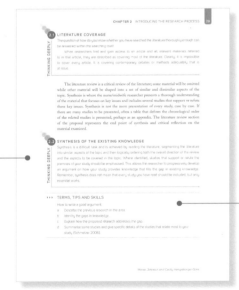

Thinking deeply encourages further discussion and critical reflection of a topic, and takes students beyond a basic level of understanding

Terms, tips and skills help students build their understanding of research methods terminology and provide guidance on key aspects of the research process

Research in practice/evidence-based practice provide research examples and practical cases to enable students to link the importance and application of research to clinical practice

END OF CHAPTER MATERIAL

Summary and Implications for evidence-based nursing and midwifery consolidate learning and highlight the significance of the issues discussed

Problem solving and Practice exercises help students apply their learning and stimulate critical thinking

Further reading and Weblinks provide valuable resource materials encouraging students to extend their knowledge further

Pathways to Evidence-based Practice

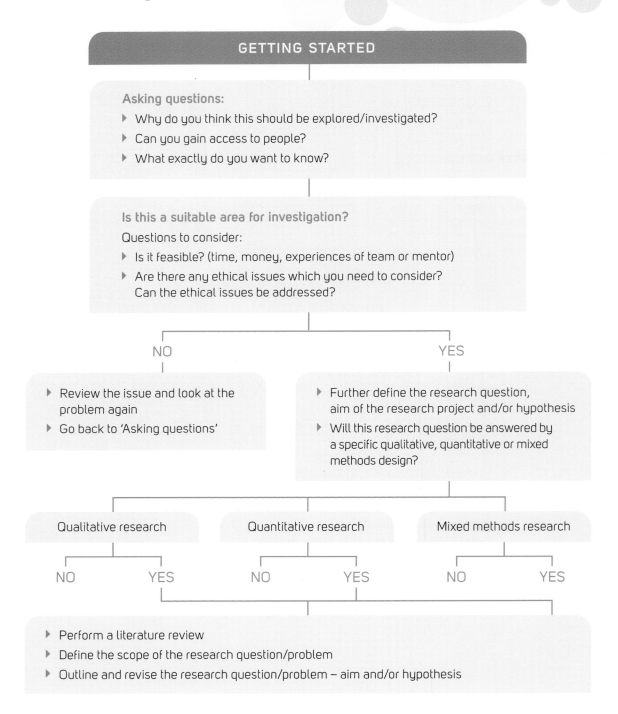

GETTING STARTED

Asking questions:
- Why do you think this should be explored/investigated?
- Can you gain access to people?
- What exactly do you want to know?

Is this a suitable area for investigation?

Questions to consider:
- Is it feasible? (time, money, experiences of team or mentor)
- Are there any ethical issues which you need to consider? Can the ethical issues be addressed?

NO
- Review the issue and look at the problem again
- Go back to 'Asking questions'

YES
- Further define the research question, aim of the research project and/or hypothesis
- Will this research question be answered by a specific qualitative, quantitative or mixed methods design?

| Qualitative research | Quantitative research | Mixed methods research |
| NO   YES | NO   YES | NO   YES |

- Perform a literature review
- Define the scope of the research question/problem
- Outline and revise the research question/problem – aim and/or hypothesis

▶ What is the lived experience of patients who present to the ER with chest pain?

Qualitative research

▷ Select the research design
See Chapter 5 – Qualitative Research Design

▷ What type of data is to be collected?
See Chapter 5 – Qualitative Research Design and Chapter 9 – Data Collection: Qualitative Research

▷ What data collection approaches and processes will be used? For example, face-to-face interview, focus group interview, observation, document search
See Chapter 9 – Data Collection: Qualitative Research

Data analysis
Qualitative research

▷ Is the analysis process descriptive, interpretive, critical or theory building?

▷ What processes will be used? Thematic analysis, content analysis, coding (using manual or computer programs)
See Chapter 9 – Data Collection: Qualitative Research and Chapter 11 – Qualitative Data Analysis

▷ Interpret and present the findings

▸ What is the lived experience of patients who present to the ER with chest pain?
▸ Will patients with self-management tools have fewer presentations to the ER than patients who do not use such tools?

Quantitative research

▸ Select the research design
  See Chapter 6 – Quantitative Research Design
▸ What is the sample?
  See Chapter 8 – Populations and Sampling
▸ What is the study setting?
  See Chapter 3 – Ethical and Legal Considerations in Research
▸ How will data be collected?
  See Chapter 10 – Data Collection: Quantitative Research

Data analysis
Quantitative research

▸ What is the form of the data?
▸ Is it a nominal, ordinal or a continuous measure?
▸ Will the research question and the data be answered by univariate, bivariate or multivariate analysis?
  See Chapter 12 – Quantitative Data Analysis

▸ Interpret and present the findings

▸ What are the experiences of patients with chest pain attending an
ED and how does this affect their future ED attendances?

Mixed methods research
▸ Outline the research questions, aims and/or hypothesis

Selecting the methods

▸ Check again whether both qualitative and quantitative research is
needed for the study?

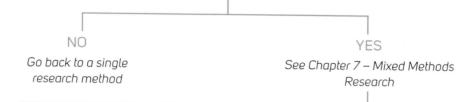

NO
*Go back to a single
research method*

YES
*See Chapter 7 – Mixed Methods
Research*

▸ Does the qualitative or quantitative component have a complementary
or unique contribution to the study?
▸ Are the qualitative and quantitative components of equal or unequal
importance in the study?
▸ In what order does the research question need to be answered or the
data collected? Nested, parallel, sequential?

Select research design
▸ What is the sample?
▸ What is the study setting?
▸ What data is to be collected?
▸ How will data be collected?
See relevant chapters for both quantitative and qualitative research

Data analysis for both qualitative and quantitative data
See relevant chapters for both quantitative and qualitative research

▸ Interpret and present the findings

Interpreting and presenting the findings
▶ Qualitative, quantitative, mixed methods research

▶ Are conditions and factors that may affect the findings identified and described?

▶ Have the research questions been answered or has the hypothesis been tested? Is it statistically significant or non-significant?

▶ Are key findings from the quantitative research presented?

▶ Are themes, conceptual understandings or other findings from the qualitative analysis presented?

▶ Have the findings been compared and contrasted with findings from other studies?

▶ Are further research studies identified?

▶ What are the implications for patients, clinicians, educators, managers, and other health care professionals?

PART 1

Getting Started in Research

ANN AND BOB are registered nurses working in a busy emergency department (ED) of a large referral hospital. They observe that many patients who present with chest pain are discharged after a few hours of observation. However, it is also observed that half of these patients repeatedly re-present to the ED. Ann and Bob would like to explore why this group of patients continue to re-present to ED and what additional services can be provided after discharge to help them manage their condition better and therefore reduce the rate of re-presentations. Ann and Bob are aware that a number of research publications are available, including systematic reviews and guidelines for pain management, and so they decide to review what is known about pain management before deciding how to go about researching this issue. As this is their first project, Ann and Bob want to ensure that the project will be conducted to the best of their ability—in a systematic and rigorous manner. As the hospital has links with a local university Ann and Bob decide first to consult experienced researchers for direction and guidance. The decision to undertake this project sets them on the path of research.

Chapter 1 gives important information about beginning the research journey: the processes involved in starting your first piece of research, for example, identifying a researchable question, and working with experienced researchers as mentors. Chapter 2 introduces the reader to the processes involved in developing a research proposal: selecting the topic, developing a researchable question, reviewing the research literature to identify what is already known about the topic, establishing aims and objectives for the project, and exploring an appropriate research design.

Undertaking research in health means that information, that is, data, is obtained either directly from individual participants or from health records of individuals held by health or health-related organisations. It is not uncommon for researchers to have access to sensitive information about people. To ensure that such information is treated with respect, and in confidence, legal and ethical regulations and guidelines for conducting research have been drawn up. Chapter 3 discusses what the researcher needs to consider in order to achieve research credibility. Issues addressed in this chapter include confidentiality, privacy, benefits, potential for harm and how to obtain ethics approval.

Chapter 4 provides in-depth information about various research issues when vulnerable and disadvantaged groups are research participants. You may want to combine information provided in this chapter with the information in Chapter 3 as they are clearly linked with each other.

After reading the four chapters of Part 1, Ann, Bob, and you the reader, will have sufficient information to get started in putting together ideas about the actual focus of the intended study. The pathway shown in the front of the book summarises the major steps involved at this early stage of the research journey.

CHAPTER 1

The Importance of Research in Nursing and Midwifery

Sansnee Jirojwong and Anthony Welch

Chapter learning objectives

After reading this chapter you will be able to:

▶ recognise the importance of research and evidence-based practice in nursing and midwifery

▶ differentiate major philosophical approaches in the conduct of research and its use in nursing and midwifery services

▶ understand developments in nursing and midwifery research in the context of society, politics and history

▶ understand the links between nursing and midwifery services, education and research

▶ recognise the importance of nursing research and its contribution as a part of interdisciplinary research and health care services.

KEY TERMS

Deductive approach

Inductive approach

Model

Naturalist

Paradigm

Positivist

Theory

Introduction

There are various ways by which we as human beings come to know and understand our everyday world (Streubert & Carpenter 1995). Over the centuries different forms of knowledge have been developed and valued by individuals and societies. As a young child we come to value the knowledge of our parents. We go to them for information and for guidance. As we move into our teens we begin to question what they know and start to seek out our own way of understanding our world and what is important to us. At high school and university we enrol in different subjects to acquire particular forms of knowledge for our future career pathway such as nursing, teaching, architecture or psychology. Within your nursing program you study different subject areas to gain particular forms of knowledge: science, to understand the molecular world of the cell; biology, to learn about the workings of the human body; psychology, to understand human behaviour and the way people think and interact; and research, to learn how to determine what is the most appropriate form of knowledge or the best evidence on which to make clinical decisions about, for example, aseptic technique, pain management, caring for a person with a mental illness and their family, or deciding whether breastfeeding or bottle feeding is best for a mother and her new baby.

Over the past six decades scientific knowledge and technology have expanded. The health of populations has improved significantly, with an increase in life expectancy and a reduction of morbidity and mortality from infectious diseases (Beaglehole & Bonita 2004). Changes to nursing and midwifery services, education and research have occurred in many developed and developing countries such as the USA, UK, Australia, New Zealand, Thailand, Indonesia and Malaysia.

In Australia, nurses and midwives were formally recognised as health care professionals in the early 1980s. This was the result of political, social and professional forces such as scientific discoveries, the use of technologies in medicine and public health services, the expansion of Australian universities, the increasing number of nursing and midwifery leaders with postgraduate qualifications in education, and the requirement of graduate education for beginning nurse clinicians (Greenwood 2000). Nursing and midwifery education is now located in the tertiary education sector. Knowledge of the practice of nursing and midwifery has expanded as the professions have become increasingly cognisant of the need for clinical practice to be underpinned by research. Clinical practice informed by research is increasingly demanded by the general public, who expect practising nurses and midwives to provide care that is evidence-based (International Council of Nurses 2006; Nursing and Midwifery Board of Australia 2010).

The professions of nursing and midwifery will experience ongoing changes in response to an increasingly ageing population, rising health care costs, and the use of technology in the health care sector. The shift towards empowering health consumers to be active participants in managing their health, and the increasing expectation of the consumer to self-manage, challenges nurses and midwives to be responsive and adaptable to these trends.

In this chapter, the importance of nursing and midwifery research and evidence-based practice is emphasised. The identification of existing and emerging problems in nursing and midwifery are from the perspectives of two major philosophical approaches, positivism and naturalism. Both approaches will be described in the context of nursing and midwifery research. The future of nursing and midwifery research and evidence-based practice will be presented in the context of ongoing changes in Australian social, political and professional environments.

The place of research in generating knowledge

Let us reflect on how health knowledge was generated in traditional societies. People observed that certain behaviours would have certain outcomes. Women who were carers would encourage sick people to rest and drink plenty of fluid because they saw that the recovery process was faster when the sick attempted to do something rather than doing nothing. The use of trial and error as an approach to problem solving was the most common means of identifying what worked and what did not. Communities and individuals depended on cultural beliefs, social customs, traditional healers or acknowledged experts as the main sources of knowledge for decisions about health and quality of life. Over time, trial and error has been replaced with a more effective way of generating knowledge and applying it systematically.

As nurses and midwives, we have improved our practices as new knowledge of what is more effective has become available from convention, custom and tradition, the opinion of experts, observations, the experiences from trial and error, and research (Burns & Grove 2009). Examples are early ambulation among post-operative patients, and the use of pets in providing emotional support for residents in long-term care. Planned investigations help consumers of research—nurses, midwives, researchers and educators—to apply research results to their work environment. The result will be improved practice.

We all use research results in one form or another. For example, clinical guidelines based on the synthesis of research results are used in our daily working life. We care for patients and their families who vary in their knowledge and the management of their illness. It is our business to ensure that our clients have the most up-to-date and appropriate knowledge with which to make informed decisions about their care and management. To be effective in improving health outcomes for clients and their families, we need knowledge that is evidence-based. We, as nurses and midwives, also need to be competent in evaluating the strengths and weaknesses of research studies, and the applicability of their findings to our work environment.

The importance of evidence-based nursing and midwifery practices

As mentioned earlier, health professionals such as nurses and midwives use different sources of information for the delivery of services. In the 1960s Archie Cochrane found that much of clinical practice in health services lacked evidence of effectiveness, resulting in wastage of health care resources and sub-optimal outcomes. Cochrane was a strong advocate of randomised controlled trials (RCTs) (Cochrane 1972; Cochrane Collaboration 2010). In 1976 the first systematic review of controlled trials in perinatal medicine began in the UK. The Cochrane Centre opened in Oxford in 1992 with registration of the Pregnancy and Childbirth Group and its Subfertility Group. In 1993 at a conference in New York, the concept of the Cochrane Collaboration was presented by the New York Academy of Sciences. Since that time there has been rapid and extensive adoption of the concept. By January 2009 there were 5676 completed Cochrane reviews and protocols (see the approach used for this research in Chapter 14), which are available to health care workers and consumers.

Sackett and his colleagues (1996), pioneers of the Cochrane Collaboration and the Centre for Review and Dissemination, defined evidence-based medicine as 'a conscientious, explicit and judicious use of current best evidence in the decision making about the care of individual patients' (p. 2). In 2000, the definition was expanded further to include client values and clinical expertise. The evidence needs to be generated by systematic investigation. Patients' illness condition, rights and preferences are considered when making clinical decisions about their care. Clinicians use their personal expertise and the best available evidence in the delivery of care. The definition of evidence-based medicine is also applied to evidence-based nursing (EBN) and midwifery (EBMid) (see Chapter 14).

Since the early 1990s evidence-based nursing and midwifery practices have been actively promoted by York University and McMaster University (Craig & Smyth 2007). Over these two decades, there has been a growth of publications of EBN and EBMid practices by different organisations including the International Council of Nurses, the Australian Nursing and Midwifery Council, and the Joanna Briggs Institute (JBI) (see Greenwood 2000; Usher & Fitzgerald 2008). These publications are as brief as a one-page summary or a comprehensive document of more than 40 pages. The range of formats accommodates the needs of consumers who may wish to access such evidence.

Levels of evidence are classified according to the validity and reliability of research (NHMRC 2009). Comprehensive criteria used to assess the quality of quantitative research have been well developed (see Chapter 14). Analysis and synthesis of experimental research are considered to be level I evidence. It should be noted that the Australian National Health and Medical Research Council (NHMRC) does not allocate any level to the opinions of experts (see Table 1.1).

Table 1.1   Levels of evidence according to the type of intervention

Level	Intervention
I	A systematic review of Level II studies
II	A randomised controlled trial
III-1	A pseudo-randomised controlled trial (i.e. alternate allocation of some other method)
III-2	A comparative study with concurrent controls: • Non-randomised, experimental trial • Cohort study • Case-control study • Interrupted time series with a control group
III-3	A comparative study without concurrent controls: • Historical control study • Two or more single-arm studies • Interrupted time series without a parallel control group
IV	Case studies with either post-test or pre-test/post-test outcomes

Source: National Health and Medical Research Council (2009).

However, Polit and Beck (2010, p. 37) have included levels V, VI and VII:

Level V: Systematic review of descriptive, qualitative or physiologic studies
Level VI: Single descriptive, qualitative or physiological study
Level VII: Opinions of authorities or expert committees.

Compared to quantitative research, qualitative research has been classified at levels V and VI evidence, based on qualitative evaluation of reliability and validity. Currently the Cochrane Collaborative Research Groups and the Joanna Briggs Institute are developing criteria for evaluating evidence from the perspective of qualitative research.

Purposes of research

What is research? We do research because we are curious and interested in solving problems. 'Research is a systematic investigation which aims to discover new knowledge or to validate and refine existing knowledge' (Burns & Grove 2009, p. 2). The professions of nursing and midwifery are committed to generating new knowledge that informs their practice and to validating best practice for health care delivery.

Nurses and midwives are in a good position to generate research questions because they provide direct and continuous care to individuals, families and communities. New knowledge can be initiated through our observations. For example, a nurse in Sydney was the first to observe an increase in congenital malformations in newborn children of mothers who had been treated with thalidomide during pregnancy. Subsequent investigations confirmed that this was a world-wide phenomenon (McBride 1962; Smithells & Newman 2009).

Nursing and midwifery care vary across a broad range of contexts from illness prevention, health promotion, acute and chronic care settings and school health, to terminally ill persons who are receiving palliative care at home or in a hospice. Our clients can also be a community, such as people in rural and remote areas or disadvantaged people.

Like other professionals, nurses and midwives need to be aware of new knowledge about emerging trends and innovations in health care delivery that are informed by research. It is quite common to find a single issue investigated by many researchers. Of these, few projects may have findings that corroborate each other, while others may have findings that contradict those of other projects. The question that needs to be asked is, Which study gives the most credible findings and provides the best outcomes that we can use? The process used to critically analyse a large number of research studies concerned with exploring the same issue is called 'systematic review' (Cochrane Collaboration 2010; Craig & Smyth 2007; see Chapter 14).

Knowledge development is an ongoing process. It occurs in response to a continual advance in technology and the changing health care needs of clients and society. As part of a multidisciplinary health care team, it is important to be aware that knowledge in nursing and midwifery can be improved or confirmed through the synthesis of knowledge from other health disciplines' research.

THINKING DEEPLY

1.1 PATIENT INFORMATION

Nurses observe that a few post-operative patients require pain relief medication more than others. They start talking to patients in order to explain why. One possibility is the patients' fear of surgery and the post-operative situation. The nurses know that fear can be reduced by providing the patient and their family with knowledge about the operation and what is to be expected post-operatively.

To investigate the problem, two approaches can be used: quantitative research and qualitative research. The choice of approach depends on the philosophical orientation of the nurses. Aspects of both approaches are often used on the same problem. Qualitative research is based on enquiry into human quality and action and should consider all circumstances in which that quality and action occur. There must be an endeavour to extract some general observations with regard to these (Law 2007; Rée & Urmson 2004). Open-ended questions (qualitative) provide an opportunity to explore a broad sweep of experiences such as What does it mean to care for another who is in pain? The knowledge generated from such a study can provide information that can be tested by quantitative research. The latter is based on the premise that real knowledge must preclude the possibility of error and logic (Law 2007; Thompson 2003).

Quantitative and qualitative research have arisen from worldviews on how knowledge can be discovered. Characteristics of both research methods are summarised in Table 1.2.

The philosophical approach of quantitative research is that knowledge is good, that it accumulates through time and that it builds on previous knowledge. If the knowledge is true, it needs to stand the scrutiny of time or be tested in different environments and groups of people. An event cannot occur without preceding events, so it has to occur as the result of previous events. A particular event needs to be precisely observed or measured without any interference from other events. The hypotheses of the occurrence of an event can be tested in different environments and different groups of people. Hypotheses can never be proved absolutely because no event in the world can be proved at once, since there could be alternative hypotheses not considered. A hypothesis is only capable of being falsified (Susser 1986).

THINKING DEEPLY

1.2 SYSTEMATIC RESEARCH

People in European countries always see white swans. It would be incorrect to state that 'All swans are white' as there are black swans in Western Australia. A better way to make such a statement is, 'Not all swans are white' and testing this statement in different locations. Researchers or testers can falsify their statement and have more and more confidence that a swan is likely to be white. When they come across a black swan, then the statement is accepted as true.

This indicates that researchers are unable to check an event that occurs all over the world. The best they can propose is to 'falsify' that the event is not true.

You can apply this situation to many health issues. For example, we may assume that patients with terminal illness may want to know the prognosis so they can plan their life or activities. This may not be true in certain cultures as there may be a cultural belief that the psychological health of patients with terminal illness should be maintained by not letting them know about imminent death. This knowledge will not be confirmed if no systematic investigations or research are conducted among different cultural groups.

RESEARCH AND EVIDENCE-BASED PRACTICE 1.1

1.1 QUANTITATIVE RESEARCH—THE CONCEPT

Based on observations described in Thinking deeply 1.1, a team of nurses plan to assess the influence of fear and social support on some patients' perceived pain so that their care can be improved. If they can provide evidence that fear has more impact on the level of pain than social support, interventions can be made in order to reduce fear before the operation. If social support has more impact, supporters of patients may need to be included in the pre-operative care so that their support can be enhanced, potentially reducing the patients' pain. The literature provides information that fear, social support and pain can be investigated and measured. Based on the team's philosophical approach, quantitative research is likely to be used.

The use of quantitative research to explore human behaviours has been criticised because it includes phenomena that have been predetermined by researchers and separated from their overall context, and also because the control applied in quantitative research does not allow the voice of participants to be heard.

Nurse and midwife researchers who want to focus on human experience and ways by which humans come to understand and interpret their everyday world therefore prefer a qualitative approach to enquiry. Qualitative research generates information that produces understanding of the human condition in all its manifestations.

More than 40 terms are used to explain qualitative research. Among them are research frameworks or designs (ethnography, phenomenology, grounded theory), theoretical perspectives (naturalistic, constructivist, humanbecoming, humanistic) and methods (interviewing, observation, document analyses) (Goodrick 2010). Chapter 5 discusses various qualitative research designs and theoretical perspectives. Readers are advised to seek detailed information from advanced qualitative research textbooks.

The foundation of qualitative research is the philosophical stance that reality is constructed by individuals as part of their everyday experience of living. Lincoln and Guba (1985) support such a notion by suggesting that a constructed reality 'fosters the idea that there are multiple realities…and [therefore] there is more than one way to know something and that knowledge is context bound' (Streubert & Carpenter 1995, p. 9). In the context of research, 'ideas and knowledge belong to participants (agents) rather than the researcher (spectator)' (Flew 1971, p. 258). The characteristics of qualitative research as shown in Table 1.2 reflect the nature of the research paradigm.

Note that the term 'naturalistic' has a range of meanings. It may mean that data collection is conducted in a natural setting where participants feel comfortable about providing information on their experiences devoid of any control by the researcher. It is holistic in that the context of the experience is captured. The results of qualitative studies can generate hypotheses that can form the basis of both qualitative and quantitative studies.

Qualitative research—the concept

Based on the scenario in Thinking deeply 1.1, the team of nurses discuss the problem and find out that their patients are from several social and demographic backgrounds. Their responses to pain also vary. Long-term illness and previous use of analgesics appear to affect patients' perceived level of pain. The team concludes that the experience of pain from the perspectives of their patients needs to be explored. They expect that the results of their research will help provide care that meets the needs of an individual patient.

Table 1.2   Major characteristics of qualitative and quantitative research

Characteristic	Qualitative research	Quantitative research
Philosophical approaches to knowledge development	Naturalistic, interpretive, humanistic, metaphysic	Logical positivism
Focus	Broad, subjective, holistic	Concise, objective, reductionist
Reasoning	Dialectic, inductive	Logistic, deductive
Basis of knowing	Meaning, discovery, understanding	Cause and effect relationship
Theoretical orientation	Generates theory	Tests theory
Researcher involvement	Shared interpretation, subjective	Control, objective
Methods of measurement	Unstructured	Structured
Data	Words	Numbers
Analysis	Interpretive	Statistical analysis
Findings	Understanding of phenomena	Generalisation

Source: Modified from Burns & Grove (1997)

Inductive and deductive reasoning in research

Inductive and deductive reasoning are applied in human reason and enquiry (Thompson 2003). Inductive reasoning works from 'a set of specific facts to a general conclusion. Specific phenomena are observed and a general statement is later formed' (Burns & Grove 1997, p. 6). Inductive reasoning is applied in qualitative research.

In contrast, deductive reasoning begins from a general premise with logical consequence to a specific conclusion. If the premise is false, generally the conclusion is also false. Deductive reasoning is used in quantitative research. The hypothesis testing and probability used in quantitative research have been developed from the argument that true understanding can be achieved by testing whether a premise is false. If the premise can be tested and is shown to be not false, it remains as probable but is never confirmed. Therefore, it is more accurate to use deductive reasoning to observe the falsifiability of a premise (Susser 1986). Table 1.3 gives a schematic representation of differences between inductive and deductive reasoning.

Table 1.3   Examples of inductive and deductive reasoning

	Inductive reasoning	Deductive reasoning
Characteristic	From specific to general	From general to specific
Example	Specific: Bleeding during pregnancy is stressful to pregnant women. Having high blood sugar during pregnancy is stressful to pregnant women. General: All symptoms during pregnancy are stressful to pregnant women.	General: All humans are mortal. Specific: John and Mary are human. Therefore, John and Mary are mortal.

The hypothesis to be tested in quantitative research (see Chapters 6 and 12) is stated as, 'No relationship between two variables (null hypothesis)'. If it is proved that this null hypothesis is false, the relationship between both variables is probable. In other words, an alternative hypothesis which stated that 'There is a relationship' is likely to be valid, given a good study design, lack of bias, appropriate sample and adequate sample size.

Two examples of hypotheses used in quantitative research are:

- *Null hypothesis:* There is no relationship between health care workers' perceived risk of infection and their hand washing.
- *Alternative hypothesis:* There is a relationship between health care workers' perceived risk of infection and their hand washing.

Quantitative research is considered a scientific approach. Original hypotheses may result from observations, intuitions and human imagination. Observations and subsequent systematic investigations can provide information that refutes traditionally held beliefs such as stress causing peptic ulcer (Marshall & Warren 1984; Marshall et al. 1988) and shoes causing a higher prevalence of *Hallux valgus* in women (MacLennan 1966). Possible hypotheses may be proposed and considered so that the most likely hypothesis can be formally investigated to explain a phenomenon (Thompson 2003). Demonstrating that a hypothesis is false may lead to the generation of another hypothesis.

One requirement of the knowledge generated from scientific investigations is that it needs to be scrutinised. New knowledge may refute or support currently held knowledge. Acceptance of new knowledge by others in the profession may take years, as in the research by Marshall and Warren (1984). Traditional beliefs held by medical practitioners were that stress and acidity caused peptic ulcer. An alkali was one of the treatments. Marshall and Warren reported research results that bacteria cause peptic ulcer, which challenged standard clinical practice and greatly reduced the cost of treatment.

Paradigms for nursing and midwifery research

A paradigm is the thought pattern in a scientific discipline or the theory of knowledge (Flew 1971). Historically, knowledge was gained through observations and trial and error. An individual who accumulated knowledge or expertise on particular issues was another source. The truth of this knowledge could be tested.

Since the late 19th century, technologies and scientific enquiries have been used to improve the health of populations. This improvement was gained through scientific methods such as laboratory experiments and field trials. This theory of generating knowledge is referred to as the positivist paradigm (see Table 1.2) and it underpins quantitative research.

The application of a positivist approach to research, especially in the area of human behaviour, was criticised for its apparent inability to explore human experience from a holistic perspective. The limitations of the positivist paradigm to conduct research in this complex area of human existence has led to the development of another research paradigm, the 'naturalist paradigm'.

Qualitative research methods are still evolving and need to be consolidated. However, researchers such as Kleinman (1980) and Leininger (1988), pioneers in using qualitative research in health, proposed conceptual frameworks that have been used in many nursing and midwifery research studies (Fawcett 2002).

Recently the combination of qualitative and quantitative approaches, referred to as a mixed methods approach to research, has been applied to many disciplines, including nursing and midwifery. Understanding the principles behind this approach is necessary because it is not a simple matter of combining quantitative and qualitative approaches in a study. Chapter 7 explains mixed methods research in detail.

The role of theory in nursing and midwifery research

Increasing death and illness due to chronic diseases, the increasing cost of technology in health care, and the shift towards a holistic view of the aetiology of illness have led to the development of models and theories to explain individual health and illness in families and communities. The development of such theories in nursing and midwifery has a similar history. The Nightingale theory, which emphasised cleanliness in individuals and environments (Geison 1995), was developed at a time when infectious diseases were the leading causes of death. Poor nutrition, environment and public health infrastructure were discovered to be major contributing factors to illness and death.

The growth of current nursing theories began in the early 1980s, initially in the USA and the UK. Professionalism and nursing education at tertiary level were major factors leading to the development of nursing theories. More than 27 theories have been proposed, falling into four classes: philosophy, grand theory, middle-range nursing theory and micro theory (Marriner-Tomey 1994; Marriner-Tomey & Alligood 2006) (Table 1.4). As research and evidence-based practices grow, new knowledge is being generated. New theories such as Trans-cultural Dynamics in Nursing and Cultural Safety theory have been developed and tested, while some theories such as the Behavioural System by Johnson have been found to have limited use. Some theories such as the Cultural Care Theory and the Pender Health Promotion Model have been reviewed and revised as the result of their use in research projects. Readers who are interested in learning more about nursing theories are recommended to read other sources that focus on these matters (see Further reading).

Table 1.4 Examples of theories and research using some of these theories

Major levels of nursing and midwifery theories or models	Examples of theories or models
Philosophy of Nursing	F Nightingale: Modern Nursing E Wiedenbach: The Helping Art of Clinical Nursing V Henderson: Definition of Nursing L Hall: Core, Care and Cure Model J Watson: Philosophy and Science of Caring P Benner: From Novice to Expert-Excellence and Power in Clinical Nursing Practice
Grand Theory	DE Orem: Self-Care Deficit Theory of Nursing MR Rogers: Unitary Human Beings C Roy: Adaptation Model B Neuman: System Theory I King: Theory of Goal Attainment
Middle Range Theory	IJ Orlando: Nursing Process Theory RT Mercer: Maternal Role Attainment KE Bernard: Parent-Child Interaction Model M Leininger: Cultural Care Theory NJ Pender: The Health Promotion Model
Micro Theory	Stress-Strain-Coping Theory Pain Gate Theory

Sources: Greenwood 2000; Marriner-Tomey 1994

What is the purpose of theory for research and evidence-based practice?

In the early 1970s recognition of nursing and midwifery as health professions in North America and the UK led to changes in education, research and practice. Nurses, midwives and other health professionals clearly indicated their need to have a body of knowledge relevant to their specific disciplines. The educational backgrounds of leaders have also influenced the development of theories. Early theories were originally used as philosophical frameworks of educational programs in tertiary education institutions (Gruending 1985; Tompkins 2001;

Walsh 1998). These theories included Philosophy and Science of Caring, From Novice to Expert—Excellence, Power in Clinical Nursing Practice, and Humanbecoming, each of which has been used in educational and clinical practice research. Research projects have been conducted to evaluate the application of selected elements of theories to the world of clinical practice. These theories are still evolving. Some of the theories have proved useful in their application to clinical practice, while others have had limited success (see also Greenwood 2000).

While educators and researchers have focused on the conduct of primary research, many practising nurses and midwives have questioned the relevance or applicability of research in light of the complex and ongoing changes occurring in clinical environments. Socio-cultural and political backgrounds and contexts of health care systems, communities, clinicians and clients influence the application of research. At an individual level, barriers to using research include lack of time, lack of interest, and inability to access or understand research publications (Usher & Fitzgerald 2008).

The implementation of research in a specific location or organisation depends on the development of professional relationships between researchers and clinicians. Many strategies have been established to link researchers and clinicians in research endeavours. Some of these include in-service training programs, creation of research positions in health organisations, and joint appointments between universities and hospitals.

The emergence of the evidence-based practice movement and the establishment of organisations such as the Cochrane Systematic Review Groups, the Joanna Briggs Institute (JBI) and the Evidence-Based Nursing Institute at York University have facilitated the translation of research findings to the actual points of care by practising nurses and midwives. These organisations have devoted resources to reviewing and summarising the findings of research publications that identify best practice outcomes (see also Chapter 14). Many journals, for example *Australian Journal of Advanced Nursing*, *Journal of Advanced Nursing* and *Advance in Nursing Sciences*, have also published results of systematic reviews of research publications. Organisations such as the International Council of Nurses and the World Health Organization Nursing and Midwifery program (WHO 2002) also provide evidence-based information for nurses and midwives.

Qualitative research has become increasingly accepted as a philosophical approach to knowledge development. Meta-synthesis has been developed to identify evidence from the results of such research. However, ongoing assessments are needed of the translation of the evidence to actual care in clinical areas. Health care systems, health care professions, and social and cultural characteristics of clients are major factors that can influence the applicability of evidence. Details of the systematic review including meta-analysis and meta-synthesis can be found in Chapter 14.

The future use of nursing and midwifery theories and frameworks in research

Changes in societies will influence the advancement of theories and frameworks in research and evidence-based practices. An ageing population, increased health care costs, high expectation of health care services and empowerment of health care consumers are some factors to which nurses and midwives must respond. Health information is now widely available to consumers through the internet and many commercial publications. Increased understanding of genetics and its use in screening and the provision of care has the potential to impact significantly on future health care. Health care personnel also have to increase their evidence-based knowledge so that credible, valid and effective care is provided. All of these factors will influence the use of theories and frameworks in nursing and midwifery research.

Developments in Australian nursing and midwifery research

As professions, nursing and midwifery have made significant advances in Australia and New Zealand over the past four decades. The evolution of these advances is integral to contemporary nursing and midwifery practice, research and education. The relocation of nursing education from the vocational and hospital sectors to universities has been instrumental in achieving recognition of nursing and midwifery as professions. Nursing and midwifery education in Australia is underpinned by a strong focus on research and evidence-based practice.

Acknowledgment of the importance of research to advancing clinical practice and the increasing interest in nurses and midwives engaging in research is evidenced by the number of research journals and research institutes now in existence, and the number of universities offering undergraduate and postgraduate studies in nursing and midwifery.

The Joanna Briggs Institute has reviewed and issued more than 57 nursing and midwifery best practice publications (JBI 2010). There are more than 30 nursing schools/departments/faculties that offer undergraduate and postgraduate programs (Hobsons 2009), and more than six refereed journals that publish both quantitative and qualitative research findings. In the Australian tertiary education sector, there is a demand on student places for higher degrees by research. The collaboration between education and practice sectors in the development of clinical guidelines has been a significant advancement in the provision of quality patient care.

Looking ahead: Research and its application in nursing and midwifery care

Nurses and midwives are parts of a health care team. Their roles and responsibilities in contributing to community health are well recognised. Support has been provided by the Federal Government, which has allowed nurse practitioners and midwives to access Medicare benefits and PBS prescribing (Medicare Australia 2010).

Increasing control of local health care services requires nurses and midwives to be responsive to local needs and to be accountable for their services. For this, research-based knowledge and evidence-based practice are required.

The social and demographic characteristics of health care consumers are continually changing. The proportion of aged persons from culturally and linguistically diverse (CALD) backgrounds will increase faster than the aged population from Anglo-Saxon backgrounds (Aged and Community Services Australia 2008; Australian Institute of Health and Welfare 2007). Varying health care needs of different population groups such as the disadvantaged Indigenous, long-term unemployed and homeless people must be met. Socially and culturally appropriate care is needed. The complexity of the health care workforce, the high turnover rate and the lack of health care workers in certain locations will continue to be problems. Research leading to evidence-based practice and the provision of quality holistic health care seem the only solutions.

1.2   RESEARCH AND EVIDENCE-BASED PRACTICE 1.2

Caring for the elderly

Elderly people constipate more often than younger people. This is related to lack of mobility, no roughage in their diet such as vegetable or fruit, and inadequate fluid intake. One of the guidelines developed by the Joanna Briggs Institute focused on caring for elderly people who are at risk of constipation. The guideline recommended that 'For persons unable to walk or who are restricted to bed or otherwise incapacitated, exercises such as low trunk rotation, pelvic tilt and single left lifts are advised' (JBI 2008, p. 1).

Use your own words to explain why this guideline generates nursing knowledge based on research studies.

Mentoring

Maria is a third-year nursing student who has her clinical placement at a medical ward. She is mentored by Yvonne, a registered nurse. Maria observes that Yvonne has drawn up heparin in advance before checking the prescriptions of their patients. Yvonne explains that it is a routine that medical patients receive heparin to reduce the chance of deep vein thrombosis. Does Yvonne use the results of research correctly? Why/Why not?

Comments: There are at least two major issues relating to the use (or incorrect use) of research findings by Yvonne. The first is that not all patients have equal risk of having deep vein thrombosis. The second is that Yvonne is not complying with the rules of medication administration. She is introducing a health risk to patients because of her practice.

Summary

Over more than six decades, significant advances have taken place in nursing and midwifery that have seen both professions providing leadership in the development of policy and global health care practices. These advances can be attributed to developments in nursing and midwifery education, research and practice. Theory development informing practice, paradigm shifts in philosophical beliefs about what constitutes professional practice, and the increasing complexity of health care needs of individuals, families and communities have been key elements influencing the changing patterns of professional practice. One of the main challenges for nursing and midwifery is to recognise the importance of research evidence as an integral component of professional practice.

IMPLICATIONS FOR EVIDENCE-BASED NURSING AND MIDWIFERY

Not all health issues can be investigated by quantitative research methods. Descriptive research and qualitative research can also provide quality evidence. It is important that researchers and research users are aware of reasons for the use of a particular research design. Systematic reviews such as meta-analysis and meta-synthesis are used to evaluate the results of quantitative and qualitative research. Different sources ranging from refereed journals, professional organisations and health care organisations provide many evidence-based practices and practice guidelines. Nurses and midwives need to gain access to information applicable to their practices.

In Australia, evidence-based nursing and midwifery have great potential because of their contributions in the educational and health care sectors. It is important that they continue to be responsive and proactive to emerging health issues in society.

Practice exercise 1.1

a   Based on your personal experiences, list three major changes in Australian nursing and midwifery professions. To what extent have education and research influenced these changes?

b   You may come across a health issue that can lead to a research question. Reflect on your personal view of this issue. What will be the research approach you use: quantitative, qualitative or mixed methods? Why?

Practice exercise 1.2

Write a few sentences of your opinion of the following conversations over dinner among friends:

Jane: Nurses have to have knowledge in both health sciences and the arts. They also have to develop the knowledge of their own disciplines because they can't keep on borrowing knowledge from other disciplines. Their patients also want to know more and start asking questions about their care.

Peter:	I won't argue about that. But nurses mainly use their skills during their day-to-day work. Very little of their work needs any scientific knowledge.
Jane:	If you are sick, do you want to receive care from a nurse who has both knowledge and skills or a nurse who has very good skills?
Peter:	You got me!

Practice exercise 1.3

a   In Australia, a number of Vietnamese pregnant women with gestational diabetes are admitted to a hospital to have their blood sugar controlled. The rate is approximately 11%, which is three times higher than the rate in Australian-born women (3.5%) (AIHW: Thow & Waters 2005). Midwives at a maternity unit observe that Vietnamese women tend to eat very little and appear very concerned when insulin is given.

   The midwives would like to know how the women interpret their illness and the impact of lifestyle modification and use of insulin on their own health and the baby's health. Is qualitative research or quantitative research suitable to gain answers for the research questions? Explain.

b   Despite strict procedures used to administer medication to patients by nurses, medication errors still occur. At a medical unit, there are at least four reports of medication error. The clinical nurse manager observes that the errors tend to happen between 3 a.m. and 7.30 a.m. and involve at least a casual or agency nurse. Does this observation warrant research? If yes, does it require a lot of money to conduct the research?

Answers to practice exercise 1.3

a

Qualitative research. It is possible that culture and beliefs may influence the concern and fear that Vietnamese women have and which has been observed by the midwives.

b

Yes, the issue potentially will have an impact on patients' health outcomes. The clinical nurse manager may review patients' records systematically using an audit (see Chapter 6), which can be conducted at a low cost (see also Chapter 2).

Further reading

Chang, E., & Daly, J. (eds). (2007). *Transitions in Nursing: Preparing for Professional Practice.* Sydney: Elsevier Churchill Livingstone.

Greenwood, J. (2000). *Nursing Theory in Australia: Development and Application.* Sydney: Pearson Education.

Weblinks

International Council of Nurses:

<www.icn.ch>

World Health Organization, Nursing and Midwifery program:

<www.who.int/hrh/nursing_midwifery/en>

Selected list of qualitative research journals:

<www.slu.edu/organizations/qrc/QRjournals.html>

Journal of Research in Nursing:

<www.jrn.sagepub.com>

References

Aged and Community Services Australia. (2008). Fact sheet 1: An ageing Australia. Retrieved 9 October 2010, from <www.agedcare.org.au/PUBLICATIONS-&-RESOURCES/General-pdfs-images/ACSA%20Fact%20Sheet%201%202008-%20An%20Ageing%20Australia.pdf>

Australian Institute of Health and Welfare (AIHW). (2007). *Older Australians at a Glance.* Canberra: Australian Institute of Health and Welfare.

Beaglehole, R., & Bonita, R. (2004). *Public Health at the Crossroads: Achievements and Prospects.* Cambridge: Cambridge University Press.

Burns, N., & Grove, S. K. (1997). *The Practice of Nursing Research: Conduct, Critique, and Utilization.* Philadelphia: W. B. Saunders.

Burns, N., & Grove, S. K. (2009). *The Practice of Nursing Research: Appraisal, Synthesis, and Generation of Evidence.* St Louis, MI: Saunders Elsevier.

Cochrane, A. L. (1972). *Effectiveness and Efficiency: Random Reflections on Health Services.* London: Nuffield Provincial Hospitals Trust.

Cochrane Collaboration. (2010). History. Retrieved 9 October 2010, from <www.cochrane.org/about-us/history>

Craig, J. V., & Smyth, R. L. (2007). *Evidence-Based Practice Manual for Nurses.* Edinburgh: Churchill Livingstone.

Fawcett, J. (2002). The nurse theorists: 21st-century updates—Madeleine M. Leininger. *Nursing Science Quarterly* 15(2), 131–6.

Flew, A. (1971). *Introduction to Western Philosophy: Ideas and Argument from Plato to Sartre.* London: Thames & Hudson.

Geison, G. L. (1995). *The Private Science of Louis Pasteur.* Princeton, NJ: Princeton University Press.

Goodrick, D. (2010). Qualitative research: Design analysis and representation. Workshop note, Australian Consortium for Social and Political Research Incorporated (ACSPRI) Summer program. Victoria: ACSPRI. (manuscript).

Greenwood, J. (2000). *Nursing Theory in Australia: Development and Application*. Sydney: Harper Educational Publisher.

Gruending, D. L. (1985). Nursing theory: A vehicle of professionalization? *Journal of Advanced Nursing* 10(6), 553–8.

Hobsons. (2009). *The Good Universities Guide to Education, Training and Career Pathways*. Melbourne: Hobsons.

International Council of Nurses. (2006). The ICN code of ethics for nurses. Retrieved 9 October 2010, from <www.icn.ch/images/stories/documents/about/icncode_english.pdf>

JBI (Joanna Briggs Institute). (2008). Management of constipation in older adults. *Best Practice* 12(7), 1–4.

JBI. (2010). *The Joanna Briggs Institute*. Best Practice series. Retrieved 9 October 2010, from <www.joannabriggs.edu.au/pubs/best_practice.php>

Kenny, A. (2001). *The Oxford Illustrated History of Western Philosophy*. Oxford: Oxford University Press.

Kleinman, A. (1980). *Patients and Healers in the Context of Culture: An Exploration of the Borderland Between Anthropology, Medicine, and Psychiatry*. Berkeley, CA: University of California Press.

Law, S. (2007). *Philosophy*. London: Dorling Kindersley.

Leininger, M. M. (1988). Leininger's theory of nursing: Cultural care diversity and universality. *Nursing Science Quarterly* 1(4), 152–60.

Lincoln, Y. S., & Guba, E. G. (1985). *Naturalistic Inquiry*. Beverly Hills, CA: Sage.

MacLennan, R. (1966). Prevalence of hallux valgus in a neolithic New Guinea population. *Lancet* 1(7452), 1398–400.

Marriner-Tomey, A. (ed.) (1994). *Nursing Theorists and Their Work*. St Louis, MO: Mosby.

Marriner-Tomey, A., & Alligood, M.R. (eds) (2006). *Nursing Theorists and Their Work*. St Louis, MO: Mosby.

Marsh, H. W., & Perry, C. (2005). Self-concept contributes to winning gold medals: Causal ordering of self-concept and elite swimming performance. *Journal of Sport & Exercise Psychology* 27, 71–91.

Marshall, B. J., & Warren, J. R. (1984). Unidentified curved bacilli in the stomach of patients with gastritis and peptic ulceration. *Lancet* 1(8390), 1311–15.

Marshall, B. J., Goodwin, C. S., Warren, J. R., Murray, R., Blincow, E. D., Blackbourn, S. J., Phillips, M., Waters, T. E., & Sanderson, C. R. (1988). Prospective double-blind trial of duodenal ulcer relapse after eradication of Campylobacter pylori. *Lancet* 2(8626–8627), 1437–42.

McBride, W. G. (1962). Thalidomide and congenital abnormalities (letter), *Lancet* 2, 1358.

Medicare Australia. (2010). *Nurse practitioner and midwives*. Retrieved 9 October 2010, from <www.medicareaustralia.gov.au/provider/other-healthcare/nurse-midwives.jsp>

NHMRC (National Health and Medical Research Council). (2009). *NHMRC Levels of Evidence and Grades for Recommendations for Developers of Guidelines*. Retrieved 9 October 2010, from <www.nhmrc.gov.au/_files_nhmrc/file/publications/synopses/cp30.pdf>

Nursing and Midwifery Board of Australia. (2010). *Competency Standard*. Retrieved 9 October 2010, from <www.nursingmidwiferyboard.gov.au/Codes-and-Guidelines.aspx>

Polit, D. F., & Beck, C. T. (eds). (2010). *Essentials of Nursing Research: Appraising Evidence for Nursing Practice*. Philadelphia: Wolters Kluwer.

Rée, J., & Urmson, J. O. (2004). *The Concise Encyclopaedia of Western Philosophy and Philosophers*. London: Routledge.

Russell, B. (2004). *History of Western Philosophy*. New York: Simon & Schuster.

Sackett, D. L., Rosenberg, W. M. C., Gray, J. A. M., Haynes, R. B., & Richardson, W. S. (1996). Evidence based medicine: What it is and what it isn't. *British Medical Journal* 312, 71.

Smithells, R. W., & Newman, C. G. H. (2009). *The Thalidomide Story*. Retrieved 9 October 2010, from <www.thalidomide.org.uk/Thalidomide.aspx>

Streubert, H. J., & Carpenter, D. R. (1995). *Qualitative Research in Nursing*. Philadelphia: J. B. Lippincott Company.

Susser, M. (1986). The logic of Sir Karl Popper and the practice of epidemiology. *American Journal of Epidemiology* 124(5), 711–18.

Thompson, M. (2003). *Teach Yourself Philosophy of Science*. Abingdon: Bookprint Ltd.

Thow, A. M., & Waters, A. M. (2005). *Diabetes in Culturally and Linguistically Diverse Australians: Identification of Communities at High Risk*, AIHW cat. no. CVD 30. Canberra: Australian Institute of Health and Welfare.

Tompkins, C. (2001). Nursing education for the twenty-first century. In E. Rideout (ed.), *Transforming Nursing Education Through Problem-Based Learning* (pp. 1-20). Sudbury, MA: Jones & Bartlett Publishers.

Usher, K., & Fitzgerald, M. (2008). Introduction to nursing research. In S. Borbasi, D. Jackson & R. W. Langford (eds), *Navigating the Maze of Nursing Research: An Interactive Learning Adventure*. Sydney: Elsevier.

Walsh, M. (1998). What is the basis for nursing practice? In *Models and Critical Pathways in Clinical Nursing* (pp. 1–25). London: Baillèire Tindall.

WHO (World Health Organization). (2002). *The Nursing & Midwifery Programme at WHO: What Nursing and Midwifery Services Mean to Health*. Retrieved 9 October 2010, from <www.who.int/hrh/nursing_midwifery/leaflet.pdf>

CHAPTER 2

Introducing the Research Process

Maree Johnson and Cecily Hengstberger-Sims

Chapter learning objectives:

By the end of this chapter you will be able to:

▶ define the tasks in the research process

▶ discuss the essential aspects of a research proposal

▶ develop and present a logical argument to support a research problem

▶ demonstrate awareness of the differences between aims, research questions and hypotheses

▶ appraise the feasibility and ethical aspects of a research problem

▶ outline aspects of budgeting in research

▶ develop a study timeline.

KEY TERMS
Hypothesis
Problem statement
Research proposal plan
Research question
Variable

Introduction

As student nurses or midwives, when we first learnt to give an injection in our nursing courses, we were given a set of discrete tasks that we followed. The order of the tasks was defined, and we could not do the second task unless the first was completed. With practice, we gained confidence and knew the order of the tasks, and could complete the entire process safely and competently.

Giving an injection is a practical skill, and the conduct of nursing research and the research process is similar. Readers and novice researchers should first understand all the tasks, learn how to complete each task and how to carry out these tasks in a logical order to completion. With practice, understanding or doing, research can become very manageable. Research has a unique language and its own set of terms, which will require some attention before they are grasped. Continue to revise the key terms throughout this chapter as often as you wish. Research is a subject that requires ongoing reading to remain conversant with the contemporary changes in methods; it is a subject of lifelong learning.

In this chapter, we introduce readers to the key steps and the overall plan for research. By exploring key aspects of the research process, you will become familiar with the language and logical order of research. Subsequent chapters will provide more detail on each of the steps in the process.

The research process is a complex series of sequential activities that are carried out to allow nurses and midwives to develop new knowledge and skills for nursing and midwifery practice, management or education. The research process consists of 13 major steps in three main stages: planning the research, executing the research plan, and informing the scientific and clinical community.

Stage 1—Planning the research

- Select a suitable research problem and topic.
- Review and synthesise the existing literature and topic.
- Identify a frame of reference and define terms.
- Develop aims, objectives, research questions and hypotheses.
- Choose the appropriate methods (design, sampling, data collection and analysis) to answer the research questions and hypotheses posed.
- Consider feasibility and ethical issues.
- Finalise the research proposal or plan (budget, timeline, dissemination strategies, research time profile).

Stage 2—Executing the research plan

- Obtain ethical approval.
- Obtain funding (optional).
- Collect the data.
- Analyse the data.

Stage 3—Informing the scientific and clinical nursing and midwifery community of the research

- Write up the study findings.
- Disseminate the findings.

The focus of this chapter is on Stage 1 of the process.

Planning the research

The research proposal, plan or protocol is the initial plan developed by the researcher to explain the research process to be undertaken to other team members, funding bodies and other interested parties such as ethics committees. The proposal 'forces the investigator to create, define, and refine the research project…[This] time to fully conceptualise and synthesise the proposal will enhance the investigator's ability to conduct a better study and will provide the framework for future reports of the work' (Inouye & Fiellin 2005). A proposal that is perceived as meeting a 'good' standard is described by Harper (2007, p. 15) as one that answers the following questions:

- What is this research trying to find out: what questions is it trying to answer?
- How will the proposed research answer these questions?
- Why is this research worth doing?

The research proposal required for service managers, ethics committees, funding bodies or other health professional reviewers can have slightly differing components to be completed by the researchers (Harper 2007). We present here the most common format (see Box 2.1) of the proposal and strongly advise researchers to read the specific instructions for the particular committee or persons requiring the proposal (Harper 2007). As Endacott (2008) notes, the research plan or proposal must 'convince others that the work is necessary, soundly constructed and expects to generate outcomes worthy of pursuing' (p. 212).

BOX 2.1

KEY COMPONENTS OF A PROPOSAL

- Synopsis (often in layperson's language)
- Problem
  - Aim of the study
  - Background (introduction/literature review/definition of terms/frame of reference)
- Aim/specific objectives
  - Hypotheses/research questions
- Methods
- Design
- Sample and setting
- Data collection tools
- Data collection procedures
- Analysis procedures
- Ethical considerations
- Timeframe
- Budget
- Funding sources
- Dissemination strategies
- References
- Profile of researchers or research team

RESEARCH AND EVIDENCE-BASED PRACTICE 2.1

2.1 RESEARCHING THE COST:BENEFIT RATIO

Alison Thompson, Clinical Nurse Consultant (CNC) for Ambulatory Care, had visited the Clinical Nursing Research Unit at Raymond House Hospital. Alison was seeking advice from the Senior Research Fellow for Nursing and Midwifery Research. Alison said that she had been changing the intravenous cannulae for community clients receiving antibiotic therapy every 96 hours or when required, while other services were changing them every 48 hours or when required. Alison believed there was no difference in the patient outcomes and wanted to compare the two approaches as she thought there were considerable benefits for the patients and cost savings for the health service.

Task 1: Select the topic and research problem

The first step in any research study is to select the topic. There are many approaches to this. Clinicians often identify topics from problems experienced during their clinical practice, as in the case study above. Occasionally new technologies or health policies may prompt nurses and midwives to explore the merit of new treatments or policies within their practice. Other authors suggest that even casual conversations with patients and their families can be a rich source of research topics (Ayres 2007). For experienced nurse and midwifery researchers, national health priorities may influence the selection of topics because these topics are likely to be funded. Vivar and associates (2007) define the topic as 'what specific situations have been observed that require a research question to be answered' (p. 71).

Shaping the research topic into a manageable research problem

Shaping the research topic is a process whereby a broad research topic is narrowed into a researchable question (Houser 2008).

The word 'problem' is often used to reflect the focus of the study similar to the topic. The problem is often presented in a research proposal in terms of the issue or the impact or scale of the problem. In a study of coping styles of pregnant adolescents, the problem is presented in the introduction in terms of the rate of pregnancy in adolescent populations in Australia and other countries (Myors et al. 2001). The problem should be presented in a manner that engages the reader, or convinces the reader that the study is important because of the nature of the problem (Francis et al. 1979).

However, a problem statement is considerably more precise and is used to describe what the situation is that requires changing or understanding and how the study will address these problems (Francis et al. 1979). Similarly, Houser (2008) defines the problem statement as a 'declaration of disparity; the difference (gap) between what is known and what needs to be known about a topic' (p. 113). For example, a problem statement may be as follows:

> There is considerable research comparing intermittent versus continuous naso-gastric feeding of patients undergoing gastro-intestinal surgery. However, there is little research comparing these feeding methods in patients experiencing facial surgery. This study will use a randomised clinical trial to compare the benefits of intermittent versus continuous naso-gastric feeding in patients undergoing facial surgery.

The problem could be understood as feeding in patients undergoing facial surgery; the problem statement is a series of related statements positioning the research within existing knowledge.

Reviewing the literature or exploring the background to the problem will help to shape the research problem. Aspects such as the definition of terms, limiting the scope of study for sampling, defining how the methods might influence the problem or directing which outcomes are likely, are all important components of shaping the problem (Vivar et al. 2007).

Task 2: Review and synthesise the literature

The purpose of undertaking the literature review is, first, to collect all the recent literature on the topic area. A comprehensive review of viewpoints, debates, methods, findings or areas for further research is the focus of the review; seminal literature also can be used. Second, the researcher should synthesise the literature and develop an argument reflecting the omissions or 'gaps' in the literature (Endacott 2008). The researcher needs to read the literature and to comprehend, summarise and synthesise it.

The literature should be read in a systematic manner. You may find it helpful to place readings from authors with similar viewpoints together or similar methods together, or sources that focus on instruments or measurement tools. Synthesis, or the bringing together of like-minded positions, or similar or dissimilar methods or findings, should be carried out before writing the literature review.

A suitable database or table can be invaluable to the novice and advanced researcher when managing volumes of papers or monographs. Once the scope of the aspects to be discussed is identified, the researcher can develop a logical order to the presentation in the literature, such as from general to specific issues. In Figure 2.1, for example, articles related to similar positions or methods can be located together when writing the material and important differences in the works noted for the literature review. The use of the spreadsheet is to organise material logically before putting down what is similar and what is contrasting literature. This gives researchers a balanced presentation of the material examined and allows them to position their own study in relation to the existing material, in other words to begin shaping their argument. Chapter 13 presents a thorough discussion on searching through databases, the scope of literature to be examined, and sorting the literature.

It is important to decide on a 'line of argument or discussion to be taken to support or enhance the research [that] introduces the literature at strategic points to support that argument...[and] establishes the "case" for the research' (Hamilton & Clare 2004, p. 9).

How much literature should be considered in the literature search? For some topics with extensive literature, such as HIV, researchers may choose to do a random selection of literature. A general guide for topics with extensive literature is to ensure coverage within the past five years; for more obscure topics you may need to search literature dating back to the 1960s when databases commenced.

2.1 LITERATURE COVERAGE

THINKING DEEPLY

The question of how do you know whether you have searched the literature thoroughly enough can be answered within the searching itself.

When researchers find and gain access to an article and all relevant materials referred to in that article, they are described as covering most of the literature. Clearly, it is impossible to cover every article. It is covering contemporary debates or methods adequately that is at issue.

The literature review is a critical review of the literature; some material will be omitted while other material will be shaped into a set of similar and dissimilar aspects of the topic. Synthesis is where the nurse/midwife researcher presents a thorough understanding of the material that focuses on key issues and includes several studies that support or refute these key issues. Synthesis is not the mere presentation of every study, case by case. If there are many studies to be presented, often a table that defines the chronological order of the related studies is presented, perhaps as an appendix. The literature review section of the proposal represents the end point of synthesis and critical reflection on the material examined.

2.2 SYNTHESIS OF THE EXISTING KNOWLEDGE

THINKING DEEPLY

Synthesis is a difficult task and is achieved by reading the literature, segmenting the literature into similar aspects of the topic and then logically ordering both the overall direction of the review and the aspects to be covered in the topic. Where identified, studies that support or refute the premises of your study should be emphasised. This allows the researcher to progressively develop an argument on how your study provides knowledge that fills the gap in existing knowledge. Remember, synthesis does not mean that every study you have read should be included, but only essential works.

▶▶▶   TERMS, TIPS AND SKILLS

How to write a good argument:

a   Describe the previous research in the area.

b   Identify the gaps in knowledge.

c   Explain how the proposed research addresses the gap.

d   Summarise some studies and give specific details of the studies that relate most to your study (Schmelzer 2006).

The literature review is often summarised in two paragraphs in a proposal, revising the key aspects covered and reiterating the problem being addressed by the study (Falk 2006). Readers should see Chapter 13 for a detailed discussion on the literature review. Researchers often use wording like 'this study uniquely contributes to knowledge in the area of…' or 'this study examines for the first time key issues of…'

Now back to our case study…

RESEARCH AND EVIDENCE-BASED PRACTICE 2.2

2.2   DEVELOPING THE PROPOSAL

CNC Alison Thompson has searched numerous databases at the hospital library and located 200 articles relating to cannula, peripheral cannula or IV antibiotics in the English language from 2000 to 2010. On reading the abstracts of these articles, Alison decided that only clinical trials would be included in the literature review and some papers on methodologies, which resulted in 60 articles remaining. Alison set up a spreadsheet outlining the authors and year of publication, design, sample and setting, outcome measures, results and conclusions. She noted that 13 studies suggested that 96 hours before replacement had no harmful effects, while eight studies suggested 48-hour replacement of cannula was required. She began shaping the literature review to reflect the trials and any reviews of the several studies found in the literature.

Alison provided a clinical context for her proposal in that there were no studies on community living populations such as the ambulatory care setting. She summarised similar and dissimilar studies, including the outcome measures used, and noted the gaps in existing knowledge that her study would fill. She has proposed a similar study to others using similar outcome measures but using a community-residing population and sample. Alison developed the argument from the literature.

Other aspects of managing the literature

There are many bibliographic software packages available. Weblinks at the end of this chapter includes several products the reader can explore.

One example is EndNote. This computer software can be used to locate references by exporting the reference details directly from library search engines and also allows for material to be inserted as an electronic file directly within the reference listing. Figure 2.1 opposite demonstrates a computer screen capture of an EndNote library relating to patient safety.

Considerable time and energy is saved by the use of bibliographic software. These packages include embedding the reference directly in the text when writing the literature review and locating the article with the reference in the library. The ability to alter the reference format from American Psychological Association (APA) or Harvard or other forms (depending on the requirements of journals or other parties) will save time.

Figure 2.1 EndNote Library relating to patient safety

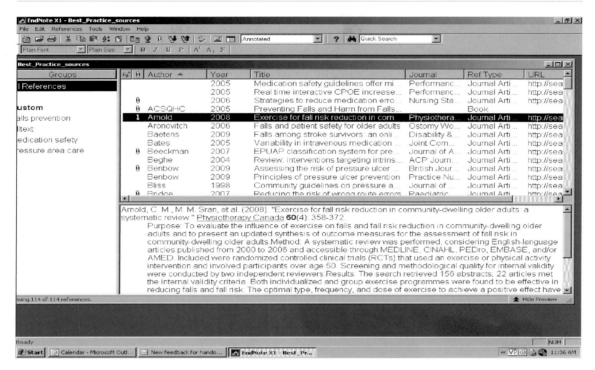

Task 3: Identify a frame of reference and/or define terms

The frame of reference or the way the researcher understands aspects of a study can inform the research aims, methods and interpretation of the data.

Not all studies will use or require a conceptual framework or a set of related general concepts. In nursing and midwifery research, a conceptual or theoretical framework or established theory 'provides the structure to guide the development of the study' (Engberg & Bliss 2005, p. 157).

In some cases, the researcher is studying the theory or its components or relationships in a specific group of patients or clinical settings (Engberg & Bliss 2005). Theories in nursing, psychology, social sciences or biology have all been applied to nursing and midwifery research.

We advise the reader to review Chapter 1 on the use of theory in nursing and midwifery research. In theory-testing research, the research aims, questions or hypotheses test the relationships between components of the theory as defined by the theory or conceptual framework (Engberg & Bliss 2005). The following example emphasises the use of a theoretical framework that influenced the design of an instrument to measure nurses' self-concept.

Contemporary self-concept research has established that self-concept is a multidimensional construct (Craven et al. 2003; Marsh & Perry 2005), particularly when related to adult populations (Marsh & Ayotte 2003). When studying self-concept in an adult population such as registered nurses, it would be expected that multiple dimensions of self-concept will be related to behavioural outcomes, such as job satisfaction (Cowin et al. 2008).

Throughout the literature review, it is important to identify any key terms. In the example above, the term 'self-concept' can mean many things to many readers. However, for the purposes of the study, Marsh and Perry (2005) defined self-concept as 'a person's self-perceptions that are formed through experience with and interpretations of one's environment' (p. 72).

All terms should be defined in clear language and these should appear early in a research proposal to avoid misinterpretation by the readers. Definitions can be obtained from existing literature such as dictionaries, books of synonyms and technical glossaries (Francis et al. 1979) or from other research studies. The form of the definition taken by the researcher is often referred to as the 'operational definition' (Francis et al. 1979). The following example demonstrates the operational definition for the biological measure of heat gain:

> Heat gain (°C) refers to the number of degrees of temperature the subject had to gain to reach 36°C (i.e., 36°C minus arrival temperature at recovery) (Clevenger 1994).

Operational definitions are also portrayed as the way the construct (abstract interpretation) is measured within the study: 'Depression, as measured by the Edinburgh Post-natal Depression scale (Cox et al. 1987).

··

▶▶▶ TERMS, TIPS AND SKILLS

- Terms should be specific to the field in which the study is being conducted.
- Use everyday language that will not cause confusion.
  - Terms are related to the conceptualisation of the study or to the methodology (Francis et al. 1979).

··

Having reviewed the literature and developed the argument in support of the study to be undertaken, the researcher presents a case for the significance of the study and then refines the research question further to form aims or specific objectives, hypotheses or research questions.

▶▶▶   TERMS, TIPS AND SKILLS

The term 'research question' is often used in a broad or general sense and means the broad topic of the research; 'question' here is roughly equivalent to 'problem' or 'matter', as in 'the question of fever management in children'. For example, 'refining the research question' means that the researcher reduces the topic or aspects of the topic to a more precise definition of the problem that is to be researched. Specific research questions are a set of questions to be answered by the data that will be collected by the researcher. This is often confusing to novice researchers. We will look at a few examples to help understand the use of the term. Research questions are not the questions the researchers will ask in a survey or at an interview.

Task 4: Develop aims, objectives, research questions and hypotheses

Research studies, whether undertaken by quantitative (using numbers) or qualitative (using text) methods, all have research aims or purposes. A research aim is a general statement about the research: 'The aim of this study is to compare differing warming procedures for post-surgical patients' or 'The aim of this study is to explore how carers experience living with partners with chronic heart disease'. Specific objectives are clear statements of what is to be achieved by the study, or they provide detail on what is expected as outcomes (Parahoo 2006). Examples of specific objectives may include describing the characteristics of carers, outlining the procedures used in techniques that use warmed blankets, or developing an education program for nurses using technology-based warming devices.

Research questions and hypotheses are the most precise statements of a research proposal. Polit and Beck (2010) define research questions as 'specific queries researchers want to answer in addressing the research problem' (p. 46). They qualify this statement by noting that when researchers can make 'specific predictions about answers to research questions [they] pose hypotheses that are tested empirically'.

Hypotheses are statements about the relationship between two variables: independent variable and dependent variable (factors in a study). In some cases, there can be independent variables or factors that cause change in the dependent variables and outcome factors (Polit & Beck 2010).

▶▶▶   TERMS, TIPS AND SKILLS

Researchers use the terms 'aim' and 'purpose' interchangeably. Readers can easily locate the aim or purpose of a study when reading a research paper by simply looking for the specific word (aim or purpose). In an exploratory study, where little is known on the topic, the researcher may choose to include only the aim or purpose and no research questions.

Research questions are used in both quantitative and qualitative research, although the use of a hypothesis is preferred when testing of relationships or differences in interventions are to be examined.

What are the characteristics of a 'good' research question?

Research questions and hypotheses should have the following components: the participants, the clinical context, the phenomenon of concern (if applicable in qualitative studies), intervention (if applicable in quantitative studies), comparison group (if applicable in quantitative studies) and outcomes (if applicable in quantitative studies).

▸▸▸ TERMS, TIPS AND SKILLS

An easy way to remember the difference between a research question and a hypothesis is that research questions ask the question of the study and hypotheses answer the question (Nieswiadomy 2008).

In a qualitative study the aim and the research question appear very similar:

The primary aim of the study was to explore how decisions about care and support were made following brain injury… (McCluskey et al. 2007, p. 294).

A research question that could be written for this study would be:

What are the decision-making processes that carers use to provide care and support to persons experiencing brain injury?

Hypotheses are not used in qualitative research and many qualitative researchers believe that only research aims or objectives should be used.

Specific types of hypotheses

For quantitative research, depending on what is known about a research topic and question, hypotheses may take the form of a directional, non-directional or null hypothesis.

A directional hypothesis is by far the most common. The researcher reviews the literature and then develops the hypothesis based on those findings, often concluding that a new intervention of X will result in improved patient outcomes, for example, increased time to wound healing, reduced depression, reduced readmission rates. The hypothesis predicts that there is a direction of the change either increasing or decreasing the dependent or outcome measure (Houser 2008; Nieswiadomy 2002, 2008; Polit & Beck 2010).

Houser (2008) defines the directional hypothesis as 'a one-sided statement of the research question that is interested in only one direction of change' (p. 126).

Mild (35.5–36.0°C) or moderate (34.5–35.4°C) hypothermic patients who have undergone surgery for greater than 20 minutes, and who received Bair-Hugger™ warming, will achieve normothermia in less time (increased rewarming rate) than hypothermic patients receiving only warmed cotton blankets. (Stevens et al. 2000, p. 270)

A non-directional hypothesis is likely when the literature suggests that there will be a change in the dependent variable or outcome measure, but there is no clear direction as to whether outcomes will improve or deteriorate. In this situation a non-directional hypothesis is posed.

Houser (2008) defines a non-directional hypothesis as 'a two-sided statement of the research question that is interested in change in any direction' (p. 126).

> There is a relationship between mothers' first birthing methods and their satisfaction with subsequent birthing methods.

A null hypothesis is posed when the literature and the researcher believe there will be no difference between the groups receiving the intervention. This is relevant when there is a change in interventions in a clinical context where there is little harm evident, such as childbirth. Houser defines a null hypothesis as 'a statement of the research question that declares no difference between the groups' (p. 126).

> Similar numbers (proportion) of infants with Apgar scores less than 7 at 5 minutes will be demonstrated for low risk mothers receiving primary health midwifery care and [mothers receiving] standard hospital care. (Johnson et al. 2005, p. 23)

RESEARCH AND EVIDENCE-BASED PRACTICE 2.3
2.3 HYPOTHESES ARE MOST APPROPRIATE FOR CNC ALISON'S STUDY

Community-living clients, receiving a short course of intravenous antibiotic therapy with reinsertion of cannulae every 96 hours, will have a similar incidence of thrombophlebitis as clients having their cannulae replaced every 48 hours or when required.

This is a null hypothesis or a no difference hypothesis as developed in the argument from the literature: the research problem seeks to confirm that no harm (or no difference in the rate of harm) occurs when the cannula is changed less frequently.

Some researchers also distinguish between simple and complex hypotheses. A simple hypothesis includes one independent variable (factor or intervention being manipulated) and one dependent variable (factor or outcome of the study). Complex hypotheses include more than one independent variable and/or one or more dependent variables.

Task 5: Choose appropriate methods to address the research questions or hypotheses

In this section the researcher defines the research design and overall methodology or approach. Every method has strengths and weaknesses and your study will fall into general areas.

> Your choice should be based upon careful consideration of how appropriate each available methodology fits your purpose [aim], and the feasibility of each method depending on the limits of your time and resources. (Francis et al. 1979)

Choosing the best or most appropriate design is a challenging task and is largely reliant on the research questions or hypotheses posed and the type of data (numbers or text) that are to be collected. Method includes the design of the study, the sample and setting, the data collection instrument or tools, data collection procedures and analysis approaches. The choice of qualitative or quantitative approaches can be made with a thorough understanding of the range of designs, sampling, data collection procedures and tools available in both these paradigms (see Chapters 5 and 6 and 7 on design, Chapter 8 on populations and sampling, Chapters 9 and 10 on data collection for quantitative and qualitative methods, and Chapters 11 and 12 on data analysis).

In general terms, qualitative research is frequently used when little is known about a topic, when factors cannot be easily defined or 'theories are not available to explain behaviour' (Vivar et al. 2007, p. 64), and the collected data collected is usually text. Qualitative research examines the human experience and is concerned with description and understanding. Quantitative research is appropriate when there is measurable information and defined relationships or there is prediction between variables, and data collected is usually numeric (Vivar et al. 2007).

2.4

RESEARCH AND EVIDENCE-BASED PRACTICE 2.4

RESEARCH METHODOLOGY

Alison's study compares two groups of community clients using two time periods between replacement of intravenous cannulae. Incidents of thrombophlebitis can be measured and much is known about this topic. Existing literature tells us that both periods are valid. Data to be collected is numeric. The chosen method is quantitative and the design is a non-randomised experimental design. (See Chapters 5, 6 and 7 for further details on design and methods.)

Other considerations when choosing a method may relate to the researcher's method of choice; for example, a Masters student may have quantitative skills and is seeking to develop qualitative research skills in their doctorate.

Some data collection methods such as face-to-face interviews may be more in keeping with the philosophical position of the researcher. In some rare cases, there may be only a small number of cases with a specific research condition and so quantitative methods may not be possible or suitable.

Task 6: Defining the significance and outcomes of the research

One of the most important aspects of any proposal is outlining the significance or likely outcomes or products from the study. This is the 'So what?' aspect of the study (Nieswiadomy 2008, p. 78).

The significance statement emphasises the importance of your study 'as distinct from any and all other studies that might address the same topic' (Francis et al. 1979, p. 25). Your study may address or inform key state or national policies, use innovative methods or instruments/technology, affect specific health care groups or clinicians, test theories in differing settings or samples, or provide knowledge for health consumers, nurse managers, educators or others. Often the social and economic benefits of research are set out in this section. Falk (2006) states that 'the significance of the grant should clearly point out why the problem addressed is important and how scientific knowledge will be advanced by the proposed study' (p. 511). As far as possible, the study's outcomes should be specifically defined.

Scope and limitations

Outlining the scope and limitations of a research study can be just as important as identifying the topic. Containing the study allows it to become more manageable or allows a more precise comparison study than would otherwise be possible. For example, a study may be proposed to examine all older people receiving oral medications. Some older people take two medications per day while others may be prescribed 12 doses per day and may be more vulnerable to adverse events.

The researcher can define or contain the scope of the study as older people, living in the community, receiving 12 medication doses or more per day. Hence the study, or more particularly in this case the sample and setting, is constrained. Similar constraints may be applied to methods, instruments or other methods used to collect data, and indeed, analysis procedures. Disclosure of the scope and limitations of the study allows others to determine whether the study has been thoroughly considered by the researcher.

Task 7: Consider the feasibility and ethical issues

How can novice nurse researchers evaluate whether the research question or problem they have selected is an important one that is feasible and ethical? One approach is to apply the FINER (an acrostic) model to the question as proposed by Houser (2008, p. 122):

- Feasible: Adequate subjects, technical expertise, time and money are available; the scope is narrow enough for the study.
- Interesting: The question is interesting to the investigator.
- Novel: The study confirms or refutes previous findings or provides new findings.
- Ethical: The study cannot cause unacceptable risk to participants and does not invade privacy.
- Relevant: The question is relevant to scientific knowledge, clinical and health policy, or further research directions.

Nurses and midwives can apply this model to their research questions and problems in order to clarify the issues of appraisal of a research problem inclusive of feasibility and ethical considerations. A comprehensive discussion on the issues of concern relating to ethics is presented in Chapter 3.

Task 8: Finalise the research proposal plan

Budget

Estimating the budget required to conduct a project is an important task of the lead researcher. There are two major categories of grants available: project funding or researcher development support (Inouye & Fiellin 2005). For project funding there are several major components of a budget: personnel, consultants or technical/support staff, supplies, equipment, services, computer hardware and software, survey formatting and printing, postage, photocopying, travel, incentives/compensations for subjects and other support technology such as telephones, mobiles and faxes (Bliss 2005).

Personnel may include research assistants with Masters degrees, or post-doctoral qualifications as required by the project. Personnel often reflect the major cost of the budget and the cost is determined by the level of research officer support required, the hourly rate and the number of weeks they will be required. Consultants are often budgeted on an hourly rate and can be used for statistical support, design, analysis of data, or occasionally to collect data. Specialised equipment required for the study or consumables such as dressings should always be precisely costed within the budget.

As a guide, small studies such as a qualitative study of 20 people would be expected to cost around $20 000 to $60 000 while large studies such as multicentre trials may cost from $500 000 to $1 million. Research projects should always be properly funded.

There are various funding sources to be considered, such as external grants (e.g. Australian Research Council or National Health and Medical Research Council [NHMRC] grants), internal grants (small funding provided by the university or the health service) or in-kind funding (such as health staff allocated to data collection for a short period, or facilities such as office space, equipment, computers). The budget and funding body are selected depending on the level of funding being sought and the priorities of the funding bodies.

Table 2.1   Research budget

Item	Description	Cost
Salary	Clinical Nurse Educator (engaged in research) with a Masters qualification in nursing or a related discipline	$7718 for 170 hours ($45.40 per hour: base rate with on-costs for superannuation and casual allowances) Data collection and entry/data analysis/ report writing/assistance with coaching and education material preparation
Administration	Workshop materials (photocopying/ printing and binding) x 100 workbooks	$500
Research Materials	NVivo 8 software for data analysis	$800
Miscellaneous	Transcription services for two focus groups of one hour duration	$360
Miscellaneous	Use of telephone/fax and other services	$600
Equipment	Digital recorder (popular brand)	$500
Total		$10 398

Justification of the budget is important. Each item identified in the study will need to have an explicit and clearly related role in the potential completion of the study and this should be made immediately apparent to potential funding bodies. Inclusion of budget items that are unrealistic, poorly justified or unrelated may threaten the possibility of securing funding.

Timeframe

A timetable of the specific tasks to be completed throughout the process informs the reviewers and the study team of the required time in which to complete tasks.

Realistic timelines are always recommended. All the tasks described in this chapter would usually appear in the timeline: finalising the literature and proposal, ethics approval, development of survey or interview schedule, recruitment of participants, data collection, data analysis, and writing up or reporting on the study. Most of these tasks require between one and six months each. Be generous with your time allocations as in some cases you will be required to comply with them or give reasons for any non-adherence. Table 2.2 suggests a timeframe for a simple survey research study.

Table 2.2   Timeframe for tasks in a simple research study

DATE	ACTIVITY
January–March	Finalise literature review and proposal
March–May	Secure ethics clearance and approval
May–June	Identify potential survey recipients Finalise print survey instrument and prepare for mail dissemination
July	Commence data collection with dissemination of mail survey. Develop code for data entry
August–September	Data entry of returned survey responses
September–November	Analysis of data responses
November–December	Write up findings and identify potential sources for dissemination of findings (journals/conferences)
January–February	Finalise written report and send these to funding authorities/ethics committee and identified prospective disseminators of study results

Dissemination of findings

As noted at the start of this chapter, informing the scientific and clinical nursing and midwifery community of the research findings is the final and very important part of the process. Nurses and midwives can present their findings to their local community, or at national or international conferences. Unfortunately, conference proceedings are not widely available to the international research community and researchers should always strive to publish their research in national or international refereed journals.

A thorough discussion on the procedures to follow to present a paper at a conference or to publish a paper is provided in Chapter 15.

When writing a proposal, the nurse researcher is required to detail when and where papers from this study will be presented for review by the scientific community. Many funding bodies request substantial detail on this topic and some may judge the proposal on the ability of the study to be published in high-ranking academic journals.

Writing the synopsis

Finally, the synopsis is a summary of key aspects of a research proposal or plan. The synopsis is the final section of the proposal to be written but appears first in the proposal or may appear separate from the main proposal. Aspects of the plan are included briefly: the problem, aim, method or methodology, and likely outcomes of the research. Many funding bodies and ethics committees require that this section be written in plain English or layperson's language; in other words, don't use complex health terms.

The length of this section is between 150 and 250 words and is often the most difficult to write.

Summary

We have introduced you to the key aspects of the research process across three major stages: planning the research, executing the plan and informing the scientific community of the findings. Although the process contains many intricate tasks, the novice researcher has an opportunity to commence a new and wonderful journey into nursing and midwifery research. For some clinicians, the ability to understand the whole process will enable them to critique research and discern which findings can be used in their practice. For other nurses and midwives, their first study may be the beginnings of a long and productive career as a nurse researcher or academic.

IMPLICATIONS FOR EVIDENCE-BASED NURSING AND MIDWIFERY

Readers of this chapter will be able to understand the key components of a research study that is outlined in any research paper. Both clinicians and users of research information, together with creators of research, will understand how the tasks defined in this chapter influence the way findings are interpreted and how conclusions are understood by nurse and midwife researchers.

▶▶▶ **PROBLEM SOLVING 2.1**

a

Ann and Bob want to explore why a number of patients with chest pain return to the emergency department (ED) at the hospital within six months. Ann is interested in studying this health problem within the environment context of a patient, such as their understanding of chest pain, the meaning of chest pain to their life and death, and what sources of information are being accessed. Write at least one research question arising from Ann's interest.

b

Bob wants to assess whether or not giving instruction and printed health education materials relating to self-management of chest pain will reduce the proportion of patients who re-present to the ED with chest pain within six months. Write at least one research question arising from Bob's interest.

Maree Johnson and Cecily Hengstberger-Sims

Practice exercise 2.1

Access your library and locate a research article that you find interesting, easy to read and understand.

Write down the headings of each major section in the article.

Compare these headings with those in the research process listed above.

What is similar?

What is different?

Practice exercise 2.2

Access your library and locate a simple research article that you find interesting, easy to read and understand. This may be the same one used in the previous exercise.

Read the article and locate the following:

    Research aim or purpose.

    Research question(s) and/or hypothesis(es).

Are the hypotheses directional, non-directional or null, and why? Note that sometimes only the aim is presented, particularly in descriptive studies.

Answers to problem solving 2.1

a

What is the meaning of chest pain perceived by patients who re-present to a hospital emergency department?

OR

What is the lived experience of patients with chest pain who re-present to a hospital emergency department?

b

Is intervention by giving instruction and printed health education materials relating to self-management of chest pain to patients with chest pain reducing their return to the ED within six months?

OR

Is the proportion of patients with chest pain who receive instruction and printed health education materials on self-management of chest pain and return to the ED within six months less than the proportion of patients who receive routine care and return to the ED within the same period?

Appendix 2.1
Example of a Quantitative Research Proposal

Title: Outcomes with home follow-up visit after postpartum hospital discharge
Researchers: Dr Sansnee Jirojwong, Ms Barbara Ritchie, Ms Erin Russell, Ms Sandra Walker

Aims and objectives

The major aim of this comparative study is to identify the health outcomes of home follow-up visits provided by midwives to women after the births of their infants.

Specific objectives are to:

- describe and compare characteristics of mothers who receive home follow-up visits and those who do not
- assess the relationship between the home follow-up visits and mothers' physical health outcomes
- assess the relationship between the home follow-up visits and mothers' psychological health outcomes
- assess the relationship between the home follow-up visits and mothers' satisfaction with health care after discharge
- assess the relationship between the home follow-up visits and infants' physical health outcomes
- assess the relationship between the home follow-up visits and breastfeeding
- describe mothers' comments relating to home follow-up visits and other early postpartum care.

Expected outcomes

This study will include all postpartum women who meet the study criteria and give birth at Hospital ABC. It will identify characteristics of postpartum women who receive home follow-up visits and those who do not. The difference in maternal and infants' health outcomes between these two groups of women will be evaluated. The results of this study will help strengthen or broaden existing home follow-up visits provided to postpartum women by midwives. Health information given to women may be formalised in a systematic approach. A booklet containing essential information which can be used widely can be developed. A summary of methods of assessing current health education provided to early discharge patients including postpartum women can be developed.

Background and significance

Background

The introduction of casemix and diagnostic-related groups (DRG) in Australia has reduced the average length of hospital stay of patients admitted for treatments and procedures. This casemix and DRG has been used as a tool to compare hospital performance, provide a basis for funding and charging for hospital services, and aid interpretation of other aspects of care such as cost and quality (AIHW 1996). Patients affected by the DRG systems also include postpartum women who have normal births and births with complications. The length of postpartum stay in hospital among mothers has decreased over the decade. Annual Australian Institute of Health and Welfare (AIHW) reports (1994, 1996, 1999) showed that the average duration of postnatal hospital stay was reduced from 5.3 days in 1991 to 4.1 days in 1997. The figures include all postpartum women regardless of the types of birth, maternal medical and obstetric complications, neonatal morbidity and specific hospital policies of early discharge. Queensland and New South Wales have a relatively shorter stay on average (4.0 days) than other states. The latest data show that in Queensland public-insured postpartum women stay in hospitals for a shorter period (3.2 days) compared with private-insured women (5.4 days) (AIHW 1999).

In order to prevent and detect complications early among postpartum women and their infants, many hospitals and community health centres have introduced home follow-up services by midwives. There is a variation of practices from one locality to another relating to the number of visits, time of initial and subsequent visits after the hospital discharge and the range of protocol of services. However, the services generally include physical, psychological and social assessment, health education and anticipatory guidance (Ghilarducci & McCool 1993; Grullon & Grimes 1997; Williams & Cooper 1993). If required, women or their infants are referred to other health professionals such as social workers or paediatricians for appropriate care.

Studies of home follow-up visits after postpartum discharge and its outcomes

Studies in many countries including the United Kingdom, the United States, Canada, and Australia have assessed the outcomes of home follow-up visits after postpartum discharge (Carty & Bradley 1990; Frank-Hanssen et al. 1999; Ghilarducci & McCool 1993; Johnson et al. 1999; Lieu et al. 2000). Comparing the results of one study with others is problematic due to the difference in outcome measures, study designs, period between hospital discharge and data collection, protocol and content of home visit, and types of health care providers (Frank-Hanssen et al. 1999; Johnson et al. 1999; Lieu et al. 2000). For example, Johnson et al. assess the success or continuation of breastfeeding, while Lieu et al. assessed a number of mothers' and infants' outcomes including newborn hospitalisation, newborn urgent clinic visit, maternal re-hospitalisation and maternal postpartum depression. Only women who had vaginal births were included in the study by Meikle et al. (1998) while Armstrong et al. (1999) included high risk women in their study.

In the 1980s and 1990s many studies were conducted to evaluate the maternal and infants' health outcomes of postpartum women who were discharged early with home follow-up visit compared with women who had a longer hospital stay (Armstrong et al. 1999; Brooten et al. 1994; Brumfield at al. 1996; Carty & Bradley 1990; Serwint et al. 1991). The results of these have supported the provision of home visits to postpartum women; particularly first-time mothers, single mothers and mothers who intend to breastfeed their infants. A wide range of outcomes have been measured including maternal depression (Carty & Bradley 1990), satisfaction with care, and the reduction of readmission (Brooten et al. 1994). Another common and consistent outcome derived from these studies is that mothers who received the home visit were more likely to be satisfied with the postpartum care (Brooten et al. 1994) or to be confident to seek help from health care providers (Ghilarducci & McCool 1993) than women who did not receive the home visit. However, these studies were conducted in major hospitals. Women who lived in rural and remote areas were not included in the studies.

Social support during postpartum period

During the early postpartum period, women may receive support from many sources including their partners, family members, friends, general practitioners, paediatricians and midwives (Jirojwong 1995). As mentioned earlier, midwives provide a range of support such as information and psychological support during the home follow-up visits. The women's supporters may also provide similar types of help as midwives, particularly to those who do not have any home visits. This important factor has not been taken into account in many studies which assess the outcomes of home follow-up visits (Carty & Bradley 1990; Frank-Hanssen et al. 1999; Ghilarducci & McCool 1993; Johnson et al. 1999; Lieu et al. 2000). It also should be noted that outcomes of social support assessed by researchers were also similar to outcomes of home follow-up visits by midwives.

Hospital ABC and home follow-up visits

Hospital ABC is a major hospital which serves the population in a large geographical area that includes Central Queensland, Central Highlands and Central West Queensland. Publicly insured and privately insured women can receive care during all stages of their perinatal period. After the birth of their child, a home follow-up visit or extended midwifery services (EMS) are offered to postpartum women who meet the criteria of being women who live in Town XYZ and nearby geographical area and are willing to have a midwife visit their homes. Approximately 90% of women who meet the criteria receive at least one home visit. Other women, who are not eligible to receive the EMS services, may or may not receive home follow-up visits depending on the policies of the hospital located nearest to them.

No systematic investigation was conducted to assess a range of potential outcomes of EMS, although the hospital EMS was initiated in 1991. Despite anecdotal data of beneficial effects to the health of both the women and their infants, only one systematic evaluation has been conducted to assess the continuation of breastfeeding between women who have a home visit and women who do not. Preliminary results indicate no difference in breastfeeding between two groups (Personal communication 2000). The lack of EMS effects can be explained by women's intention to breastfeed before their child is born. This clearly indicated the need to demonstrate the beneficial effects of health care resources provided to women in the community.

This study aims to assess the EMS outcomes by comparing the difference of health measures among women who receive the EMS and those who do not. The results of this study will help strengthen or broaden the existing services. Similar services such as access to health care personnel by telephone may be initiated or formalised for postpartum women who live in rural and remote communities. A referral system between hospital ABC and smaller health care organisations may be established as a result of this project.

Two major aspects of social support will be included in this study: sources of support and types of support. The sources of support include significant individuals who help a postpartum woman in various ways. The types of support can be categorised as emotional, material, information and appraisal supports (Cronenwett 1985a,b; Weiss 1974). These support persons can be included in health education sessions provided to women early in their pregnancy.

Methodology and timing

A prospective study will be conducted at Hospital ABC. All postpartum women will be invited to participate in the study. If a woman is younger than 18 years old, permission will be sought from her parents or guardian.

Informed consent will be sought from all women regarding access to their hospital records and willingness to be contacted again following discharge. The objectives of the study, namely potential benefits to women, will be explained to them. They can refuse to participate in the study at this time and will be informed that their refusal will not have any effect on the EMS services. Ethical clearance is being sought from Central Queensland Health District and from Central Queensland University.

Sample selection and sample size

There are approximately 90 births per month at the study hospital (Queensland Health 1999). Based on information from a study previously conducted at the hospital, it is anticipated that 15% will decline to participate in the study. Data collection will be categorised in two stages. Over a period of six months, a total of 450 women are to be included in the first stage of the study. The second stage will comprise two groups of women: a sample of women who have home visits (an EMS group, 90 women) and a sample of those who do not (a non-EMS group, 90 women). As far as possible, the two groups will be of similar age and parity. Other variables which may influence outcomes will not be matched but will be included in analyses. Information from hospital records and the initial interviews will be used for selecting women for the second stage of the study.

Data collection

All women: Information relating to obstetrics and sociodemographic characteristics of all participants will be based on hospital records. The first stage will include all participants, limited descriptive data on the recipient, and number of home follow-up visits. Demographic and obstetrics history will also be collected. These will be followed up by telephone interviews two weeks after hospital discharge. The following information will be gathered from the telephone interview: physical health, psychological health and overall satisfaction with postpartum care.

EMS and non-EMS groups: Outcomes of women with home follow-up visits will be compared with women without the visits. The following data will be gathered by telephone interviews, two weeks after their hospital discharge: sources of support (health care personnel including midwives, family members, non-family members), types of support provided to women and their infants (emotional, material, information, appraise support), overall satisfaction with the support, knowledge of available health resources during the early postpartum period, breastfeeding and postpartum check-up.

Variables and their measurements

Measurements used by four studies will be modified to design data collection tools: Jirojwong (1995); Jirojwong and Skolnik (1990); Lieu et al. (2000); Serwint et al. (1991). The study variables and measurement are as follows:

- Independent variables: home follow-up visits (no visit, 1–2 visits, 3 or more visits)
- Dependent variables: physical health (selected items of SF-36, emergency visit or re-hospitalisation of mother or infant)
- Psychological health (postpartum depression measure and feeling confidence in maternal roles)
- Knowledge (information relating to health care resources)
- Overall satisfaction with postpartum care
- Breastfeeding
- Postpartum check-up.

Other variables (confounding variables) are: obstetrics factors (number of antenatal clinic attendances and obstetrics abnormality); sociodemographic factors (age, types of health care insurance, education level, occupation of main income earner); and sources and types of social support during the postpartum period.

Data analyses

Quantitative data will be analysed using the SPSS program. Number percentage, range and mode will be used to analyse and present descriptive data. In order to assess group differences, a chi-square test for categorical variables and the student t-test or the Wilcoxon rank-sum test for continuous variables will be used. Multivariate logistic regression analyses adjusted for any confounding variables will be used in the final analyses in order to assess the group differences in outcome variables.

Research timeline

Personal in-depth interview (1–2 months): The design questionnaire will be validated by personal in-depth interviews among 10 postpartum women. The researchers will explore factors included in the questionnaire and their applicability. If required, the questionnaire will be modified.

Pilot study (1–2 months): When the questionnaire is completed, it will be used in a pilot study among 20 postpartum women. Differences between the information gained from personal interviews and telephone interviews will be explored. The extent of variation between two data collection methods will be assessed using the correlation coefficient. When applicable, records will be used as a principal source to validate the data collected from the women.

Sample recruitment (6 months) with additional follow-up of the second stage data collection period (2 months).

Data analyses (1 month).

Report writing (2 months).

Limitation of the study design

During the postpartum period, it is unlikely that women would be able to take part in an interview for more than 20 minutes. Limited information will be gathered from participants during this period. Statistical methods will be used for controlling the influence of confounding variables on the association between home visits and health outcomes. The study does not intend to conduct an experimental study but aims to strengthen or broaden ongoing follow-up visit services.

Composition and justification of budget

The major cost will be in data collection: interview time and telephone costs. Each interview is expected to take approximately 15–20 minutes to complete.

Personnel: research assistant (RA): The RA will review hospital records to obtain information relating to obstetrics history and home follow-up visits. She will be employed to conduct telephone interviews and data entry using the SPSS program. Initial training will be provided. She will be required to assist in communicating with relevant organisations and to conduct administrative tasks.

Maintenance: Telephone and fax will be used to communicate with community organisations and key persons. Data will be collected by using a telephone interview method. Postage is needed for a summary of the study results to be mailed out to the participants, if requested.

Travel and others: Travel is required to conduct a pilot study using a personal interview method during the initial stages of the study.

Benefits of the study

Results of the study will be presented to the Hospital ABC staff at their departmental monthly meeting. A paper will be presented at the annual Australia Public Health Association conference. Research articles will be submitted to be published in international journals such as the *Journal of Advanced Nursing* and *Midwifery*. Grants will be sought from external sources.

If a difference in health outcomes between private-insured and public-insured women is identified, the implications for health care insurance will justify the grants to be sought from private health care insurers such as MBF. Any materials developed as the result of this project can be licensed with a commercial value.

Budget

Budget item	Amount ($)
Personnel (RA step 2, $24.52 p.hr total 467 hours)	12 162.00
Maintenance (telephone and facsimile)	819.00
Travel	282.00
Postage	90.00
Printing questionnaires	648.00
GST (applied to selected non-personnel items only)	184.00
Total	**14 185.00**

References

Armstrong, K. L., Fraser, J. A., Dadds, M. R., & Morris, J. (1999). A randomized, controlled trial of nurse home visiting to vulnerable families with newborns. *J Paediatr Child Health* 35(3), 237–44.

Australian Institute of Health & Welfare. (1994). *Australia's Mothers and Babies 1991.* Sydney: AIHW National Perinatal Statistics Unit.

Australian Institute of Health & Welfare. (1996). *Australia's Mothers and Babies 1993.* Sydney: AIHW National Perinatal Statistics Unit.

Australian Institute of Health & Welfare. (1999). *Australia's Mothers and Babies 1997.* Sydney: AIHW National Perinatal Statistics Unit.

Brooten, D., Roncoli, M., Finkler, S., Arnold, L., Cohen, A., & Mennuti, M. (1994). A randomized trial of early hospital discharge and home follow-up of women having cesarean birth. *Obstet Gynecol* 84(5), 832–8.

Brumfield, C. G., Nelson, K. G., Stotser, D., Yarbaugh, D., Patterson, P., & Sprayberry, N. K. (1996). 24-hour mother-infant discharge with a follow-up home health visit: Results in a selected medicaid population. *Obstet Gynecol* 88(4 Pt 1), 544–8.

Carty, E. M., & Bradley, C. F. (1990). A randomized, controlled evaluation of early postpartum hospital discharge. *Birth* 17(4), 199–204.

Cox, J., Holden, J. M., & Sagovsky, R. (1987). Detection of post-natal depression. Development of the 10-item Edinburgh Postnatal Depression scale. *British Journal of Psychiatry* 150, 782–6.

Cronenwett, L. R. (1985a). Network structure, social support, and psychological outcomes of pregnancy. *Nursing Research* 34, 93–9.

Cronenwett, L. R. (1985b). Parental network structure and perceived support after birth of first child. *Nursing Research* 34, 347–52.

Frank-Hanssen, M. A., Hanson, K. S., & Anderson, M. A. (1999). Postpartum home visits: Infant outcomes. *J Community Health Nurs* 16(1), 17–28.

Ghilarducci, E., & McCool, W. (1993). The influence of postpartum home visits on clinic attendance. *J Nurse Midwifery* 38(3), 152–8.

Grullon, K. E., & Grimes, D. A. (1997). The safety of early postpartum discharge: A review and critique. *Obstet Gynecol* 90(5), 860–5.

Jirojwong, S. (1995). Psychosocial factors relating to the use of antenatal services among pregnant women in Southern Thailand. PhD dissertation, Faculty of Medicine, Dentistry and Health Sciences, University of Melbourne.

Jirojwong, S., & Skolnik, M. (1990). Types of antenatal care and other related factors associated with low birth weight in Southern Thailand. *Asia Pacific Journal of Public Health* 4(2–3), 132–41.

Johnson, T. S., Brennan, R. A., & Flynn-Tymkow, C. D. (1999). A home visit program for breastfeeding education and support. *J Obstet Gynecol Neonatal Nurs* 28(5), 480–5.

Lieu, T. A., Braveman, P. A., Escobar, G. J., Fischer, A. F., Jensvold, N. G., & Capra, A. M. (2000). A randomized comparison of home and clinic follow-up visits after early postpartum hospital discharge. *Pediatrics* 105(5), 1058–65.

Meikle, S. F., Lyons, E., Hulac, P., & Orleans, M. (1998). Rehospitalizations and outpatient contacts of mothers and neonates after hospital discharge after vaginal delivery. *Am J Obstet Gynecol* 179(1), 166–71.

Personal communication, anonymous. (2000). Rockhampton, 6 July 2000.

Queensland Health. (1999). *1998 Annual Report*. Brisbane: Queensland Health.

Serwint, J. R., Wilson, M. H., Duggan, A. K., Mellits, E. D., Baumgardner, R. A., & DeAngelis, C. (1991). Do postpartum nursery visits by the primary care provider make a difference? *Pediatrics* 88(3), 444–9.

Weiss, R. S. (1974). The provision of social relationships. In Z. Rubin (ed.), *Doing Unto Others*. Englewood Cliffs, NJ: Prentice-Hall.

Williams, L. R., & Cooper, M. K. (1993). Nurse-managed postpartum home care. *J Obstet Gynecol Neonatal Nurs* 22(1), 25–31.

Appendix 2.2
Example of a Qualitative Research Proposal

Title: Health literacy and self-management of gestational diabetic: a study among Vietnamese, Cambodian, Thai and Laotian women in Sydney.

Researchers: Dr Sansnee Jirojwong, Associate Professor Virginia Schmied, Dr Jane Cioffi, Professor Maree Johnson, Professor Rhonda Griffiths, Associate Professor Hannah Dahlen.

Aim

This is a qualitative in-depth study that aims to explore Southeast Asian migrant women's health literacy relating to gestational diabetes. It will describe how Vietnamese, Cambodian, Thai and Laotian women use information from health professionals to self-manage their illness during the perinatal period. The impact of information from other sources including their family and community to self-manage the illness also will be explored.

Background

Gestational diabetes and Southeast Asian migrant women

Gestational diabetes (GDM) is a form of diabetes which develops during pregnancy in some women. Women with the disease will have high blood sugar for the first time during their pregnancy and this high blood sugar will disappear after birth. The symptom can recur in later pregnancies (AIHW 2006).

For pregnant women who appropriately manage the illness, complications including cesarean birth and having a large baby can be reduced (Koklanaris et al. 2007; Lee et al. 2007). They also have reduced risk of developing diabetes later in life (Gomez et al. 2008). Studies have shown that women who have gestational diabetes have a greater risk of developing type 2 diabetes. Many researchers (AIHW: Thow & Waters 2005; Hoffman et al. 1998; Lee et al. 2007) have found that approximately 10% of women with gestational diabetes will be diagnosed with type 2 diabetes within five years after the birth of their child and 50% will develop the diabetes within 25 years following the birth.

Southeast Asian-born women tend to have a higher rate of gestational diabetes than the rate in Australian-born women (Doery et al. 1989; Cheung et al. 2001; AIHW: Thow & Waters 2005). The rate of some migrant groups can be up to three times higher than the rate of GDM in Australian-born women. For example, the rate of gestational diabetes in Cambodian (6%) and Filipina (7%) migrant women in Australia was found to be twice the rate of all pregnant women (3.5%), while Vietnamese born women have a rate of 10%, which is three times higher than the rate of all pregnant women (Doery et al. 1989; Beischer et al. 1991; Moses et al. 1994).

Early detection and lifestyle modification are important strategies to reduce the severity and complications of gestational diabetes. Insulin or its derivatives is also used to control the GDM in some groups of women. If there are options, Asian-born women tend to choose oral medication rather than injectable insulin to control their blood sugar (Jacobson et al. 2005). Little is known about how Southeast Asian women understand and experience gestational diabetes. No published information describes how women gain information to manage their illness and how women understand the influence of the illness on the pregnancy, birth and health outcomes for both mother and infant. No published information explains how these women interpret their symptoms and use this to change their lifestyles. One small study using survey design in Victoria was reported recently at the Population Health Congress. This study found that Vietnamese and Arabic women with gestational diabetes had less knowledge about the disease, its management and impact when compared to Indian migrants and a group of Australian-born women (Razee et al. 2008). The influence of the women's family members and their communities on the management of the women's health is also reported.

This study is informed by the concept of health literacy. Health literacy is defined by the US National Library of Medicine as the degree to which individuals have the capacity to obtain, process and understand basic health information and services needed to make appropriate health decisions. It includes the ability to understand instructions on prescription drug bottles, appointment slips, medical education brochures and doctor's directions. Tasks include locating health information, evaluating information for credibility and quality, and analysing relative risks and benefits of various options of managing their illness.

Statement of the problem

Vietnamese, Cambodian, Thai and Laotian women have a high risk of having gestational diabetes (Doery et al. 1989; Cheung et al. 2001; AIHW: Thow & Waters 2005). There is a gap of knowledge about how these women interpret their symptoms and use their interpretation to monitor or reduce the severity of diabetes. The impact of information gained from health care professionals, their family and their community on their perception of the disease and self-management is not known.

Significance of the problem

Diabetes is one of the national chronic diseases priorities. Southeast Asian pregnant women have a higher rate of gestational diabetes. They also have a higher risk of having type 2 diabetes than Australian born women (AIHW 2006; AIHW: Thow & Waters 2005). Early and appropriate self-management of the disease by the women will have long-term effects on reducing the severity of the disease and its complications (Gomez et al. 2008).

The results of this study will help identify barriers and facilitating factors that influence the ability of Southeast Asian-born pregnant women to understand and use information to manage their illness. These self-managements include their diet, physical activities and medication, when applicable. Their understanding of illness management on their infant's health will also be explored. This is particularly important because cultural beliefs and practices are known to strongly influence disease management and outcomes (Kleinman 1980). This study's results will be used to improve the quality of health promotion and disease prevention information so that women can use it to effectively manage their current illness. It will also have long-term effects if women can modify their lifestyles, which then reduce the risk of having the diabetes later in their life.

Research questions

The participants of this study are Vietnam, Cambodia, Thailand and Laos-born pregnant women. Specific research questions are:

- What are Vietnamese, Cambodian, Thailand and Laos-born pregnant women's knowledge, attitudes and cultural beliefs about gestational diabetes and its impact on their health and their infant's health?
- How do Vietnamese, Cambodian, Thai and Laos-born pregnant women seek, locate and understand health information about gestational diabetes from different sources (for example, health professionals, family and community)?
- How do the women interpret and evaluate information from different sources and ignore it or use it to manage their symptom during the perinatal period?
- To what extent do these women modify their lifestyles including diet and physical activities during pregnancy and following birth because of gestational diabetes and how has this been influenced by information from different sources?

Research method

Study design

A qualitative in-depth research method will be used.

Study participants and recruitment

Four major migrant groups (Vietnamese, Cambodian, Thai and Laotian women) will be recruited from Liverpool and Fairfield Hospitals. Women who receive care at a special antenatal clinic (endocrinology clinic) will be invited to participate in the study. We will also work with the bilingual early parental educators in this area who provide education for Vietnamese, Cambodian, Thai and Laotian women during pregnancy to identify and approach women who have gestational diabetes.

The first investigator will also use her well-established link with community organisations such as Buddhist temples to recruit additional participants by the use of a snowball method (personal contact or word of mouth). This method is effective in studies among Australian minority groups (Jirojwong & Manderson 2001). Bilingual research assistants together with Chief Investigator (CI 1) will recruit women and conduct the interview in their own language.

Sampling procedure and sample size

There will be 10–12 women of each migrant group included in the study. They will be the first or the second generation migrant women from Vietnam, Cambodia, Thailand and Laos. The total of 50 participants will have gestational diabetes and will be interviewed in their own language either during their pregnancy or within three months after birth.

Women will be recruited at the Liverpool and Fairfield Hospitals endocrinology antenatal clinic. Hospital staff will identify women who are eligible to be included in the study. The researcher will approach and invite women to take part in the study. Arrangements will be made to interview participants at a time and location convenient to them. An interview will be tape-recorded and will be no longer than one hour.

In addition, personal contact through community organisations such as Buddhist temples and community organisations will be used. The number of participants will be sufficient to saturate the data and identify themes.

Collection of data

Three research assistants (RAs) who are bilingual in Vietnamese-English, Khmer-English or Laotian-English will be employed to assist with data collection. The first CI is an accredited interpreter in Thai-English and will interview Thailand and Laos-born women. Training of the RAs will be conducted prior to the data collection. Personal interviews will be audio-recorded and transcribed verbatim. Field notes and diary will be used to record observation information.

The participants will participate in a personal in-depth interview at the hospital clinic, their own home or a location nominated by them. The interview will explore how women understand gestational diabetes and its impact on their health and their infant's health, what are the sources of information that they use to manage the symptom and the impacts of their environments including home, work, social gathering and community organisations on their self-management. Their beliefs, relating to lifestyle modification and medication when applicable to their health and their baby's health during their perinatal period, will be explored. Field notes and diary will be used as other sources of information.

Data will be analysed using content analysis to identify themes and categories (Miles & Huberman 1994). The steps described by Miles and Huberman will be used. The study results will be presented to relevant organisations and individuals. The results will be further used to design structure a questionnaire which will be applied in a larger study among Asian-born pregnant women.

Budget

The requested project budget is $16 360.00.

Request	Amount $
Personnel	13 441.30
Bilingual research assistants (Vietnamese, Cambodian, Thai and Laotian) (300 hr will be used to conduct interviews and also transcribe the recordings) HEW 5.1 rate/hr = $34.34, plus on cost 16.5% (total = $40.01/hr) (a) Interview 50 participants, 1 hr/person = 50 hr (b) Recruitment of participants (additional 30 min/participant, total = 25hr) (c) Communication with team members and meetings = 20 hours & attend training sessions for reliability = 5 hours (total = 25 hr) (d) Transcribe the recorded interviews – verbatim, 4 hr / 1 hr interview (200 hr)	12 001.83
Administrative assistance 40 hours (help with filing and communications) HEW 4.1 rate/hr = $30.89, plus on cost 16.5% (total = $35.99/hr)	1 439.47
Travel	1 320.00
Interview each participant 40 km round trip x 50 participants x $0.66/km	1 320.00
Maintenance	1 600.00
Computer accessories (memory sticks, disks)	400.00
Consumables	200.00
Fax, mail and other communication, $50/mth x 4 mth	200.00
Digital recorder (Each $200.00 x 4)	800.00
TOTAL Requested	16 360.00 (note 1)

Note 1 Round to the nearest absolute figure.

Timeline for funds to be expended in 2008

Activities	Month											
	1 July 08	2	3	4	5	6	7 Jan 09	8	9	10	11	12
Literature review	X	X	X	X	X	X	X	X	X	X		
Gaining ethical clearance, confirmation of the study with participating organisations and key contact persons	X	X										
Employing and training research assistants	X	X										
Data collection (RAs and SJ)			X	X								
Data analysis (SJ and the team)					X	X	X	X	X			
Writing grant application for external fund (SJ and the team)						X	X	X	ARC linkage	X		
Writing the final report (SJ and the team)								X	X	X		
Writing manuscripts for publication (SJ and the team)					X	X	X	X	X	X	X	

Projected outcomes of the project

By mid-2009, the following outcomes will be achieved:

- The results of this study will support an external grant application. Targeted grant agencies are Diabetes Australia, the Kidney Foundation and ARC linkage grant.
- At least two research manuscripts will be submitted to refereed journals.
- The results of the study will be presented at two international conferences (Public Health Association of Australia and International Council of Nurses Conference).
- The ongoing work will attract at least one new higher degree research student for 2009.
- An interdisciplinary collaborative research team will be formed with researchers from Victoria University and Monash University.
- Links will be strengthened with community organisations including Khmer Workers Forum, Lao Buddhist Society, Australia and Health Promotion Service, Sydney South West Area Health Service.

References

Australian Institute of Health & Welfare: Thow, A.M., & Waters, A.-M. (2005). *Diabetes in Culturally and Linguistically Diverse Australians: Identification of Communities at High Risk.* AIHW cat. no. CVD 30. Canberra: Australian Institute of Health and Welfare.

Australian Institute of Health & Welfare. (2006). *Australia's Health 2006*. Canberra: Australian Institute of Health and Welfare.

Beischer, N. A., Oats, J. N., Henry, O. A., Sheedy, M. T., & Walstab, J. E. (1991). Incidence and severity of gestational diabetes mellitus according to country of birth in women living in Australia. *Diabetes* 40 Suppl 2, 35–8.

Cheung, N. W., Wasmer, G., & Al-Ali, J. (2001). Risk factors for gestational diabetes among Asian women. *Diabetes Care* 24(5), 955–6.

Doery, J. C. G., Edis, K., Healy, D., Bishop, S., & Tippett, C. (1989). Very high prevalence of gestational diabetes in Vietnamese and Cambodian women (letters to the editor). *Med J Aust* 151, 111.

Gomez, M., Colagiuri, R., Buckley, A., Eigenmann, C., & Thomas, M. (2008). Evaluating type 2 diabetes prevention programs in culturally and linguistically diverse communities (CALD)— What's needed? Paper presented at the Population Health Congress 2008: A Global World, Practical Action for Health and Well-being, 6–9 July 2008, Brisbane, Queensland.

Hoffman, L., Nolan, C., Wilson, J. D., Oats, J. J., & Simmons, D. (1998). Gestational diabetes mellitus: Management guidelines. The Australasian Diabetes in Pregnancy Society. *Med J Aust* 169(2), 93–7.

Jacobson, G. F., Ramos, G. A., Ching, J. Y., Kirby, R. S., Ferrara, A., & Field, D. R. (2005). Comparison of glyburide and insulin for the management of gestational diabetes in a large managed care organization. *Am J Obstet Gynecol* 193(1), 118–24.

Jirojwong, S., & Manderson, L. (2001). The feeling of sadness: Migration and subjective assessment of mental health among Thai women in Brisbane, Australia. *Transcultural Psychiatry* 38(2), 167–86.

Kleinman, A. (1980). *Patients and Healers in the Context of Culture*. Berkeley: University of California Press.

Koklanaris, N., Bonnano, C., Seubert, D., Anzai, Y., Jennings, R., & Lee, M. J. (2007). Does raising the glucose challenge test threshold impact birthweight in Asian gravidas? *J Perinat Med* 35(2), 100–3.

Lee, A. J., Hiscock, R. J., Wein, P., Walker, S. P., & Permezel, M. (2007). Gestational diabetes mellitus: Clinical predictors and long-term risk of developing type 2 diabetes: A retrospective cohort study using survival analysis. *Diabetes Care* 30(4), 878–83.

Miles, B. M., & Huberman, A. M. (1994). Introduction: Three approaches to qualitative data analysis. In B. M. Miles & A. M. Huberman (eds), *An Expanded Sourcebook: Qualitative Data Analysis*. London: Sage Publications, pp. 8–12.

Moses, R. G., Griffiths, R. D. & McPherson, S. (1994). The incidence of gestational diabetes mellitus in the Illawarra area of New South Wales. *Aust N Z J Obstet Gynaecol* 34(4), 425–7.

Razee, H., Cheung, W., Ploeg, H., Smith, B., Blignault, I., & McLean, M. (2008). Physical activity and nutritional behaviour in women with recent gestational diabetes. Paper presented at the Population Health Congress 2008: A Global World, Practical Action for Health and Well-being, 6–9 July 2008, Brisbane, Queensland.

Sources: Modified from

Jirojwong, S., Ritchie, B., Russell, E., & Walker, S. (2000). *Outcomes with Home Follow Up Visit After Postpartum Hospital Discharge*. Research proposal submitted to Central Queensland University, Rockhampton.

Jirojwong, S., Schmied, V., Cioffi, J., Johnson, M., Griffiths, R., & Dahlen, H. (2008). *Health Literacy and Self Management of Gestational Diabetic: A Study Among Vietnamese, Cambodian, Thai and Laotian Women in Sydney*. Research proposal submitted to College of Health and Science, University of Western Sydney, Sydney.

Further reading

Allen, D., & Lyne, P. (2006). *The Reality of Nursing Research Politics, Practices, and Processes.* London and New York: Routledge.

Brinkmann, S. (2009). Literature as qualitative inquiry: The novelist as researcher. *Qualitative Inquiry* 15(8), 1376–94.

Burns, N. P. D., & Grove, S. K. (2007). *Understanding Nursing Research: Building an Evidence-Based Practice.* St Louis, MI: Elsevier Saunders.

Chung, K. C., & Shauver, M. J. (2008). Fundamental Principles of Writing a Successful Grant Proposal. *Journal of Hand Surgery* 33(4), 566–72.

Darbyshire, P., Downes, M., Collins, C., & Dyer, S. (2005). Moving from institutional dependence to entrepreneurialism: Creating and funding a collaborative research and practice development position. *Journal of Clinical Nursing* 14(8A), 926–34.

Weblinks

EndNote

<www.endnote.com>

Reference Manager

<www.refman.com>

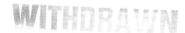

Zotero

<http://libguides.mit.edu/zotero>

Comparison of the major bibliographic software products

<http://libraries.mit.edu/help/bibliography/comparison.html>

References

Avery, D. (2005). A modest proposal for research. *Bulletin of the World Health Organization* 83(7), 484.

Ayres, L. (2007). Qualitative research proposals—Part I: Posing the problem. *Journal of Wound, Ostomy and Continence Nursing* 34(1), 30–2.

Beitz, J. M., & Bliss, D. Z. (2005). Preparing a successful grant proposal—Part 1: Developing research aims and the significance of the project. *Journal of Wound, Ostomy and Continence Nursing* 32(1), 16–18.

Bliss, D. Z. (2005). Writing a grant proposal—Part 6: The budget, budget justification, and resource environment. *Journal of Wound, Ostomy and Continence Nursing* 32(6), 365–7.

Bliss, D. Z., & Savik, K. (2005). Writing a grant proposal—Part 2: Research methods—Part 2. *Journal of Wound, Ostomy and Continence Nursing* 32(4), 226–9.

Clevenger, L. (1994). The effect of head covering on rewarming and shivering in cardiac surgical patients. *Critical Care Nursing Quarterly* 17, 73–85.

Colwell, J. C., Bliss, D. Z., Engberg, S., & Moore, K. N. (2005). Preparing a grant proposal—Part 5. Organization and revision. *Journal of Wound, Ostomy and Continence Nursing* 32(5), 291–3.

Cowin, L., Johnson, M., Craven, R. G., & Marsh, H. W. (2008). Causal modeling of self-concept, job satisfaction, and retention of nurses. *International Journal of Nursing Studies* 45, 1449–59.

Craven, R. G., Marsh, H. W., & Burnett, P. (2003). Cracking the self-concept enhancement conundrum: A call and blueprint for the next generation of self-concept enhancement research. In H. W. Marsh, R. G. Craven & D. McInerney (eds). *International Advances in Self Research*, vol. 1 (pp. 91–126). Greenwich, CT: Information Age Publishing.

Devine, E. B. (2009). The art of obtaining grants. *American Journal of Health-System Pharmacy* 66(6), 580–7.

Dickson, G. L., & Flynn, L. (2009). *Nursing Policy Research: Turning Evidence-Based Research into Health Policy.* New York: Springer.

Endacott, R. (2005). Clinical research 6: Writing and research. *Intensive and Critical Care Nursing* 21(4), 258–61.

Endacott, R. (2008). Clinical research 6: Writing and research. *International Emergency Nursing* 16(3), 211–14.

Engberg, S., & Bliss, D. Z. (2005). Writing a grant proposal—Part 1: Research methods. *Journal of Wound, Ostomy and Continence Nursing* 32(3), 157–62.

Falk, G. W. (2006). Turning an idea into a grant. *Gastrointestinal Endoscopy* 64(suppl.), S11–S13.

Farthing, M. J. G. (2006). Authors and publication practices. *Science and Engineering Ethics* 12(1), 41–52.

Fitzpatrick, J. J., & Wallace, M. P. R. N. (2006). *Encyclopedia of Nursing Research.* New York: Springer.

Flaherty, A. (2007). A brief proposal, 150 words [3]. *Nature* 450(7173), 1156.

Francis, B. J., Bork, E. C., & Carstens, P. S. (1979). *The Proposal Cookbook. A Step by Step Guide to Dissertation and Thesis Proposal Writing*, 3rd edn. USA: Action Research Associates.

Fridlund, B. (2006). Writing a scientific manuscript: Some formal and informal proposals. *European Journal of Cardiovascular Nursing* 5(3), 185–7.

Gerrish, K., & Lacey, A. (2006). *The Research Process in Nursing.* Oxford, UK and Malden, MA: Blackwell Publishers.

Grieger, M. C. A. (2005). Authorship: An ethical dilemma of science. *Sao Paulo Medical Journal* 123(5), 242–6.

Haber, J., LoBiondo-Wood, G., Cameron, C., & Singh, M. D. (2009). *Nursing Research in Canada: Methods and Critical Appraisal for Evidence-Based Practice.* Toronto: Mosby Elsevier.

Hamilton, H., & Clare, J. (2004). Reviewing the literature: making 'the literature' work for you. *Collegian: Journal of the Royal College of Nursing Australia* 11(1), 8–11.

Harper, P. J. (2007). Writing research proposals: Five rules. *HIV Nursing* 8(2), 15–17.

Houser, J. (2008). *Nursing Research: Reading, Using, and Creating Evidence*. Sudbury, MA: Jones & Bartlett Publishers.

Inouye, S. K., & Fiellin, D. A. (2005). An evidence-based guide to writing grant proposals for clinical research. *Annals of Internal Medicine* 142(4), 274–82.

Jenicek, M. (2006). How to read, understand, and write 'Discussion' sections in medical articles. An exercise in critical thinking. *Medical Science Monitor* 12(6), SR28–SR36.

Johnson, M., Stewart, H., Langdon, R., Kelly, P., & Yong, L. (2005). A comparison of the outcomes of partnership caseload midwifery and standard hospital care in low risk mothers. *Australian Journal of Advanced Nursing* 22(3), 22–8.

Kelly, J. E. (2008). Getting funded. *Journal of Hospital Librarianship* 8(4), 469–78.

Kilbourn, B. (2006). The qualitative doctoral dissertation proposal. *Teachers College Record* 108(4), 529–76.

Klopper, H. (2008). The qualitative research proposal. *Curationis* 31(4), 62–72.

LoBiondo-Wood, G., & Haber, J. (2010). *Nursing Research: Methods and Critical Appraisal for Evidence-Based Practice*. St Louis, MO: Mosby Elsevier.

Macnee, C. L., & McCabe, S. R. N. (2008). *Understanding Nursing Research: Using Research in Evidence-Based Practice*. Philadelphia, PA: Wolters Kluwer Health/Lippincott Williams & Wilkins.

Marsh, H. W., & Ayotte, V. (2003). Do multiple dimensions of self-concept become more differentiated with age? The differential distinctiveness hypothesis. *Journal of Educational Psychology* 95(4), 687–706.

Marsh, H. W., & Perry, C. (2005). Self-concept contributes to winning gold medals: Causal ordering of self-concept and elite swimming performance. *Journal of Sports Exercise Psychology* 27, 71–91.

McCluskey, A., Johnson, M., & Tate, R. (2007). The process of care management following brain injury: A grounded theory study. *Brain Impairment* 8(3), 293–311.

McLaughlin, M. M. K., & Bulla, S. (2010). *Real Stories of Nursing Research: The Quest for Magnet Recognition*. Sudbury, MA: Jones & Bartlett Publishers.

Moule, P., & Goodman, M. (2009). *Nursing Research: An Introduction*. Los Angeles and London: Sage.

Myors, K., Johnson, M., & Langdon, R. (2001). Coping styles of pregnant adolescents. *Public Health Nursing* 18(1), 24–32.

Nieswiadomy, R. M. (2002). *Foundations of Nursing Research*. Upper Saddle River, NJ: Prentice Hall.

Nieswiadomy, R. M. (2008). *Foundations of Nursing Research*. Upper Saddle River, NJ: Pearson/Prentice Hall.

Parahoo, K. (2006). *Nursing Research: Principles, Process and Issues*. Basingstoke: Palgrave Macmillan.

Parker, B., & Steeves, R. (2005). The National Research Service Award: Strategies for developing a successful proposal. *Journal of Professional Nursing* 21(1), 23–31.

Polit, D. F., & Beck, C. T. (2008). *Nursing Research: Generating and Assessing Evidence for Nursing Practice*. Philadelphia: Wolters Kluwer Health/Lippincott Williams & Wilkins.

Polit, D. F., & Beck, C. T. (2010). *Essentials of Nursing Research: Appraising Evidence for Nursing Practice*. Philadelphia: Wolters Kluwer Health/Lippincott Williams & Wilkins.

Schmelzer, M. (2006). How to start a research proposal. *Gastroenterology Nursing* 29(2), 186–8.

Schneider, Z., Whitehead, D., & Elliott, D. R. N. (2007). *Nursing and Midwifery Research: Methods and Appraisal for Evidence-Based Practice*. Sydney: Elsevier Australia.

Sonis, J. H., Triffleman, E., King, L., & King, D. (2009). How to write an NIH R13 conference grant application. *Academic Psychiatry* 33(3), 256–60.

Stevens, D., Johnson, M., & Langdon, R. (2000). A comparison of two warming techniques in surgical patients with mild or moderate hypothermia. *International Journal of Nursing Practice* 6(5), 268–75.

Vivar, C. G., McQueen, A., Whyte, D. A., & Armayor, N. C. (2007). Getting started with qualitative research: Developing a research proposal. *Nurse Researcher* 14(3), 60–73.

Watson, R. (2008). *Nursing Research: Designs and Methods*. Edinburgh: Churchill Livingstone.

CHAPTER 3

Ethical and Legal Considerations in Research

Keri Chater

Chapter learning objectives

By the end of this chapter you will be able to:

▸ explain the historical development of human research ethics committees

▸ define and delineate key terms in ethics such as beneficence, non-maleficence, confidentiality, anonymity, risks and rights of participants in the research process

▸ discuss the process of gaining informed consent

▸ recognise the needs of vulnerable groups in research

▸ appreciate the need to examine potential power relationships in research.

History of ethics committees

In many countries, including Australia, all research undertaken has to adhere to a strict set of legal and ethical guidelines, and nursing research is no different. Ethical comportment in research had its genesis in the Nuremberg Trials after the Second World War (Annas & Grodin 1992). The main reason for this was a response to the Nazi experimentation on innocent people who did not consent to participation in some of the atrocious experiments that took place during the Third Reich (Caplan 1992).

Although the Nuremberg Trials were held to try criminals for different types of war crimes, the 'Doctors' trial' proved to be exceptionally complex because the judges were not only concerned with the criminal element of the medical experiments but also with the much broader ethical elements of the research that was carried out. In the opening address for the Doctors' Trial on 9 December 1946 it was stated:

> The defendants in the dock are charged with murder, but this is no mere murder trial… To kill, to maim, and to torture is criminal under all modern systems of law. These defendants did not kill in hot blood, nor for personal enrichment…They are not ignorant men. Most of them are trained physicians and some of them are distinguished scientists. Yet these defendants, all of whom are fully able to comprehend the nature of their acts, and most of whom are exceptionally qualified to form a moral and professional judgment in this respect, are responsible for wholesale murder and unspeakably cruel tortures. (Taylor 1992, p. 67)

The Nuremberg Code was a document that arose from the findings of these trials, which listed 10 points for the conduct of ethical research. Point one was that research participants need to be able to give 'free, voluntary, and informed consent' (Grodin 1992, p. 135) and this has been the guiding ethical principle adopted today.

The Nuremberg Code was formalised in law in the International Covenant on Civil and Political Rights and adopted by the United Nations General Assembly in 1976. The Nuremberg Code also informed the Declarations of Helsinki I and II (Perely et al. 1992), which emphasised informed consent and relationships of dependency between a researcher and a participant and a participant's competence to decide to take part in the research.

Subsequently, these legal and ethical guidelines for undertaking research have formed the bases of international and national human research ethics committees (HRECs). In Australia, the overriding committee is called the Australian Health Ethics Committee (AHEC), which is a sub-committee of the statutory body, the National Health and Medical Research Council (NHMRC). In New Zealand, the National Ethics Advisory Committee (NEAC) has a statutory function to advise the New Zealand Minister for Health on issues relating to ethical conduct of research, and the Health Research Council of New Zealand (HRC) reviews and assesses ethical applications for undertaking research.

Roles of research councils and the conduct of health research

Both Australia and New Zealand have national ethics committees that formulate policies and oversee the implementation of ethical conduct in human research. These committees are statutory and exist by act of Parliament. They also provide guidelines for the various levels of HRECs, which are found in many tertiary education, health and social organisations.

For the purpose of nursing research, the main committees nurse researchers will come into contact with are those based in universities or hospitals. All universities and major hospitals have an ethics committee. Many government departments, including those associated with social services, have their own ethics committees.

The role of the human research ethics committee

Generally, a HREC is composed of a minimum of eight people with equal representation of men and women, with the majority of membership being from outside the institution. The external membership of the committee should represent the community, have an interest in health and medical research, but not undertake research. One member should represent health professions, for example, a nurse or allied health person. Another member should represent and perform pastoral care in the community, for example, a religious leader or an Indigenous leader. Other membership includes a lawyer and representatives of researchers who are currently undertaking research and submitting or reviewing research proposals (NHMRC 2007).

There are two major roles of a HREC at an organisational level: first, to protect the public, and second, to support and encourage research. In order to protect the public, all proposed research must be approved by an ethics committee. Research that involves humans and collects data by interviewing, reviewing health records or surveying will require approval from a HREC of the relevant institution. If patients are participants and the research is conducted by nurses, an ethical clearance application will need to be submitted to the hospital or health organisation where the nurses are working or the patients are being treated.

For a novice researcher, it is recommended to limit the research project to one organisation only. For example, a qualitative research project may limit participants to being recruited from one educational institution or a location outside their place of employment. Therefore, only one ethics application will need to be submitted to the ethics committee of the researcher's employment organisation. If the study participants are patients, the ethics committee of the relevant health organisation needs to approve the study. The more organisations required to approve the project, the greater the number of ethics applications that will have to be submitted. Researchers need to be aware of the time required for the review process and take this into account in their project management.

In Australia, the National Ethics Application Form is completed online. HREC members often access the form electronically. For multicentre studies, a lead HREC reviews the ethics application and approves the project at the initial site, and then the researcher seeks approval from each of the other sites by supplying evidence of the initial approval from the lead committee. Although this does reduce the number of applications to be processed depending on the number of sites, the timeframe for ethical approval from multiple HRECs could still be one year or more depending on the number of sites involved.

To submit an application to the ethics committee, some relevant protocols have to be followed. Large organisations will have these available in electronic form at their relevant websites. A small organisation will have an administrative unit to review and approve a research project conducted in the organisation. Examples of ethics authorities in Australia and New Zealand that have protocols for seeking research ethics approval and their links are listed later under Weblinks. The main protocol or form required will have detailed information on the research project. The researcher needs to outline the nature of the research question and details of the research method. It is important to describe how research participants' confidentiality will be protected, what risk and benefit are associated with participating in the research, and how participant consent will be obtained. Information in the participant information sheet must include the participants' right to ask questions relating to the study, the researcher's name and contact details, the right of the participant to withdraw from the research without any negative effect on care provided to them, and how data will be managed and used by the researcher (Shamoo & Khin-Maung-Gyi 2002).

▶▶▶ TERMS, TIPS AND SKILLS

If you are receiving funding to support your research, this must be clearly stated in the research application. The HREC will want to know who is the funding body and the amount of funding, in particular if this will impact on the study's findings. If you are carrying out research in other countries as well as your own, you will need to provide evidence that ethics approval has been sought and gained in those locations.

Aside from the actual ethics application there are two additional forms the researcher will need to submit to the ethics committee. The first is called a plain language statement (PLS). The PLS outlines, in simple language, exactly what the research is about. More importantly, it outlines what the person will be participating in, what is expected of the participant and how the researcher will protect the participant's privacy. Once the potential participant has read and understood what the study is about and their level of involvement, they may agree to participate. If the person agrees to participate this is where the second form, the consent form, becomes important. The consent form is a standardised form that can be modified to reflect the nature of the research.

Box 3.1 is an example of how a PLS can be set out. It also covers all the areas that need to be addressed in the process of informing a potential participant. At the bottom of the PLS, there is a statement regarding the participant's right to contact the ethics committee that approves the research project. Examples of a PLS and a consent form are shown in Appendices 3.1 and 3.2.

BOX 3.1

INVITATION TO PARTICIPATE IN A RESEARCH PROJECT

(Fill in the project title)

Who is conducting this research?

What is the research project about?

Why am I being asked to participate?

What do I need to do when participating in this project?

What are the benefits for me?

Will there be a future benefit?

Will my participation be confidential?

What are my rights and risks as a participant?

Contact details of the researcher

Contact details of the ethics committee

Ethical principles and research conduct

Informed consent

Informed and voluntary consent to participate in research is the first principle of the Nuremberg Code (Katz 1992) and remains a cornerstone of research ethics. Consent to participate in research or indeed any nursing or medical intervention is based on the principle of autonomy (Jackson 2006). For a potential participant to be informed, there needs to be a set of requirements in place. First, all the information about the research, including risks and benefits, must be provided to the participant, the same as for carrying out a nursing procedure. Second, the participant needs to understand what the study involves. This is particularly important for people whose first language is not English. Third, the participant must have the capacity to consent to the research, which has implications for minors or people with cognitive impairment. Fourth, consent must be voluntary; this means that the participant freely consents to be part of the study and has the right to withdraw at any time (Leedy & Ormond 2010). Finally, the actual consent form must be signed by the participant and witnessed by the researcher.

As researchers, how do we ensure that our participants are informed and able to consent? Generally there are a number of steps to be followed. The researcher makes contact with each potential participant through the chosen methodological strategies. These can include making contact by telephone or emailing the person to give a brief overview of the research. If the person is interested, the researcher makes a time to meet and mail or email the research information to them before the meeting. The PLS is either read out or given to the participant before gaining their consent.

Once the potential participant has been informed and is aware of all the risks and benefits of participating in the research, they will be asked to sign a consent form (see Appendices 3.1 and 3.2). Consent forms contain standardised information with some variation depending on each organisation's requirements. Specific information in the consent form has to be modified to fit with the research protocol, such as methods used to collect the data from participants and how the data will be used.

Beneficence and non-maleficence

When undertaking research there needs to be a favourable risk:benefit ratio. This means that the benefit to the participant will outweigh the risk of being involved in the research. The researcher has the obligation to maximise the benefit of participation and minimise the risk. In ethical terms, this is called beneficence (Katz 1992). The word 'beneficence' comes from the Latin *beneficus* from *bene* meaning 'good' or 'well', so beneficence means doing good, generosity, etc. During the research process the researcher needs to be aware that what they are asking the participant to do will be of benefit.

However, the benefit of research to the participant may not be immediately obvious and this needs to be made clear to the participant. For example, what the researcher is asking the participant to do is to contribute to the growing body of knowledge of nursing. In addition, by their participation they will be contributing to the improvement of nursing care and health outcomes of future clients who have a health condition similar to theirs. Their participation is thus of benefit to the discipline of nursing and to society in general.

It is important that the researcher also ensures that they do no harm. In ethics, this is termed non-maleficence. 'Maleficence' comes from the Latin *maleficus* meaning 'doing evil', 'wicked'. The researcher needs to ensure that the person participating in the research will not be harmed or will be able to weigh up the benefits and risks associated with the research. Non-maleficence therefore means doing no harm.

Beneficence and non-maleficence are not the same, although they are often confused or used interchangeably. The confusion is mostly due to individual interpretation (Burkhardt & Nathaniel 2002). Simply put, beneficence is the act of doing a good or beneficial act whereas non-maleficence means that as nurses we consciously do not act to harm a person. The complexity of this can be very easily demonstrated below.

As nurses, we all have to give someone a potentially painful injection or carry out a painful procedure. We know that our nursing action may cause pain (maleficence) and we also know that the action will be beneficial (beneficence). But as nurses we also know that our patients need to be informed about the procedure we are about to undertake and also need to consent to it as well as being aware of the risks and benefits. This is the same with research.

RESEARCH IN PRACTICE 3.1

BENEFICENCE AND MALEFICENCE

I was undertaking a qualitative research project examining older people's decision-making as they followed health-related instructions. People I was interviewing were attending a day-based rehabilitation clinic and the interviews were conducted either at the clinic or in the participant's home. While I was interviewing a male participant, he became visibly distressed. At that time I was tape-recording the interview and the data were potentially excellent. I recognised that the questions I was asking were distressing.

My choices were to continue with the interview or stop and allow the participant some time to regain his composure. The decision was easy. I turned the recorder off and stopped the interview. It was an act of beneficence as I was trying to minimise harm. On the other hand, if I had continued with my questioning, my participant might have become even more distressed and this would have constituted an act of maleficence.

Rights

The rights of the participant are based on the broader notion of human rights, which include the right to respect for human dignity. There are two aspects to this (Johnstone 2009). First, the participant has the right to full disclosure. This means that the researcher must disclose all aspects of the research including what is to be involved in it: the risk and benefits; protection of the participant's identity; persons who will access the data; time commitment to the research; the right to withdraw at any time without prejudice; and who to contact if they have any further questions. One other aspect to be included is the methods used to handle and store the data. The participant will also need to know if the researcher is going to publish the findings or present them at a conference. All this information should be verbally explained and contained in the PLS.

Second, human dignity includes the right to be free from coercion. The participant must feel free to withdraw without penalty. Likewise there must not be any excessive reward for participating. Along with this, the researcher and the participant should not be in a dependent relationship because this could be misconstrued as coercion. Dependent relationships can also be seen as power relationships (NHMRC 2007). Examples are nurse researchers researching their patients or nurse academics researching their students. Both forms of research are legitimate, but researchers will have to take extra care in explaining how they will address the issues of dependency and power relationships.

Privacy and confidentiality

Participants also have the right to privacy. They have the choice of what information to share and what not to share. As well as this, they need to know that what is shared will be treated with respect and kept in confidence.

There are two common ways to maintain participant confidentiality. One is to assign a number to each participant's data—participant 1, 2, 3 and so on. Another is to give each participant a pseudonym. The name of each person will be replaced with another name so that they will not be recognised in any research report. The issue of confidentiality is less likely to occur in quantitative research when the number of participants is large and the data are presented in an aggregated form.

In addition, the researcher needs to assure the participant of anonymity. Anonymity is generally assured when a survey technique is used to gather data. Survey techniques are commonly used with quantitative research. If the survey has no identifying marker and the researcher does not know who returned the survey then the participant is truly anonymous to the researcher.

A major interesting methodological and ethical issue is found when a focus group interview or a group observation is used to collect qualitative data. Generally, participants in a focus group are people considered to be key stakeholders, meaning people who have a recognised expertise in a specific area of nursing (Perry 2007). This creates an interesting ethical issue because not only does the researcher hear and collect information from the participants but so do the other members of the group, who may or may not know each other.

In order to ensure confidentiality and anonymity here, the researcher will have to outline in the PLS the 'ground rules' for participating as well as reiterate the rules at the beginning of the focus group. These rules are about human dignity, maintaining privacy of the information shared by participants, and not discussing the membership of the group outside that forum; they include respect for the comments of others in the group, and allowing each member to have equal time when discussing the issue under research.

One mistake that researchers often make is to assure both anonymity and confidentiality when submitting ethics protocols for approval. Anonymity and confidentiality are different. If your research method involves participants filling out a survey and posting it back or delivering it to an assigned spot, and if the survey has no identification markers, then the participant will be anonymous. This means that the researcher has no way of identifying the participant.

On the other hand, if your research method is face-to-face interviews, the researcher knows who the participant is. In this situation anonymity cannot be guaranteed. What the researcher has to assure the participant in the PLS is how the participant's confidentiality will be ensured.

Data management throughout the research study and beyond

Another aspect of rights is that participants need to know how the information collected will be managed. There are two aspects to management of data. The first is how the researcher, particularly in qualitative research, will faithfully interpret the participant's views and the second is the physical management of the data (Kerridge et al. 2009).

Participants need to be assured that their views will not be misrepresented or misquoted. This is both a methodological and an ethical issue. When the researcher embarks on a research project, the methodology chosen is the one most suitable to address the research question. The research methodology will have clear steps guiding how data will be analysed and interpreted.

The physical management of data refers to the approach used to secure the data during the research process as well as into the future. Ethics committees generally stipulate the period that data needs to be stored and the method used to destroy the data. If the data are interview transcripts, observation notes, diary or survey questionnaires, these must be kept for five years after the research is concluded. If the research involves higher levels of risk, for example blood samples, then generally the data or sample blood needs to be kept for 15 years (NHMRC 2007).

As well as length of time kept, it is essential to maintain the security of the data. For non-computer-based data such as transcripts, surveys, tape-recordings or photos, these data need to be kept in a locked cupboard. Signed consent forms or any other information that could identify the participant needs to be kept separately from the actual data in another locked cupboard. This information needs to be conveyed to the participants, as well as a statement of exactly who will access the data and how long the data will be kept. Organisations such as universities will have policies on these issues. For example, Central Queensland University requires data to be kept for five years. Generally, people who access the data are the research team, which may include the research assistant or the student's supervisors.

Almost all researchers use computers now and data is often stored electronically on a computer. The management of data on a computer will be stipulated by the institution in which the research will be undertaken. Generally, they will be stored on a computer and need to be protected by a password.

Technology is growing rapidly and ethics committees need to keep up with the changes in the technology for gathering data. Recently more and more people are using computer technology to gain access to participants as well as collect data. Each institution will have protocols in place for each type of data collection and storage of the collected data.

Vulnerable groups and power relationships between researcher and participant

It can be argued that any person who is in hospital is vulnerable. Being sufficiently unwell to require hospitalisation, or having test results that may influence a life-changing condition, contributes to a person's vulnerability to outside factors. As nurses, we are aware of this vulnerability and also of power relationships at play between the nurse, other health care professionals and the patient. Professional codes of conduct as well as codes of ethics guide the behaviour of professionals, including the potential for the imbalance of power relationships and how to ameliorate them.

Are these the same for research? As stated earlier, in the ethics application submitted to an institution the potential power relationships need to be explicitly identified. Each identified ethical issue needs to be addressed and strategies for managing it clearly explained.

What about conducting research with groups who are considered vulnerable because of their health status or life situation? Examples of recognised vulnerable populations include people residing in aged care facilities with mental health problems, people with dementia, the terminally ill, people who are intellectually challenged, migrants without English (Nyamathi et al. 2007), victims of violence, war or terrorism. Displaced persons are particularly vulnerable and all researchers need to be aware of the unintentional risk for this group when asking them to participate in a research project. Efforts need to be made to minimise power relationships and any element of risk to the participants, as mentioned earlier in the chapter. Chapter 4 describes the details of conducting research among vulnerable groups. Appendix 3.1 shows examples of a PLS and a consent form in English.

It should be noted that there are specific guidelines in both Australia and New Zealand (see below) about ethical conduct when undertaking research with Indigenous peoples. However, no specific guidelines are available for research with people who have mental health issues or dementia. These vulnerable populations may be left out of research for fear that ethics approval will be difficult to obtain (Keogh & Daly 2009; Lorentzon & Bryan 2007; Maas et al. 2002).

Since approval to conduct research with vulnerable groups is difficult to gain, it is up to the researcher to provide very clear guidelines on how participant consent will be obtained and how the research will be ethically conducted. Maas and associates (2002) acknowledge that gaining consent from people living in aged care facilities may be difficult. They recognise that many older people may have difficulty hearing or be visually impaired, which may prevent reading a PLS or signing a consent form. Keogh and Daly (2009) argue that the problem with researching mental health service users stems from ethics committees' differing interpretations of 'capacity to consent' given the mental health condition and its severity. Lorentzon and Bryan (2007) argue that it is the ethics committee who should investigate different ways of gaining informed consent from vulnerable groups, particularly those with cognitive impairment such as dementia.

The main point here is that working with people with diminished capacity to consent should not exclude them from participating in research. As an adjunct to this, nurse researchers need to devise strategies that can include vulnerable people in research as well as ameliorate perceived power relationships.

Keogh and Daly (2009) have devised strategies for facilitating informed consent with vulnerable populations. As well as allowing the potential participant time to read or hear the information about the research, they suggest encouraging them to ask questions and stressing the voluntary nature of the research; they add that it is helpful to use

> a professional researcher/gatekeeper to make judgements in relation to each individual's capacity to consent…[as well as]…including ongoing assessment of participant understanding, continuous information giving, repeatedly seeking permission and evaluating participant willingness to continue involvement. (2009, p. 280)

Indigenous peoples as participants in nursing and midwifery research

As stated earlier, one of the researcher's roles is to minimise power relationships in their research project. What is of particular importance is the relationship between the researcher and the vulnerable group. Nurse researchers must be especially aware of protecting the human rights of these groups.

Australia and New Zealand are multicultural societies with Indigenous populations. The need to respect the values, cultures and spiritual beliefs of clients is an integral part of nursing care (Fry & Johnstone 2008; Staunton & Chiarella 2008). Similar principles are applied in conducting research among Indigenous people. However, special considerations relating to historical context and the nature of culture and clan need to be taken into account. The Australian guidelines for conducting research with Aboriginal and Torres Strait Islander communities (NHMRC 2006) and the New Zealand guidelines for ethical conduct in research with Maori communities (Health Research Strategy to Improve Maori Health and Wellbeing 2004) have to be clearly adopted in all research protocols involving Indigenous people.

The explicit nature of the guidelines for working with both Aboriginal and Torres Strait Islanders and Maori has emanated from the knowledge that colonisation of both countries by the British had a major impact on their health and welfare. In Australia, the British considered that the country was empty—'no one's land' or terra nullius (Eckermann et al. 2006). This set the tone for less than adequate treatment of Indigenous peoples and the dispossession from the land (Australian Institute of Aboriginal and Torres Strait Islander Studies 2008). In New Zealand, the British acknowledged that the land was occupied and supported this in a document called the Treaty of Waitangi (McHugh 1991).

Regardless of the differing approaches by the British at the time of settlement, it is acknowledged that Indigenous populations in both countries have lower life expectancy, increased health risks, less access to resources (Eckermann et al. 2006; Johnstone 2009) and less control over personal life decisions than non-Indigenous populations. The poor health, social outcomes and historical context need to be acknowledged in research protocols that include Indigenous populations as participants.

In Australia, these guidelines have been extended by adding specific statements on research values. These values include acknowledging spirit and integrity, reciprocity, respect, equality, survival and protection, and lastly responsibility (NHMRC 2006). Not only do these value statements have to be present in the research application but also there has to be clear evidence of how each value will be addressed in the research process.

In New Zealand, specific guidelines are in place for research with Maori for the same reasons. The Health Research Council of New Zealand also bases their research strategy with Maori on the Treaty of Waitangi, specifically Articles Two and Three, which outline Maori control over resources as well as a fair share of benefits from society (Health

Research Strategy to Improve Maori Health and Wellbeing 2004). The implications of this for research are that there needs to be an acknowledgment of the traditional power imbalances between Indigenous and non-Indigenous peoples and that researchers and Indigenous peoples need to share in the processes and the outcomes of the research.

Summary

In summing up this chapter and the ethical implications for research that have been outlined, it is best to give a step-by-step example of starting your research and applying for ethics approval. This by no means exhausts all research ethical issues. It aims to be used as a guide to think about what you need to do.

Choosing your topic: Ask yourself what are the ethical implications of the topic. These include power relationships with potential participants and the participants' vulnerability throughout the research process.

Choosing a research design: Is it a quantitative or a qualitative research study? How are confidentiality, privacy and anonymity to be addressed? How is consent to be gained? Will potential participants understand your plain language statement? Do you need to use a language other than English so the participants can provide the data that you want?

If you choose a face-to-face interview to collect the data, how will you address ethical issues such as consent to participate, risk/benefit, harm, confidentiality, and the participant's right to withdraw consent without prejudice?

Accessing the correct forms or protocols: It is important to provide details of your research and its method so that members of the HREC can understand what you are intending to do. The methodology will determine the level of risk as well as the ethical implications of your proposed study. Ethics committees have two important mandates: protect the public while encouraging research.

Storage of data: Make sure that the data storage procedures are appropriate and it is clear who will access the data. Internal strategies need to be in place to ensure that the office and the computer are not publicly shared or accessed by others who are not involved with the project. Online surveys should not be open to being violated by hackers. The ongoing changes of computer technology need to be considered for the security of data.

Happy researching. Remember, you are not only researching as a part of your study, you are also researching to further the knowledge and practice of nursing and midwifery. Do not let your research sit on a shelf getting dusty; present your findings at conferences and get it published in journals. The disciplines of nursing and midwifery are only as dynamic as the people who pursue excellence in practice, and your research contribution is part of this.

Keri Chater

IMPLICATIONS FOR EVIDENCE-BASED NURSING AND MIDWIFERY

Evidence-based nursing research has gained popularity within the disciplines of nursing and midwifery. As has been mentioned, there are many different types of evidence-based research including, but not limited to, systematic reviews of the literature, quantitative and qualitative research, and randomised controlled trials (RCTs).

With any type of research, whether it be conducted as part of an evidence-based research project or not, all are required to go through the same ethics approval protocols and address the same type of ethical issues as mentioned in this chapter. However, there are some other ethical issues that need to be considered.

Nurse and midwife researchers need to be aware of the ethical implications associated particularly with RCTs as by the very nature of the trial one group of patients will be receiving the intervention, be it nursing, surgical or pharmacological, and the other group will be forgoing the intervention (Davies 2005). The ethical implications here are that one group might be receiving an intervention that may have a beneficial outcome while the other group is not receiving the same benefit.

If research has been carried out and there is clear evidence that the intervention or treatment has a positive or improved outcome, it will probably be implemented. With implementation the nurse and midwife researcher needs to be aware of the cost of changing one practice for another. If the cost is deemed too high the proposed change is unlikely to occur. Likewise if the change does occur and is implemented, nurses and midwives must also be aware that patient preference needs to be considered (Glenny & Gibson 2007). Participants as well as patients need to have explained to them the risks and benefits associated with participation or implementation of the intervention.

Risk and benefit are a specific aspect of all ethics applications. The researcher must explain what level of risk is involved in the research. For example, if the proposed research is an anonymous survey then the level of risk will be considered negligible or level 1 risk. This means that there is no foreseeable harm to a person filling out the survey. Low-level risk or level 2 risk is where the researcher has identified that there may be some risk to the participant. This may mean that there is the potential for the participant to experience some discomfort during an interview. If this has been identified by the researcher they will have to outline what strategies are to be implemented if discomfort occurs.

If the research process involves something more than discomfort, it is not deemed level 2 risk. Once a research strategy involves invasive procedures such as taking blood or taking a biopsy then the level of risk is deemed to be high. Section 2.1.8 of the Australian National Statement on Ethical Conduct in Human Research (NHMRC 2007) states that 'the greater the risks to participants in any research for which ethical approval is given, the more certain it must be both that the risks will be managed as well as possible, and that the participants clearly understand the risks they are assuming' (p. 18).

Practice exercise 3.1

You are in your second year in the Bachelor of Nursing degree. You are undertaking a core subject that has two pieces of assessment. A lecturer for this subject will mark your assessment papers. One day this lecturer comes to the class and describes a research project that she is about to undertake. The research will involve interviewing students. The lecturer has asked your class, including you, to participate in the project.

In this scenario, is there a power relationship between the researcher and the participant? How could the research be structured in a way that reduces or eliminates a power relationship? List two potential ethical issues and strategies for addressing them.

Practice exercise 3.2

You are about to undertake research examining the efficacy of cleansing central venous catheter sites. In your clinical experience you have witnessed two different cleansing procedures: one clinical venue uses Chlorhexidine and the other uses Betadine. You have become interested in this and you want to discover which one is more efficacious. Furthermore, what is the evidence to suggest one cleansing agent is more effective than another?

Once having decided on your methodology you will need ethics approval from your university as well as the hospital where you wish to undertake your research. At what level of risk would you classify your research?

Practice exercise 3.3

Many nursing research projects are conducted in a hospital where patients are recruited by nurses or midwives working in the same unit as the patients. What is an ethical issue that researchers need to be aware of when applying for ethical clearance application? Discuss.

Practice exercise 3.4

1 Discuss the principles of informed consent and how they apply to nursing as well as nursing research. The principle of informed consent applies equally to nursing and to nursing research and is based on the individual's autonomous ability to make an informed choice. There are five components to informed consent:
   * disclosure of all relevant information
   * comprehension or understanding of this information
   * competency to decide or make a choice
   * freedom from coercion or voluntary participation
   * the actual signed consent form.

2   Explain the difference between confidentiality and anonymity. When conducting interviews or running focus groups the researcher actually sees the participants, so the participant cannot be anonymous. Therefore the researcher has to promise confidentiality. This means that the participant's name will be replaced with a coded number or a pseudonym to protect confidentiality. Alternatively, if the research involves quantitative surveys that are not coded in any way, so that the researcher cannot identify the participant, this is considered anonymity.

3   Discuss the reasons behind the need for a plain language statement. Often a formal ethics application contains technical or medical terms that may not be understood by the average person in the street. A PLS is designed to make the research understandable to the average person. It should contain no jargon and should address all components of the proposed research.

Answers to practice exercises

3.1

A power relationship exists between the researcher and the participant because the potential participants rely on the researcher (lecturer) to guide teaching and learning as well as assessment tasks. A potential participant might feel obliged to participate because of this and therefore feel unable to say no to participation. Two possible ethical issues in the above scenario are 'dependency' and 'coercion'.

A way to diminish these potential ethical issues is for the researcher (lecturer) to ask another member of staff to collect participants' data while the lecturer is out of the room. This has the effect of ameliorating the dependency and coercion issues.

3.2

If you are using the same treatment modalities that are currently being used and you are comparing the level of infection rate, then the risk level is 2. This is because you are not introducing a change in treatment but comparing existing treatments. However, if you decide to change treatment modalities as part of your research, the risk increases to level 3.

3.3

Coercion: It is highly likely that there is an unbalanced power relationship between potential participants (patients) and researchers (nurses). Patients may be reluctant to refuse to take part in the study. To get around this problem, researchers may have to have others who are not working in the unit recruited as potential participants.

Appendix 3.1
Example of Plain Language Statement and
Consent Form in English

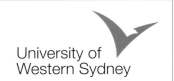

SYDNEY SOUTH WEST
AREA HEALTH SERVICE
NSW✚HEALTH

University of
Western Sydney

Dr Sansnee Jirojwong
College of Health and Science
School of Nursing, Hawkesbury Campus
Locked Bag 1797
Penrith South DC NSW 1797
Email s.jirojwong@uws.edu.au
Phone (02) 45701918, 0427733004, Fax (02) 45701420

INFORMATION SHEET
FOR WOMEN WITH GESTATIONAL DIABETES

**Health literacy and self management of gestational diabetic: a study among
Vietnamese, Cambodian, Thai and Laotian women in Sydney**

Invitation

You are invited to take part in this research which is being conducted by Drs Sansnee Jirojwong
& Jane Cioffi, Associate Professors Virginia Schmied & Hannah Dahlen, Professors Maree
Johnson & Rhonda Griffiths from the University of Western Sydney. You are being invited
as a participant because you have high blood sugar or diabetes in pregnancy.

What is the purpose of this research?

The purpose of this study is to explore how the first or second generation Australian-
Vietnamese, Cambodian, Thai and Laotian women in Sydney use information from
health professionals to self manage their blood sugar from the time they know that they
have the condition until about three months after birth of their baby. We also would like to
know other sources of information about this condition that you seek and use to self manage
your health.

It is hoped the information gained in this study will improve maternity and health services for women who have high blood sugar in pregnancy.

Who can participate in the research?

Women who can participate in this study are women who have high blood sugar in their pregnancy and were born in Vietnam, Cambodia, Thailand or Laos or their parents were born in one of these countries. We will be asking about how women understand about high blood sugar in pregnancy or gestational diabetes and its impact on their health and their infant's health. We will also ask about how women seek, locate and understand health information about this high blood sugar from different sources and use or do not use it to manage their health.

Your decision to participate is completely voluntary. If you decide to participate you can withdraw at any time without having to give a reason. If you decide not to participate, or you wish to withdraw from the project at any time, your decision will not disadvantage you. If you choose to withdraw, we will remove information from you from our record. Your decision whether or not to participate will not prejudice your present or future care or your relationship with Sydney South West Area Health Service as it will not be known to any health care provider.

What would you be asked to do?

If you agree, you will be asked to participate in an individual face to face interview. An interview will be conducted using your own language by a bilingual research team member. The aim of this interview is to explore how you manage your high blood sugar using information from various sources and how you understand about high blood sugar in pregnancy and its impact on your health and your baby's health. Key broad questions will be used to facilitate this interview. The following are examples of the questions that will be asked:

- When you were told that you have high blood sugar, what was your feeling?

- How do you feel now?

- In your opinion, what is the effect of having high blood sugar on your own health and the health of your baby?

- What do you think are long term effects of having high blood sugar on your own health and your baby's health?

- Where and how did you find information so it can be used to manage your blood sugar?

The interview will not last more than one hour. You can nominate the place and time convenient for this interview. With your permission, the interview will be audio recorded.

What are the risks and benefits of participating?

This study involves discussing, on a one to one about having high blood sugar in your pregnancy and the sources of information you use or not use to manage your health. It is possible that the discussion during this interview may relay incidents or stories that may cause you distress or discomfort. You may feel distressed talking about an incident. We feel that there is only a small chance that this may occur. If it does, we will encourage you to seek support from a counselling or support services that are available such as your church, temple or health care workers. We also will provide the contact numbers and details of support workers for additional support if you need this. If you are uncomfortable during the discussion, remember that participation in this study is completely voluntary and you can withdraw at any time without any consequences. You can also ask for the tape recording to be stopped at any time or you can review the tape and ask for your words to be changed.

Women may benefit from this study by having the opportunity to talk about issues that are important to their health and their baby's health. We hope that the knowledge generated by this study will be used to improve the quality of maternity and health services for these women.

How will your privacy be protected?

We would ask you not to identify yourself during the recording of the interview. This is to protect your privacy. No identifying information will be kept about you. The audio recordings, hand-written and transcribed notes will be de-identified, thus removing all reference to individuals and institutions. If necessary, we will use fictitious names to ensure your privacy. The audio recordings and notes will be securely stored at the University of Western Sydney and destroyed seven years after publication. Individual participants and institutions will not be identifiable in any publications arising from this project.

How will the information collected be used?

The information will be used in a report that will be submitted to the University of Western Sydney who have funded the study. A report will be provided to all participating organisations, hospitals and area health services. We also plan to write papers for publication in professional journals outlining the research and the findings and present the results at professional conferences. Confidentiality of individual participants and organisations will be assured.

What do you need to do to participate?

Please read this Information Statement and be sure you understand its contents before you consent to participate. After you have read this information, and you have questions you wish to ask, or any issues you wish to discuss, please feel free to contact Dr Sansnee Jirojwong (Principal Researcher), on Ph. 45701918, 0427733004.

You are making a decision whether or not to participate. Your signature on the consent form indicates that, having read the information provided above, you have decided to participate.

Thank you for considering this invitation

Signature ....

Dr Sansnee Jirojwong
University of Western Sydney

Date ..../......./.......

Complaints about this research

This research has been approved by the Sydney South West Area Health Service Human Research Ethics Committee (Western Zone), Reference .... Should you have concerns about your rights as a participant in this research, or you have a complaint about the manner in which the research is conducted, it may be given to the researcher, or, if an independent person is preferred, to the Ethics Secretariat (Western Zone), SSWAHS Area Health Service, Locked Bag 7017, LIVERPOOL, BC, NSW 1871, telephone (02) 96120614, fax (02) 96120611, email jennie.grech@sswahs.nsw.gov.au.

You will be given a copy of this form to keep.

Dr Sansnee Jirojwong
College of Health and Science
School of Nursing, Hawkesbury Campus
Locked Bag 1797
Penrith South DC NSW 1797

SYDNEY SOUTH WEST
AREA HEALTH SERVICE
NSW⊕HEALTH

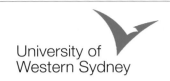
University of
Western Sydney

Email s.jirojwong@uws.edu.au
Phone (02) 45701918, 0427733004, Fax (02) 45701420

CONSENT FORM

Health literacy and self management of gestational diabetic: a study among Vietnamese, Cambodian, Thai and Laotian women in Sydney

1 I .... of ....,
aged .... years, agreed to participate as a subject in the study described in the subject information statement attached to this form.

2. I acknowledge that I have read the Subject Information Statement, which explains why I have been selected, the aims of the study and the nature and the possible risks of the investigation, and the statement has been explained to me to my satisfaction.

3. Before signing this Consent Form, I have been given the opportunity to ask any questions relating to any possible physical and mental harm I might suffer as a result of my participation. I have received satisfactory answers to any questions that I have asked.

4. I consent to participate in an individual face to face interview which will be audio-taping.

5. My decision whether or not to participate will not prejudice my present or future treatment or my relationship with Sydney South West Area Health Service or any other institution cooperating in this study or any person treating me. If I decide to participate, I am free to withdraw my consent and to discontinue my participation at any time without prejudice.

6. I agree that research data gathered from the results of the study may be published, provided that I cannot be identified.

7. I understand that if I have any questions relating to my participation in this research, I may contact the study researcher, Dr Sansnee Jirojwong, on telephone 02-45701918, 0427733004, who will be happy to answer them.

8. I acknowledge receipt of a copy of this Consent Form and the Subject Information Statement.

Complaints may be directed to the Ethics Secretariat (Western Zone), Sydney South West Area Health Service, Locked Bag 7017, LIVERPOOL BC, NSW, 1871 (phone 9612 0614, fax 9612 0611, email jennie.grech@sswahs.nsw.gov.au).

Signature of subject   Signature of witness

....

Please PRINT name   Please PRINT name

....

Date   ...... / ...... / ......   Date   ...... / ...... / ......

Signature(s) of investigator(s)   Please PRINT Name

....

Date   ...... / ...... / ......

✂ -

Where relevant to the research project, please check the box below.

I wish to have a plain English statement of results
posted to me at the address I provided below   ☐ YES   ☐ NO

Mailing Address

Name (Please print) ....

Address..

.... Postcode ....

Further reading

Courtney, M. (2005). *Evidence for Nursing Practice*. Sydney: Elsevier.

Fry, S., & Johnstone, M.-J. (2008). *Ethics in Nursing Practice*, 3rd edn. UK: Blackwell Publishing.

Health Research Strategy to Improve Maori Health and Wellbeing. (2004). Health Research Council of New Zealand, New Zealand Government.

Johnstone, M. (2009). *Bioethics: A Nursing Perspective*, 5th edn. Sydney: Churchill Livingstone.

Kerridge, I., Lowe, M., & Stewart, C. (2009). *Ethics and Law for the Health Professions*, 3rd edn. Sydney: Federation Press.

Weblinks

General

Joanna Briggs Institute:

<www.joannabriggs.edu.au/about/home.php>

The Joanna Briggs Institute is an international not-for-profit research and development organisation specialising in evidence-based resources for health care professionals in nursing, midwifery, medicine and allied health.

Cochrane Collaboration:

<www.cochrane.org>

The Cochrane Collaboration is an international not-for-profit organisation, producing and disseminating systematic reviews of health care interventions.

DARE (Database of Reviews of Effectiveness):

<www.homerton.nhs.uk/education-and-training/newcomb-library-and-information-service/our-electronic-resources/databases/dare-database-of-reviews-of-effectiveness>

DARE is located at the University of York, UK and undertakes systematic reviews of health research focusing on methodological rigour.

The Monash Centre for Ethics in Medicine and Society:

<http://cems.monash.org>

The Monash Centre for Ethics and Society is concerned with both education and research. Its focus is on ethics and cultural values.

Australia

Australian Health Ethics Committee:

<www.nhmrc.gov.au/about/committees/ahec/index.htm>

Australian Nursing and Midwifery Council (ANMC):

<http://anmc.org.au>

The ANMC is the peak body for the nursing and midwifery profession in Australia.

Keri Chater

Code of Ethics for Nurses in Australia:

<www.nursingmidwiferyboard.gov.au/Codes-and-Guidelines.aspx>

The code of ethics for nurses has been developed by the ANMC as a guide for ethical comportment in both nursing and midwifery.

Code of Professional Conduct for Nurses in Australia:

<www.nursingmidwiferyboard.gov.au/Codes-and-Guidelines.aspx>

The ANMC has also produced a Code of Conduct for Nurses and Midwifes practising in Australia.

National Statement on Ethical Conduct in Research Involving Humans:

<www.nhmrc.gov.au/publications/ethics/2007_humans/contents.htm>

The National Statement is a guide for all current and future researchers and specifies the ethical issues that need addressing when undertaking research.

Guidelines for Ethical Conduct in Aboriginal and Torres Strait Islander Health Research:

<www.nhmrc.gov.au/publications/synopses/e72syn.htm>

These guidelines, to be read in conjunction with the National Guidelines, are specific to outreaching with Aboriginal and Torres Strait Islanders.

Council for Aboriginal and Torres Strait Islander Nurses (CATSIN):

<www.indiginet.com.au/catsin>

CATSIN is specifically set up to address particular issues relating to Aboriginal and Torres Strait Islander nurses.

New Zealand

Nursing Council of New Zealand:

<www.nursingcouncil.org.nz>

This is the peak body representing nurses and midwives in New Zealand.

Code of Conduct for Nurses:

<www.nursingcouncil.org.nz/code%20of%20conduct%20March%202008.pdf>

Developed by the Nursing Council of New Zealand, this document outlines the code of conduct for nurses and midwives practising in New Zealand.

Guidelines for Cultural Safety, the Treaty of Waitangi and Maori Health in Nursing Education and Practice:

<www.nursingcouncil.org.nz/Cultural%20Safety.pdf>

These guidelines were established by the New Zealand Nursing Council and are specifically designed to raise cultural awareness of the health of Maori.

New Zealand National Ethics Advisory Committee:

<www.neac.health.govt.nz>

The National Ethics Advisory Committee (NEAC) provides advice to the Minister of Health on ethical issues relating to health and disability. It also determines nationally consistent standards for conducting research.

Health Research Council of New Zealand:

<www.hrc.govt.nz/root/About%20the%20HRC/About_the_HRC.html>

The Health Research Council of New Zealand (HRC) is responsible for managing the New Zealand government's investment in health research.

References

Annas, G., & Grodin, M. A. (eds). (1992). *Nazi Doctors and the Nuremberg Code: Human Rights and Human Experimentation*. New York: Oxford University Press.

Australian Health Ethics Committee (2009), Retrieved 18 Feburary 2009, from <www.nhmrc.gov. au/about/committees.ahec.index.htm>.

Australian Institute of Aboriginal and Torres Strait Islander Studies. (2008). *The Little Red, Yellow, Black Book*, 2nd edn. Canberra: Aboriginal Studies Press.

Burkhardt, M., & Nathaniel, A. (2002). *Ethics and Issues in Contemporary Nursing*, 2nd edn. Australia: Delmar.

Caplan, A. (1992). How did medicine go so wrong? In A. Caplan (ed.), *When Medicine went Mad* (pp. 53-92). New Jersey: Humana Press.

Courtney, M. (2005). *Evidence for Nursing Practice*. Sydney: Elsevier.

Davies, P. (2005). Teaching, learning and evidence-based health care. In M. Dawes, P. Davies, A. Gray, J. Mant, K. Seers & R. Snowball (eds), *Evidence-Based Practice*, 2nd edn (pp. 245–63). Edinburgh: Elsevier.

Eckermann, A.-K., Dowd, T., Chong, E., Nixon, L., Gray, R., & Johnson, S. (2006). *Binan Goonj: Bridging Cultures in Aboriginal Health*, 2nd edn. Sydney: Churchill Livingstone.

Fry, S., & Johnstone, M.-J. (2008). *Ethics in Nursing Practice*, 3rd edn. Malden, MA: Blackwell Publishing.

Glenny, A.-M., & Gibson, F. (2007). Critical appraisal of quantitative studies 2: Can the evidence be applied to your clinical setting? In V. Craig & R. Smyth (eds), *The Evidence-Based Practice Manual for Nurses*, 2nd edn (pp. 127–51). Edinburgh: Churchill Livingstone.

Grodin, M. A. (1992). Historical origins of the Nuremberg Code. In G. Annas & M. A. Grodin (eds), *Nazi Doctors and the Nuremburg Code: Human Rights and Human Experimentation*, (pp. 121–44). New York: Oxford University Press.

Health Research Strategy to Improve Maori Health and Wellbeing. (2004). Health Research Council of New Zealand, New Zealand Government.

Jackson, J. (2006). *Ethics in Medicine*. Cambridge, UK: Polity Press.

Johnstone, M. (2009). *Bioethics: A Nursing Perspective*, 5th edn. Sydney: Churchill Livingstone.

Katz, J. (1992). The consent principle of the Nuremberg Code: Its significance then and now. In G. Annas & M.A. Grodin (eds), *Nazi Doctors and the Nuremberg Code: Human Rights and Human Experimentation*, (pp. 227–39). New York: Oxford University Press.

Keogh, B., & Daly L. (2009). The ethics of conducting research with mental health service users. *British Journal of Nursing* 18(5), 277–81.

Kerridge, I., Lowe, M., & Stewart, C. (2009). *Ethics and Law for the Health Professions*, 3rd edn. Sydney: Federation Press.

Leedy, P., & Ormond, J. (2010). *Practical Research Planning and Design*, 9th edn. Boston: Pearson Education International.

Lorentzon, M., & Bryan, K. (2007). Respect for the person with dementia: Fostering greater user involvement in service planning. *Quarterly in Ageing: Policy, Practice and Research* 8(1), 23–9.

Maas, M., Kelley, l., Park, M., & Specht, J. (2002). Issues of conducting research in nursing homes. *Western Journal of Nursing Research* 24(4), 373–89.

McHugh, P. (1991). *The Maori Magna Carta: New Zealand Law and the Treaty of Waitangi*. Auckland: Oxford University Press.

Milton, C. (2007). Evidence-based practice: Ethical questions for nursing. *Nursing Science Quarterly* 20(2), 123–6.

NHMRC (National Health and Medical Research Council). (2006). *Exploring What Research Means: Resource Package for Aboriginal and Torres Strait Islander Communities and Organisations*. Canberra: Australian Government.

NHMRC. (2007). *National Statement on Ethical Conduct in Human Research*. Canberra: Australian Government.

Nyamathi, A., Koniak-Griffin, D., & Greengold, B. (2007). Development of a nursing theory and science in vulnerable populations research. In J. Fitzpatrick (ed.), *Annual Review of Nursing Research: Vulnerable Populations*, vol. 25, pp. 3–26.

Pearson, A., Wiechula, R., Court, A., & Lockwood, C. (2007). A re-consideration of what constitutes 'evidence' in the healthcare professions. *Nursing Science Quarterly* 20(1), 85–8.

Perely, S., Fluss, S., Bankowski, Z., & Simon, F. (1992). The Nuremberg Code: An international overview. In G. Annas & M. A. Grodin (eds), *Nazi Doctors and the Nuremburg Code: Human Rights and Human Experimentation*, (pp. 121–44). New York: Oxford University Press.

Perry, L. (2007). Implementing best evidence in clinical practice. In V. Craig & R. Smyth (eds), *The Evidence-Based Practice Manual for Nurses*, 2nd edn (pp. 267–304). Edinburgh: Churchill Livingstone.

Shamoo, A., & Khin-Maung-Gyi, F. (2002). *Ethics of the Use of Human Subjects in Research*. London: Garland Sciences.

Staunton, P., & Chiarella, M. (2008). *Nursing and the Law*, 6th edn. Sydney: Churchill Livingstone.

Taylor, B., Kermode, S., & Roberts, K. (2007). *Research in Nursing and Health Care: Evidence for Practice*, 3rd edn. Australia: Thomson.

Taylor, D. (1992). Opening statement of the prosecution December 9, 1945. In G. Annas & M. A. Grodin (eds), *Nazi Doctors and the Nuremburg Code: Human Rights and Human Experimentation*, (pp. 121–44). New York: Oxford University Press.

CHAPTER 4

Vulnerable Groups as Research Participants

Pranee Liamputtong

Chapter learning objectives

By the end of this chapter you will be able to:

▶ identify some vulnerable groups as participants in nursing research

▶ explore issues relating to accessing these vulnerable groups as research participants

▶ appreciate the reciprocity and respect involved in research

▶ discuss the implications of incentive and compensation when having vulnerable groups as research participants

▶ be sensitive to the needs of vulnerable participants

▶ recognise the moral concerns when having vulnerable groups as research participants

▶ appreciate evidence-based practice and the need for qualitative research.

KEY TERMS

Evidence-based practice
Moral concerns
Qualitative research approach
Vulnerable people

Introduction

As researchers (and human beings) we act as 'morally responsible selves'… we need to be flexible and reactive, but above all, accountable for our actions. (Hallowell et al. 2005, p. 149)

Within the global crisis that we are now experiencing, it is inevitable that nurses will have to work with many vulnerable people. It is likely that these people will be confronted with problems in their private and public lives as well as their health and well-being. As health professionals, nurses need to find evidence they can apply in their work. One source of the evidence must be from research and it must be a research approach that will allow nurses to work closely with people. However, the task of undertaking research with the 'vulnerable' presents researchers with unique opportunities and yet dilemmas. In this chapter I shall bring together salient issues for the conduct of research with vulnerable groups.

Who are the vulnerable?

The concept of the 'vulnerable' is socially constructed (Moore & Miller 1999), hence it is difficult to give a definite meaning of the term. According to Flaskerud and Winslow (1998, p. 69), vulnerable populations are 'social groups who have an increased relative risk or susceptibility to adverse health outcomes'. These include those who are 'impoverished, disenfranchised, and/or subject to discrimination, intolerance, subordination, and stigma' (Nyamathi 1998, p. 65). Based on these descriptions, we may include children, the elderly, ethnic people, immigrants, sex workers, the homeless, gay men and lesbians, and women. Historically, people suffering from chronic illness, the mentally ill and the caregivers of the chronically ill are also referred to as vulnerable populations (Nyamathi 1998).

The word 'vulnerable' is often used interchangeably with such terms as the 'hard-to-reach' and 'hidden' populations (Benoit et al. 2005; Liamputtong 2007; Melrose 2002). A 'hidden population' points to a group of people 'whose membership is not readily distinguished or enumerated based on existing knowledge and/or sampling capabilities' (Wiebel 1990, p. 6). An example is sex workers, who are likely to be legally and socially labelled as 'outcast'—'the whore stigma permeates all aspects of their life' (Benoit et al. 2005, p. 264). Because of their social stigma, sex workers tend to be isolated from the community. This often weakens any support and social networks they have, and increases their vulnerability to stress, depression and other conditions of ill health (Melrose 2002; Wojcicki & Malala 2001).

'The vulnerable' has also been defined as referring to people with 'social vulnerability' (Quest & Marco 2003, p. 1297). Some population groups, such as children, unemployed people, homeless people, drug-addicted people and ethnic and religious minority groups, face particular social vulnerability. When involving them in their research, these groups need special care from researchers. The 'vulnerable', to Stone (2003), includes those who are 'economically or educationally disadvantaged'. Punch (2002, p. 323) suggests that children are marginalised in an adult-dominated society, and as such they 'experience unequal power relations with adults in their lives'.

Some groups may be vulnerable because of their legal status. Some illegal immigrants are denied access to health and social services. Most of these groups live in poverty, and are employed in seasonal cropping industries that are prone to poor health and bad living situations (Birman 2005; Liamputtong 2007).

They are relatively invisible for many reasons—their marginality, lack of opportunity to voice their concerns, fear of their identity being disrespected, social stigma, heavy responsibilities and scepticism about being involved in research. Women from ethnic or low socio-economic backgrounds are less willing and able to participate because of their heavy responsibilities and their well-founded scepticism about the value of social research (Cannon et al. 1988). Some vulnerable groups may face pressing socio-economic needs that limit their participation (Anderson & Hatton 2000). Most illegal immigrants do not wish to be identified and will avoid participation in any research, especially if the research reveals their identification to authorities (Birman 2005). Refugees may feel vulnerable about taking part in any research because of their past experiences of dealing with authorities (Birman 2005; Liamputtong 2010a). For others, like sex workers, taking part in research can subject one to hate, scorn and prosecution. These people are therefore 'distrustful of non-members, do whatever they can to avoid revealing their identities, and are likely to refuse to cooperate with outsiders or to give unreliable answers to questions about themselves and their networks' (Benoit et al, 2005 p. 264).

There are a numer of salient issues that researchers must take into account in their attempts to conduct research with vulnerable people. These are discussed below.

Accessibility to vulnerable groups

Locating vulnerable groups is a challenging task and often problematic (Liamputtong 2007). The level of distrust keeps many people in hard-to-reach or transient populations from interacting with researchers. It becomes more difficult when the research issues are sensitive or threatening, since these people have greater need to hide their identities and involvement (Dickson-Swift et al. 2008; Melrose 2002; Renzetti & Lee 1993).

However, there are successful ways of gaining access to these potential participants. The snowball sampling method (asking an existing participant to invite others who meet the criteria of the study to take part in the research; see Chapter 8) has been extensively adopted in researching vulnerable or difficult-to-reach populations (see Barnard 2005; Benoit et al. 2005; Cooper et al. 2005; Liamputtong 2007, 2009; Van Kesteren et al. 2005; Weston 2004). Faugier and Sargeant (1997) suggest the use of snowball sampling to locate these populations. Members of such populations may also be involved in deviant activities, such as taking drugs or selling sex. Accessing these hidden groups can best be done by referrals from their acquaintances or peers rather than other more formal methods of identification such as the use of existing lists or screening. Umaña-Taylor and Bámaca (2004, p. 267) and Madriz (1998) refer to this approach as the 'word-of-mouth' technique. It is extremely useful in research with ethnic minorities as the potential participants are more likely to take part if someone they know is also participating.

With some vulnerable groups, particularly highly closed groups, it is essential to have 'a visible and respected individual who holds a position of authority, high respect, or leadership' or acts as a gatekeeper (Tewksbury & Gagné 2001, p. 78) to introduce researchers to the group. This authority person will link potential participants into a new society. They will act as guides and tell the researchers what cultural actions are locally meaningful. They are also patrons who help the researchers secure the trust of participants (Tewksbury & Gagné 2001, p. 78). In this way researchers will be successful in gaining access to their research participants and having an in-depth understanding of them.

Many researchers have used these gatekeepers (Liamputtong 2007, 2010a; MacDougall & Fudge 2001; Umaña-Taylor & Bámaca 2004). Moore and Miller (1999, p. 1038) suggest families and guardians as gatekeepers, but these may also be vigilant protectors and may present the biggest obstacle to accessing vulnerable participants. Very often, the families or the guardians believe that these participants have suffered many times and do not deserve another disruption in their lives. Some strategies to overcome this obstacle include carefully and thoughtfully giving information about the research, possible risks, and detailed involvement of the participant. The researchers may need to reveal the source of research funding and data handling (Moore & Miller 1999).

Gatekeeping agencies such as health and social care agencies may also be used as a point of access to vulnerable groups (Goodman 2004; Parnis et al. 2005; Takahashi & Kai 2005; Umaña-Taylor & Bámaca 2004). In their study of adolescents with severe burns, Moore and Miller (1999) worked with a tertiary care institution who specialised in paediatric burns. Takahashi and Kai (2005) recruited Japanese women who survived breast cancer through the assistance of surgeons in breast surgery clinics in the Tokyo metropolitan area. Goodman (2004) recruited Sudanese refugee youths from the resettlement agency that held legal guardianship of the youths.

Most often, researchers working with the vulnerable groups employ a combination of methods in gaining access to these hard-to-reach people. Wuest and colleagues (2003), in their study with single mothers who left their abusive partners in New Brunswick and Ontario, recruited their participants by placing advertisements in local newspapers, posters in grocery stores, community sites and libraries, contacting agencies and their personal contacts. Similar recruitment strategies were employed by Weaver and colleagues (2005) in their research with women who were recovering from anorexia nervosa in New Brunswick.

Interesting recruitment strategies adopted by Leipert and Reutter (2005) deserve our attention here. In their study exploring how women in geographically isolated settings in northern Canada maintain their health despite constraints caused by distance, terrain and weather, Leipert and Reutter recruited the women by television and radio interviews. They also placed advertisements about the research in local newspapers. Posters were displayed in tack-and-feed stores and auction markets. They also used word of mouth to recruit the participants. With these, they were successful in having more than 100 women across the North respond.

Reciprocity and respect for the participants

Working with vulnerable people, reciprocity and respect is essential (Corbin & Morse 2003; Liamputtong 2007). Ethical responsibility towards vulnerable groups such as young children needs to go beyond the protection of children's rights. It needs to include an emphasis on reciprocity (Eder & Fingerson 2002, p. 185), which may mean identifying what the participants can gain. By giving something in return for receiving information, researchers can reduce the power inequality between themselves and the researched (Liamputtong 2007, 2010b). Warr (2004, p. 586) advocates this reciprocity in her provocative discussion on researching vulnerable groups. She says that researchers must exert themselves to make a positive difference in the lives of the participants or the group.

Reciprocity can take various forms (Liamputtong 2007). Giving health education to participants or the group (Pauw & Brener 2003) or helping with accessibility to health and social services (Warr & Pyett 1999) are some tangible forms. Reciprocity may be social action or social changes made or recommended as a part of the project. A researcher can also be an advocate for participants when needed and appropriate (see Liamputtong 2009; Liamputtong Rice et al. 1994).

Providing feedback or results to the participants is widely used to show respect. In research with children, researchers need to provide a report of their findings to the children to check the accuracy of their interpretations. The children can then hear what the researchers say about their lives and be able to respond directly to any misinterpretations (Mayall 1999). Traditional research methodology texts advise against offering assistance to the participants. However, the moral implications of withholding needed information have been challenged by many feminist researchers (Cotterill 1992; Liamputtong 2007; Reinharz 1992; Stanley 1990; Stanley & Wise 1993). Rejecting requested help may cause harm to vulnerable participants (Bergen 1993). Bergen advocates offering assistance to participants that may take the form of emotional support, counselling or referral.

In research regarding family, Daly (1992, p. 7) asserts that researchers often ask numerous questions about families' day-to-day life. When these families have difficulties, they may expect some opinions of the researcher as part of the research exchange. Should we, as researchers, give advice, information or counselling? Daly suggests that there are many things to consider here. First, we need to remember that by inviting individuals to take part in our research, the researcher and participants have developed a relationship based on a fair exchange. Second, we can expect some requests for information or advice following the intimate disclosure of our participants. It is wise that researchers anticipate these requests and be prepared to give information the participants need or direct them to other resources such as reading materials or referrals to qualified professionals.

Compensation and incentive: A form of respect

Compensation or payment for participating in a research project is a controversial issue. Booth (1999, p. 78) argues that payment is not appropriate because it may influence participants' responses. Payment can also be seen as 'coercion' if researchers work with extremely poor people (Brody 1998; Crigger et al. 2001), the homeless (Paradis 2000) or drug users (Dunlap et al. 1990). Potential participants from poor countries are especially vulnerable to coercion. The income level is very low compared to the Western standard. Ten Australian dollars may be equivalent to a week's income for a worker in Thailand or Indonesia. Hence, these vulnerable poor people may try to be included in research, which can be seen as coercive or unethical (Paradis 2000).

Others, however, assert that the contribution, knowledge and skills of the participants should be valued and payment should be provided, particularly if they have no or little money (Beauchamp et al. 2002; Booth 1999, p. 78; Umaña-Taylor & Bámaca 2004). Payment can be seen as equalising the relationship or exchanging the research money for participant time (Holloway & Jefferson 2000). Based on this argument, compensation for participant time is crucial and should be seen as a symbol of the researchers' respect for the participation of these people (Liamputtong 2007, 2009). This stance applies particularly to researching the vulnerable, as most of these groups tend to be poor and money may assist them with their daily living (Cook & Nunkoosing 2008; Madriz 1998; Umaña-Taylor & Bámaca 2004). Beauchamp and colleagues (2002) point out that compensation from participating in a research study may be used to improve their life circumstances. Some feminist researchers also argue that money should be perceived as the compensation for being research partners in the research project (Paradis 2000).

Martinez-Ebers (1997) argues that compensation or a monetary incentive is essential in securing hard-to-reach populations. Responses to subjective questions may not be influenced by these incentives. For instance, money may be given to the participants after completing an interview (Holt & McClure 2006). Recently, we have seen more researchers who compensate their participants for their time, travel cost or absence from work (see Liamputtong et al. 2009; Pyett 2001; Van Kesteren et al. 2005; Varas-Diaz et al. 2005).

It is important that researchers assess whether the real interest of the participants is in the research or the compensation.

Incentive or compensation may not be cash. It can be a gift voucher, sample product relating to the research topic, pre-paid public telephone card, toy or educational materials (Husaini et al. 2001; Romero-Daza et al. 2003; Shelton & Rianon 2004; Takahashi & Kai 2005; Umaña-Taylor & Bámaca 2004). However, any such token of appreciation needs to be considered individually. Meadows and colleagues (2003) intended to buy traditional offerings of tobacco for their Aboriginal women in their study, but were informed by their Aboriginal assistant that the women preferred cash as they had more need of cash than tobacco. Tobacco is of course also a health risk factor.

Sensitivity to the needs and lives of the participants

It is crucial that researchers are sensitive to the needs of the participants (Jewkes et al. 2005; Meadows et al. 2003). It is a common practice in qualitative research that data collection takes place at the site where the participant feels most comfortable, which is usually their home (Dickson-Swift et al. 2008; Herzog 2005; Liamputtong 2009). In her study with visually impaired older women, Moore (2002, p. 563) conducted all interviews at the women's homes. Initially, she offered to meet the women in local libraries or quiet restaurants, but this was dismissed. It was only after the women started talking about their visual loss that Moore realised the importance of a familiar setting for people with visual impairment.

However, in some sensitive research when privacy and high confidentiality is involved, this may prove otherwise. In their study on violence, drugs and street-level prostitution among impoverished Hispanic women in the inner city of Hartford, Connecticut, Romero-Daza and colleagues (2003, p. 240) point out that most of the participants wanted to be interviewed at the Hispanic Health Council, a community-based agency that they could access easily. They were also more familiar with the agency and hence felt more comfortable being there. This setting also provided confidentiality. Very often, participants' family members did not know about the sex work in which they were involved.

Where sensitive issues exist, the research processes may be traumatic for the participants. In research relating to women's experiences of violence, for example, the women may experience distress, anxiety and flashbacks. The researchers need to be prepared for this. In case the women find the interviews to be overwhelming, the researchers need to be able to offer referrals for support such as counselling services, information, contacts and local support groups (Cutcliffe & Ramcharan 2002; Dickson-Swift et al. 2008; Liamputtong 2007), otherwise the interview may be harmful to the participants (Brzuzy et al. 1997). A list of social and health services may be prepared and given to participants when needed.

When a participant is emotional, researchers should respond humanly and kindly (Morse 2002, p. 321). Comfort and tissues to wipe the tears are offered when participants cry. The researchers may ask the participant if they wish to rest and then continue when they are ready.

Pyett (2001) points out in her study with female sex workers that she and a co-researcher were extremely cautious and sensitive about asking certain questions. The study aimed to investigate the health of women in sex work, but it would have been insensitive to ask the women about their health as 'health was too private. The women would be very sensitive about their nutrition, dental hygiene, and reproductive health, all of which were likely to be very poor' (pp. 114–15). However, the researchers could ask them about any sexual or drug-using practices. Through consultation and negotiation, the solution was to ask a simple question, 'How are you?' The women would be more likely to raise health issues, which would allow the researchers to follow up. In the same study, Warr and Pyett (1999, p. 293) point out that all interviews were carried out in a familiar site chosen by the participants, which was usually in a café or a welfare agency. During the interview, the women were told that they could stop the tape-recorder or 'stop the interview at any time if they became anxious, distressed or required reassurance on any matter'. Additionally, the interviews were done as 'conversations' to allow the participants to talk about their intimate matters. And each interview lasted only 20 minutes to one hour in order not to interrupt their working time too much.

Researchers should be aware of the time required for participating in the study. Moore and Miller (1999, p. 1039) warn that researchers must consider the time of day when they attempt to recruit participants and when they wish to obtain the data. These may influence the decisions of some participants as to whether they wish to participate or not. Older persons and those with disabilities may refuse to participate if it interferes with their routines or treatments. Logistical factors such as inaccessible research sites, cost of public transport, parking distances and weather conditions might also influence people's decisions (Meadows et al. 2003). These issues are more problematic for people with multiple issues or 'doubly vulnerable individuals'. Therefore, researchers should be particularly cautious when planning recruitment and data collection.

An interesting example with young men in crime is reported in the Jamieson study (2000, p. 68). Previous experience indicated that late morning would be a suitable time to interview young people as they were more likely to be up but not yet left home. Jamieson followed this experience; she would usually turn up at the home of these young men and find that they were out of bed but were in varying degrees of undress. This can be embarrassing for a young female researcher, but it can also be threatening, particularly if there are a few such young men in the same house.

Moral concerns

There are some debates about moral issues when researching vulnerable people. Should researchers carry out investigative work with some extremely vulnerable populations such as frail elderly, people suffering mental illness, or those who experience extreme loss, grief, or are homeless or terminally ill? These people are already vulnerable in many ways. Russell (1999) attempted to research social isolation with older people in Sydney. In order to be responsive to their vulnerability, she and her co-researchers had amended many aspects of their research, but throughout the research process they encountered 'a sense of unease about the ethicality (or even morality) of some aspects of their research'. They asked themselves, for example, 'should we be "mining the minds" of these disempowered people for our own research purposes?' (p. 404).

Morally speaking, the benefits of undertaking the research need to be measured against the risks of being involved in it (Cutcliffe & Ramcharan 2002; Hall & Kulig 2004; Liamputtong 2009; Ramcharan 2010). Flaskerud and Winslow (1998, p. 10) argue that studies of vulnerable groups should be focused first on benefiting the group. The moral issue of the questions asked of participants has also been raised and reviewed by the researchers. Some questions could result in harm to the community as a whole (Paradis 2000). Morally, researchers should not ask questions that might contribute to the stigmatisation of their participants. Harm to an individual, their relationship with others, their community and political implications for the group resulting from research need to be considered at the beginning of the research process. The moral challenge for researchers is to develop their enquiries in a way that does not make individual participants suffer further. It is also imperative that the researchers are cautious and aware that the study may potentially reinforce stereotyping and contribute to discrimination against the group.

Researchers may want to ask research questions that would reflect better on marginalised people (Paradis 2000). This essentially leads to the use of qualitative research questions, rather than hypothesis testing in positivist science (see also the next section). Within some highly sensitive and vulnerable groups, such as people with terminal illnesses and injuries, there is a debate about the moral imperative of involving them in research. Why should researchers intrude into the lives of these people at times when they are extremely vulnerable? Many may agree with this, but not Morse (2000, p. 545). She puts it bluntly that not researching these groups means that no information can be used to improve care. Their needs may not be met as their personal experiences are not explored (Beaver et al. 1999). Morse argues that conducting research with extremely vulnerable people is good morally as high-quality services can be designed and delivered to meet their needs.

Evidence-based nursing research and vulnerable people: The essence of the qualitative approach

I argue that it is only through knowledge that evidence can be generated. This evidence can then be used for our health care practice. How can we find knowledge? My answer is through research using a systematic process. Evidence-based practice or EBP necessitates that nurses are clear about what is known and not known about a given health problem and health practice that will be 'best' for their clients (Liamputtong 2010b; Mullen et al. 2008). Too often, we know little about the particular health problems of some vulnerable groups, or about treatment options that are not empirically based. Currently, EBP does not apply to many of the health concerns of vulnerable groups such as ethnic minorities, indigenous groups, recent immigrants and refugees, gays and lesbians, rural communities, and people with uncommon or particularly challenging health problems (Liamputtong 2010b).

Within EBP, the quantitative approach is seen as being empirical science and as being more systematic than qualitative research (Liamputtong 2010b), so the findings of this approach are seen as being more reliable. Nevertheless, I argue that evidence derived from the qualitative approach can help nurse researchers to understand the issues and use the findings in their practice. Qualitative research provides evidence that they may not be able to obtain from quantitative research or from a systematic review of quantitative research. Seeley and associates (2008), for example, point out that the quantitative part of their research, which involved more than 2000 participants, failed to provide a good understanding of some of their findings regarding the impact of HIV and AIDS on families. It was only through the life histories of 24 families that they were able to explain these findings in a more meaningful way. Their study clearly points to the essence of the place of qualitative evidence in health care and practice. Many researchers have argued that 'qualitative research findings have much to offer evidence-based practice' (Daly et al. 2007; Grypdonck 2006; Hawker et al. 2002, p. 1285). As Sandelowski (2004, p. 1382) puts it, 'Qualitative research is the best thing to be happening to evidence-based practice'.

I argue here that qualitative enquiry is an essential means for eliciting evidence from diverse individuals, population groups and contexts. Qualitative methods are especially appropriate to the study of vulnerable people (Liamputtong 2007, 2009, 2010a,b). Qualitative research is more 'open-ended' as 'it is more concerned with being attuned to who is being travelled with, so to speak, than with setting out a precise route for all to follow, as in survey research' (Warren 2002, p. 86). Qualitative research methods are flexible and fluid, and therefore are suited to understanding the meanings, interpretations and subjective experiences of vulnerable groups (Liamputtong 2007, 2009, 2010a,b; Warr 2004). Qualitative research methods allow researchers to be able to hear the voices of those who are 'silenced, othered, and marginalized by the dominant social order', as the methods 'ask not only what is it? but, more importantly, "explain it to me—how, why, what's the process, what's the significance?'" (Hesse-Biber & Leavy 2005, p. 28). The in-depth nature of qualitative methods allows the researched to express their feelings and experiences in their own words (Munhall 2007). In her study of rape survivors, Campbell (2002) argues that qualitative methods provide opportunities to hear survivors' stories in ways that quantitative research is unable to match. Campbell contends that 'if we as researchers provide opportunities for survivors to talk about what has happened to them…we can bring their experiences to light' (p. 120).

The qualitative approach, Bond and Corner (2001) argue, is 'well suited' to researching people living with dementia. Qualitative research commits to seeing the world from the research participants' own perspectives, and this is crucial if researchers are serious in their explanations of the personhood of those living with dementia. This commitment necessitates examining the meanings and experiences of people with dementia 'on their own terms' (Bond & Corner 2001, p. 106). Warr (2004, p. 578) too suggests that qualitative research provides 'researchers with an opportunity to listen to people tell their life stories'. The stories offer researchers a clear window into the lived experiences of the participants. A qualitative approach requires the involvement of the researchers and very often it means that they will be out somewhere on the ground. This provides the researchers with rich and complex data that no other means may offer. Warr's fieldwork clearly illustrates her argument. During her fieldwork on the health risks of street sex workers in one of the well-known red-light areas in Australia, she talked with the women on streets, often very late at night when it was really dark and cold. She also encountered police and ran the risks of being harassed by troublemakers, who often abused the workers. However, these experiences gave her a better understanding of the lives of these sex workers.

THINKING DEEPLY

4.1 IMPROVING HEALTH CARE THROUGH EVIDENCE-BASED PRACTICE

Within the emergence of evidence-based practice in health care, Grypdonck (2006) contends that qualitative research contributes greatly to the appropriateness of care. She argues that health practitioners need to have a good understanding of 'what it means to be ill, to live with an illness, to be subject to physical limitations, to see one's intellectual capacities gradually diminish, or to be healed again, to rise from [near] death after a bone marrow transplant, leaving one's sick life behind, to meet people who take care of you in a way that makes you feel really understood and really cared for' (p. 1379). Practitioners cannot obtain knowledge from existing literature in order to address these crucial health and illness issues. Such knowledge can only be gained through the integration of research into their daily work. Surely, by gaining a better understanding of the lived experience of patients and clients, health practitioners will be able to provide more sensitive and appropriate care.

Summary

Undertaking research with vulnerable people presents unique and often difficult challenges. Because of these challenges, many researchers have excluded vulnerable people from their endeavours, so the needs and concerns of such people are often ignored in the scientific literature. I argue strongly that this will make these people even more vulnerable. Some research questions and evidence can only be answered by vulnerable individuals or groups. This requires researchers to initiate research with them. As researchers, we need to find ways to bring the voices of these vulnerable people to the fore, and this chapter intends to help readers to do so. As researchers, we are committed to giving voice to vulnerable people as this will be our first attempt to empower them. This is perhaps the time that we may be able to help many vulnerable people to have better opportunities to enhance their lives and health. As Moore and Miller (1999, p. 1040) put it, 'Only when vulnerable groups receive the appropriate research attention [will] their care and quality of life be enhanced'.

IMPLICATIONS FOR EVIDENCE-BASED NURSING AND MIDWIFERY

There are at least two key points concerned with ethical values in human research. The first is that researchers and all research team members need to know and observe all ethical values such as beneficience, respect for human beings and justice throughout the research process. For example, a research assistant does not ethically conduct their tasks and make up information by filling out a questionnaire without using the research protocol; these research results cannot be 'evidence' applicable in clinical or community settings. The information cannot be used to improve health care services. Reports within Australia and elsewhere also highlight the importance of all research team members to ensure that the research values have been observed at all times (Van Der Weyden 2004). These ethical values need to be emphasised.

The second is that 'human research is conducted with or about people, or their data or [human] tissue' (NHMRC & AVCC 2007, p. 8). This underlies the importance of ethics, which researchers need to consider throughout the research process. Clinicians who want to apply evidence in nursing and midwifery practices have to consider and observe the same ethical values. Nurses and midwives need to provide services that are proved to be beneficial to health outcomes, to all clients regardless of their backgrounds or who they are. At the same time, the rights of clients need to be respected. The ethical values discussed in this chapter are useful to both researchers and clinicians providing evidence-based care.

▶▶▶ **PROBLEM SOLVING 4.1**

Ann and her team are conducting a research project that aims to explore the meaning of chest pain and the decision process patients used before presenting at the hospital emergency department. Major issues explored include social support and help-seeking behaviours of the patients. They will interview respondents at their own homes.

Ann and the team are aware that their hospital serves disadvantaged groups such as newly arrived refugees and homeless people. What are the issues arising from their research design if the researchers want to include these disadvantaged groups as their respondents?

Suggest two strategies used by the researchers that potentially increase the chance of having the disadvantaged groups as their respondents.

Practice exercise 4.1

As a student in community nursing, you need to carry out a small research project relevant to community health. You live in an area with a large number of poor immigrants. You have observed many problems that these people have experienced. You would like to learn more about their mental health and the means they use to deal with difficulties in their day-to-day life. What important issues do you need to consider before you commence your research so that you successfully complete the project? Your research must not jeopardise these people. Write up a reflective exercise using the discussions provided in this chapter.

Practice exercise 4.2

1   What is the meaning of 'vulnerable' in the context of nursing research?
2   What will be the circumstances in your profession in which you might encounter vulnerable people?
3   What are the crucial aspects of researching vulnerable people within the nursing field?
4   What kind of evidence-based practice do you need when working with vulnerable people?
5   What type of research will allow you to elicit more accurate information about the lives and needs of vulnerable people?

Answers to problem solving 4.1

Since recruitment at the hospital may not be suitable, the word 'home' may have to be extended so that other types of residences where refugees and homeless people live are included. Other types of recruitment such as the snowballing method or recommendation by others may be appropriate. Researchers may recognise that these disadvantaged groups may not take part in their study.

Further reading

Booth, S. (1999). Researching health and homelessness: Methodological challenges for researchers working with a vulnerable, hard-to-reach, transient population. *Australian Journal of Primary Health* 5(3), 76–81.

Liamputtong, P. (2007). *Researching the Vulnerable: A Guide to Sensitive Research Methods.* London: Sage Publications.

Liamputtong, P. (2009). *Qualitative Research Methods*, 3rd edn. Melbourne: Oxford University Press.

Liamputtong, P. (2010). *Performing Qualitative Cross-Cultural Research.* Cambridge: Cambridge University Press.

Morse, J. M. (2002). Interviewing the ill. In J. F. Gubrium & J. A. Holstein (eds), *Handbook of Interview Research: Context and Method* (pp. 317–28). Thousand Oaks, CA: Sage Publications.

Sandelowski, M. (2004). Using qualitative research. *Qualitative Health Research* 14(10), 1366–86.

Warr, D. J. (2004). Stories in the flesh and voices in the head: Reflections on the context and impact of research with disadvantaged populations. *Qualitative Health Research* 14(4), 578–87.

Weblinks

<www.beds.ac.uk/research/iasr/vyp>

This website provides information about the Vulnerable Young People's Research Unit (VYP). It has a focus on issues relevant to commercial sexual exploitation and drug use, with young people considered to be a 'hard to reach' group.

<www.lboro.ac.uk/research/ccfr/growing_together>

This website is about the research project which explores the use and benefits of social and therapeutic horticulture for vulnerable adults in the community. Research is undertaken by the Centre for Child and Family Research (CCFR) at Loughborough University in the UK, as part of the Centre's research theme entitled 'Promoting the well-being of adults and the community'.

<www.eurogenguide.org.uk/guidelines-cbd.htm>

This website gives guidelines for health professionals dealing with vulnerable people which can be useful for researchers conducting research with vulnerable groups.

<www.nfer.ac.uk/publications/publications_home.cfm>

This website gives information about research projects undertaken by the National Foundation for Educational Research (NFER). It is argued that vulnerable children need additional educational support to ensure they are able to achieve their potential. NFER has conducted a number of research projects related to vulnerable groups which include:

- Children in public care
- Children with medical needs
- Gypsy/traveller children

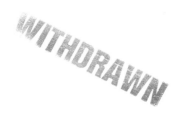

- Asylum-seeker and refugee children
- Young carers
- School refusers
- Teenage parents
- Young offenders
- Young people who are not in education or employment training.

References

Abboud, L. N., & Liamputtong, P. (2003). Pregnancy loss: What it means to women who miscarry and their partners. *Social Work in Health Care* 36(3), 37–62.

Anderson, D. G., & Hatton, D. C. (2000). Accessing vulnerable populations for research. *Western Journal of Nursing Research* 22(2), 244–51.

Barnard, M. (2005). Discomforting research: Colliding moralities and looking for 'truth' in a study of parental drug problems. *Sociology of Health & Illness* 27(1), 1–19.

Beauchamp, T. L., Jennings, B., Kinney, E. D., & Levine, R. J. (2002). Pharmaceutical research involving the homeless. *Journal of Medicine and Philosophy* 27(5), 547–64.

Beaver, K., Luker, K., & Woods, S. (1999). Research. Conducting research with the terminally ill: Challenges and considerations. *International Journal of Palliative Nursing* 5(1), 13–7.

Bender, D. E., Harbour, C., Thorp, J. M., Jr., & Morris, P. D. (2001). Tell me what you mean by 'si': Perceptions of quality of prenatal care among immigrant Latina women. *Qualitative Health Research* 11(6), 780–94.

Benoit, C., Jansson, M., Millar, A., & Phillips, R. (2005). Community-academic research on hard-to-reach populations: Benefits and challenges. *Qualitative Health Research* 15(2), 263–82.

Bergen, R. K. (1993). Interviewing survivors of marital rape: Doing feminist research on sensitive topics. In C. M. Renzetti & R. M. Lee (eds), *Researching Sensitive Topics* (pp. 197–211). Newbury Park, CA: Sage Publications.

Birman, D. (2005). Ethical issues in research with immigrants and refugees. In J. E. Trimble & C. B. Fisher (eds), *Handbook of Ethical Research with Ethnocultural Populations and Communities* (pp. 122–77). Thousand Oaks, CA: Sage Publications.

Bond, J., & Corner, L. (2001). Researching dementia: Are there unique methodological challenges for health services research? *Aging & Society* 21, 95–116.

Booth, S. (1999). Researching health and homelessness: Methodological challenges for researchers working with a vulnerable, hard-to-reach, transient population. *Australian Journal of Primary Health* 5(3), 76–81.

Brody, B. (1998). *Ethics of Research: An International Perspective*. New York: Oxford University Press.

Brzuzy, S., Ault, A., & Segal, E. A. (1997). Conducting qualitative interviews with women survivors of trauma. *Affilia* 12(1), 76–83.

Campbell, R. (2002). *Emotionally Involved: The Impact of Researching Rape*. New York: Routledge.

Cannon, L. W., Higginbotham, E., & Leung, M. L. A. (1988). Race and class bias in qualitative research on women. *Gender & Society* 2, 449–62.

Cook, K., & Nunkoosing, K. (2008). Maintaining dignity and managing stigma in the interview encounter: The challenge of paid-for participation. *Qualitative Health Research* 18(3), 418–27.

Cooper, H., Moore, L., Gruskin, S., & Krieger, N. (2005). The impact of a police drug crackdown on drug injectors' ability to practice harm reduction: A qualitative study. *Social Science & Medicine* 61, 673–84.

Corbin, J., & Morse, J. M. (2003). The unstructured interactive interview: Issues of reciprocity and risks when dealing with sensitive topics. *Qualitative Inquiry* 9(3), 335–54.

Cotterill, P. (1992). Interviewing women: Issues of friendship, vulnerability and power. *Women's Studies International Forum* 15(5/6), 593–606.

Crigger, N. J., Holcomb, L., & Weiss, J. (2001). Fundamentalism, multiculturalism, and problems conducting research with populations in developing nations. *Nursing Ethics* 8(5), 459–69.

Cutcliffe, J. R., & Ramcharan, P. (2002). Leveling the playing field? Exploring the merits of the ethics-as-process approach for judging qualitative research proposals. *Qualitative Health Research* 12(7), 1000–10.

Daly, J. (1992). The fit between qualitative research and characteristics of families. In J. F. Gilgun, K. Daly & G. Handel (eds), *Qualitative Methods in Family Research* (pp. 3–11). Newbury Park, CA: Sage Publications.

Daly, J. (2007). *Qualitative Methods for Family Studies and Human Development*. Thousand Oaks, CA: Sage Publications.

Daly, J., Willis, K., Small, R., Green, J., Welch, N., Kealy, M., & Hughes, E. (2007). A hierarchy of evidence for assessing qualitative health research. *Journal of Clinical Epidemiology* 60, 43–9.

Dickson-Swift, V., James, E., & Liamputtong, P. (2008). *Undertaking Sensitive Research in the Health and Social Sciences: Managing Boundaries, Emotions and Risks*. Cambridge: Cambridge University Press.

Dunlap, E., Johnson, B., Sanabria, H., Holliday, E., Lipsey, V., Barnett, M., Hopkins, W., Sobel, I., Randolph, D., & Chin, K.-L. (1990). Studying crack users and their criminal careers: The scientific and artistic aspects of locating hard-to-reach subjects and interviewing them about sensitive topics. *Contemporary Drug Problems* 17, 121–44.

Eder, D., & Fingerson, L. (2002). Interviewing children and adolescents. In J. F. Gubrium & J. A. Holstein (eds), *Handbook of Interview Research: Context and Method* (pp. 181–201). Thousand Oaks, CA: Sage Publications.

Faugier, J., & Sargeant, M. (1997). Sampling hard to reach populations. *Journal of Advanced Nursing* 26(4), 790–7.

Fisher, C. B., & Ragsdale, K. (2006). Goodness-of-fit ethics for multicultural research. In J. E. Trimble & C. B. Fisher (eds), *Handbook of Ethical Research with Ethnocultural Populations and Communities* (pp. 3–25). Thousand Oaks, CA: Sage Publications.

Flaskerud, J. H., & Winslow, B. J. (1998). Conceptualising vulnerable populations in health-related research. *Nursing Research* 47(2), 69–78.

Goodman, J. H. (2004). Coping with trauma and hardship among unaccompanied refugee youths from Sudan. *Qualitative Health Research* 14(9), 1177–96.

Grypdonck, M. H. F. (2006). Qualitative health research in the era of evidence-based practice. *Qualitative Health Research* 16(10), 1371–85.

Hall, B. L., & Kulig, J. C. (2004). Kanadier Mennonites: A case study examining research challenges among religious groups. *Qualitative Health Research* 14(3), 359–68.

Hallowell, N., Lawton, J., & Gregory, S. (2005). *Reflections on Research: The Realities of Doing Research in the Social Sciences*. Maidenhead, UK: Open University Press.

Hawker, S., Payne, S., Kerr, C., Hardey, M., & Powell, J. (2002). Appraising the evidence: Reviewing disparate data systematically. *Qualitative Health Research* 12(9), 1284–99.

Herzog, H. (2005). On home turf: Interview location and its social meaning. *Qualitative Sociology* 28(1), 25–47.

Hesse-Biber, S. N., & Leavy, L. P. (2005). *The Practice of Qualitative Research*. Thousand Oaks, CA: Sage Publications.

Holloway, W., & Jefferson, T. (2000). *Doing Qualitative Research Differently*. London: Sage Publications.

Holt, C. L., & McClure, S. M. (2006). Perceptions of the religion–health connection among African American church members. *Qualitative Health Research* 16(2), 268–81.

Husaini, B. A., Sherkat, D. E., Bragg, R., Levine, R., Emerson, J. S., Mentes, C. M., & Cain, V. A. (2001). Predictors of breast cancer screening in a panel study of African American women. *Women & Health* 34(3), 35–51.

Jamieson, J. (2000). Negotiating danger in fieldwork on crime: A researcher's tale. In G. Lee-Treweek & S. Linkogle (eds), *Danger in the Field: Risk and Ethics in Social Research* (pp. 61–71). London: Routledge.

Jewkes, R., Penn-Kenana, L., & Rose-Junius, H. (2005). 'If they rape me, I can't blame them': Reflections on gender in the social context of child rape in South Africa and Namibia. *Social Science & Medicine* 61, 1809–20.

Lee, R. M., & Renzetti, C. M. (1993). The problems of researching sensitive topics: Introduction. In C. M. Renzetti & R. M. Lee (eds), *Researching Sensitive Topics* (pp. 3–13). London: Sage Publications.

Leipert, B., & Reutter, L. (2005). Developing resilience: How women maintain their health in northern geographically isolated settings. *Qualitative Health Research* 15(1), 49–65.

Liamputtong, P. (2007). *Researching the Vulnerable: A Guide to Sensitive Research Methods*. London: Sage Publications.

Liamputtong, P. (2009). *Qualitative Research Methods*, 3rd edn. Melbourne: Oxford University Press.

Liamputtong, P. (2010a). *Performing Qualitative Cross-Cultural Research*. Cambridge: Cambridge University Press.

Liamputtong, P. (2010b). The science of words and the science of numbers: Research methods as foundations for evidence-based practice in health. In P. Liamputtong (ed.), *Research Methods in Health: Foundations for Evidence-Based Practice*. Melbourne: Oxford University Press.

Liamputtong, P., Haritavorn, N., & Kiatying-Angsulee, N. (2009). HIV and AIDS, stigma and AIDS support groups: Perspectives from women living with HIV and AIDS in central Thailand. *Social Science & Medicine, Special Issue: Women, Mothers and HIV Care in Resource Poor Settings* 69(6), 862–8.

Liamputtong Rice, P., Ly, B., & Lumley, J. (1994). Childbirth and soul loss: The case of a Hmong woman. *Medical Journal of Australia* 160(9), 577–8.

MacDougall, C., & Fudge, E. (2001). Planning and recruiting the sample for focus groups and in-depth interviews. *Qualitative Health Research* 11(1), 117–26.

Madriz, E. L. (1998). Using focus groups with lower socioeconomic status Latina women. *Qualitative Inquiry* 4(1), 114–29.

Martinez-Ebers, V. (1997). Using monetary incentives with hard-to-reach populations in panel surveys. *International Journal of Public Opinion Research* 9(1), 77–87.

Mayall, B. (1999). Children and childhood. In S. Hood, B. Mayall & S. Oliver (eds), *Critical Issues in Social Research: Power and Prejudice* (pp. 10–24). Philadelphia: Open University Press.

Meadows, L. M., Lagendyk, L. E., Thurston, W. E., & Eisener, A. C. (2003). Balancing culture, ethics, and methods in qualitative health research with Aboriginal peoples. *International Journal of Qualitative Methods* 2(4), 1–14.

Melrose, M. (2002). Labour pains: Some considerations on the difficulties of researching juvenile prostitution. *International Journal of Social Research Methodology* 5(4), 333–51.

Moore, L. W. (2002). Conducting research with visually impaired older adults. *Qualitative Health Research* 12(4), 559–65.

Moore, L. W., & Miller, M. (1999). Initiating research with doubly vulnerable populations. *Journal of Advanced Nursing* 30(5), 1034–40.

Morse, J. M. (2000). Researching illness and injury: Methodological considerations. *Qualitative Health Research* 10(4), 538–46.

Morse, J. M. (2002). Interviewing the ill. In J. F. Gubrium & J. A. Holstein (eds), *Handbook of Interview Research: Context and Method* (pp. 317–28). Thousand Oaks, CA: Sage Publications.

Mullen, E. J., Bellamy, J. L., & Bledsoe, S. E. (2008). Evidence-based practice. In R. M. Grinnell & Y. A. Unrau (eds), *Social Work Research and Evaluation: Foundations of Evidence-Based Practice*, 8th edn (pp. 508–24). New York: Oxford University Press.

Munhall, P. L. (2007). The landscape of qualitative research in nursing. In P. L. Munhall (ed.), *Nursing Research: A Qualitative Perspective*, 4th edn (pp. 3–36). Sudbury, MA: Jones & Bartlett Publishers.

NHMRC & AVCC (Australian Vice-Chancellors' Committee). (2007). *National Statement on Ethical Conduct in Human Research*. Canberra: NHMRC.

Nyamathi, A. (1998). Vulnerable populations: A continuing nursing focus. *Nursing Research* 47(2), 65–6.

Paradis, E. K. (2000). Feminist and community psychology ethics in research with homeless women. *American Journal of Community Psychology* 28(6), 839–58.

Parnis, D., Du Mont, J., & Gombay, B. (2005). Cooperation or co-optation? Assessing the methodological benefits and barriers involved in conducting qualitative research through medical institutional settings. *Qualitative Health Research* 15(5), 686–97.

Pauw, I., & Brener, L. (2003). 'You are just whores—you can't be raped': Barriers to safer sex practices among women street sex workers in Cape Town. *Culture, Health & Sexuality* 5(6), 465–81.

Punch, S. (2002). Research with children: The same or different from research with adults. *Childhood* 9(3), 321–41.

Pyett, P. (2001). Innovation and compromise: Responsibility and reflexivity in research with vulnerable groups. In J. Daly, M. Guillemin & S. Hill (eds), *Technologies and Health: Critical Compromises* (pp. 105–19). Melbourne: Oxford University Press.

Quest, T., & Marco, C. A. (2003). Ethics seminars: Vulnerable populations in emergency medicine research. *Academic Emergency Medicine* 10(11), 1294–8.

Ramcharan, P. (2010). What is ethical research? In P. Liamputtong (ed.), *Research Methods in Health: Foundations for Evidence-Based Practice*. Melbourne: Oxford University Press.

Reinharz, S. (1992). *Feminist Methods in Social Research*. New York: Oxford University Press.

Renzetti, C. M., & Lee, R. M. (eds) (1993). *Researching Sensitive Topics*. Newbury Park, CA: Sage Publications.

Romero-Daza, N., Weeks, M., & Singer, M. (2003). 'Nobody gives a damn if I live or die': Violence, drugs, and street-level prostitution in inner-city Hartford, Connecticut. *Medical Anthropology* 22, 233–59.

Russell, C. (1999). Interviewing vulnerable old people: Ethical and methodological implications of imagining our subjects. *Journal of Aging Studies* 13(4), 403–17.

Sandelowski, M. (2004). Using qualitative research. *Qualitative Health Research* 14(10), 1366–86.

Seeley, J., Biraro, S., Shafer, L. A., Nasirumbi, P., Foster, S., Whitworth, J., & Grosskurth, H. (2008). Using in-depth qualitative data to enhance our understanding of quantitative results regarding the impact of HIV and AIDS on households in rural Uganda. *Social Science & Medicine* 67(10), 1434–46.

Shelton, A. J., & Rianon, N. J. (2004). Recruiting participants for a community of Bangladeshi immigrants for a study of spousal abuse: An appropriate cultural approach. *Qualitative Health Research* 14(3), 369–80.

Stanley, L. (1990). Feminist praxis and the academic mode of production. In L. Stanley (ed.), *Feminist Praxis* (pp. 3–19). London: Routledge.

Stanley, L., & Wise, S. (1993). Method, methodology, and epistemology in feminist research process. In L. Stanley (ed.), *Feminist Praxis: Research, Theory and Epistemology in Feminist Sociology* (pp. 20–60). New York: Routledge.

Stone, T. H. (2003). The invisible vulnerable: The economically and educationally disadvantaged subjects of clinical research. *Journal of Law, Medicine & Ethics* 31(1), 149–53.

Takahashi, M., & Kai, I. (2005). Sexuality after breast cancer treatment: Changes and coping strategies among Japanese survivors. *Social Science & Medicine* 61, 1278–90.

Tewksbury, R., & Gagné, P. (2001). Assumed and presumed identities: Problems of self-presentation in field research. In J. M. Miller & R. Tewksbury (eds), *Extreme Methods: Innovative Approaches to Social Science Research* (pp. 72–93). Boston: Allyn & Bacon.

Umaña-Taylor, A. J., & Bámaca, M. Y. (2004). Conducting focus groups with Latino populations: Lessons from the field. *Family Relations* 53, 261–72.

Van Der Weyden, M. B. (2004). Managing allegations of scientific misconduct and fraud: Lessons from the 'Hall affair' (editorials). *Medical Journal of Australia* 180(4), 149–51.

Van Kesteren, N. M. C., Hospers, H. J., Kok, G., & van Empelen, P. (2005). Sexuality and sexual risk behavior in HIV-positive men who have sex with men. *Qualitative Health Research* 15(2), 145–68.

Varas-Diaz, N., Serrano-Garcia, I., & Toro-Alfonso, J. (2005). AIDS-related stigma and social interaction: Puerto Ricans living with HIV/AIDS. *Qualitative Health Research* 15(2), 169–87.

Warr, D. J. (2004). Stories in the flesh and voices in the head: Reflections on the context and impact of research with disadvantaged populations. *Qualitative Health Research* 14(4), 578–87.

Warr, D. J., & Pyett, P. M. (1999). Difficult relations: Sex work, love and intimacy. *Sociology of Health & Illness* 21(3), 290–309.

Warren, C. A. B. (2002). Qualitative interviewing. In J. F. Gubrium & J. A. Holstein (eds), *Handbook of Interview Research: Context amd Method* (pp. 83–101). Thousand Oaks, CA: Sage Publications.

Weaver, K., Wuest, J., & Ciliska, D. (2005). Understanding women's journey of recovering from anorexia nervosa. *Qualitative Health Research* 15(2), 188–206.

Weston, K. (2004). Fieldwork in lesbian and gay communities. In S. N. Hesse-Biber & M. L. Yaiser (eds), *Feminist Perspectives on Social Research* (pp. 198–205). New York: Oxford University Press.

Wiebel, W. W. (1990). Identifying and gaining access to hidden populations. In E. Y. Lambert (ed.), *The Collection and Interpretation of Data from Hidden Populations* (pp. 4–11). Rockville, MD: National Institute on Drug Abuse.

Wojcicki, J. M., & Malala, J. (2001). Condom use, power and HIV/AIDS risks: Sex-workers bargain for survival in Hillbrow/Jubert Park/Berea, Johannesburg. *Social Science & Medicine* 53, 99–121.

Wuest, J., Ford-Gilboe, M., Merritt-Gray, M., & Berman, H. (2003). Intrusion: The central problem for family health promotion among children and single mothers after leaving an abusive partner. *Qualitative Health Research* 13(5), 597–622.

PART 2

Making Sense of Research Methods

ANN AND BOB have had discussions with an experienced researcher at the School of Nursing and Midwifery of the local university. The constructive feedback they have received on their proposal has helped them maintain focus and direction for their intended project. They continue to maintain contact with their mentor for ongoing guidance and support.

It is now crunch time—the development of a research question/s is now required. After a review of literature relating to chest pain has been completed, and patient characteristics have been taken into account, Ann and Bob conclude that the decision by patients to re-present at the emergency department is based on their personal and socio-cultural beliefs. In order to explore the beliefs of this group of patients as to why they continue to re-present to the ED, Ann and Bob consider looking to a qualitative research design as a suitable research method. Chapter 5 describes a range of research methods used to carry out different forms of qualitative research. In deciding on which specific research design will be most appropriate, Ann and Bob will be required to review each design in relation to their research question. Choosing an appropriate research design is one aspect of the research process; knowing how to go about the correct process of data collection is another important consideration for Ann and Bob. Chapter 9 introduces you to several data collection methods from which the researcher needs to choose in order to collect the correct type of data to answer the research question.

Let us presume that after Ann and Bob have reviewed the literature for a second time, they feel that the underlying reason for patients with chest pain re-presenting to the ED is not about socio-cultural beliefs but about patients' personal demographic factors and the perceived severity of their chest pain. They would also like to generalise their research results to a wider group of patients with chest pain in other health care organisations. What is required in such a situation is a change in the research pathway from a qualitative to a quantitative approach to enquiry. The change in focus will also mean a change to the research question. Chapter 6 will be useful for Ann and Bob in deciding which research design will be the most appropriate to answer their new research question. Chapter 8 describes the methods that can ▶

be used in selecting participants and deciding on a sample size or participant numbers in order to obtain a representative sample of the participant population to be studied.

If Ann and Bob are not happy in limiting their design to either a qualitative or quantitative approach because they feel that both methods have much to offer to their project, an alternative pathway is open to them—that of taking a mixed methods approach. Chapter 7 discusses the different types of research designs or pathways that can be used in conducting mixed method research as well as issues of method and challenges that Ann and Bob will need to resolve as a result of using two different approaches in the one project.

CHAPTER 5

Qualitative Research Design

Anthony Welch

Chapter learning objectives

By the end of this chapter you will be able to:

▶ understand the philosophical foundations of qualitative research

▶ describe a range of qualitative research designs

▶ explain different methods of conducting research within particular qualitative designs

▶ list the type of questions to ask when choosing a qualitative research design.

Introduction

There are various ways by which knowledge can be generated. What constitutes knowledge has been a point of ongoing debate since the dawn of time (Streubert & Carpenter 1995). At various times in history different forms of knowledge have arisen. The desire to know has been the catalyst for the development of different approaches to research.

Two major perspectives concerning the value of knowledge to human understanding have been the natural sciences or what we call quantitative research, with its emphasis on identifying cause and effect. Such an approach to research is characterised by objectivity, the application of scientific strategies or protocols to test the validity of a particular intervention, and the use of logical deductive reasoning as a problem-solving process (Chapter 6). On the other hand, human science research, or what we call qualitative research, focuses on the exploration of people's personal accounts of their experiences, and the ways in which individuals, groups and communities construct personal and collective meaning about their everyday world (Dilthey 1977). This chapter introduces you to qualitative research. Different research pathways within the realm of qualitative research will be presented. Examples are given of various research designs and their application to health research for the professions of nursing and midwifery.

What is qualitative research?

In order to understand what qualitative research is, we first need to have some knowledge of its origins and how it has emerged as a legitimate mode of enquiry. The development of a theory of human sciences by Dilthey (1977) was motivated by a need to develop a research pathway that could explore the world of human beings in their everyday life.

Dilthey's pursuit of an appropriate method for exploring human understanding led to the emergence of the human sciences as a legitimate means of enquiry, providing a platform for the development of a system of study now referred to as qualitative research. The central aim of qualitative research is to develop an understanding of how human beings construct and make sense of the world in which they live—'a social, personal and relational world that is complex, layered, and can be viewed from different perspectives' (McLeod 2001, p. 2).

Qualitative research is characterised by six fundamental values (Streubert Speziale et al. 2007) that underpin the research process (Box 5.1).

BOX 5.1

FUNDAMENTAL VALUES OF THE PHILOSOPHICAL PERSPECTIVE OF
QUALITATIVE RESEARCH

- A belief in multiple realities—perspectives—to a given situation.
- A commitment to selecting an approach to research that is appropriate to answer the research question.
- A commitment to the participant's viewpoint—truthfully describing what is important to the participant about their experience.
- Minimising disturbance to the natural setting or context in which the study is conducted.
- Acknowledging researcher participation in the research process—the researcher is an integral part of the research.
- Presenting the findings of the study in a literary style rich with expressions and descriptions of participants' experiences.

These core characteristics or fundamental values encompass a range of theoretical approaches and research designs that fall under the umbrella of qualitative research (Patton 2002). These approaches or research designs include phenomenology, heuristics, grounded theory, ethnography, ethnonursing, critical social theory, feminisms, action research and bricolage. Each of these research designs will be discussed along with other examples.

Figure 5.1   Different qualitative research designs

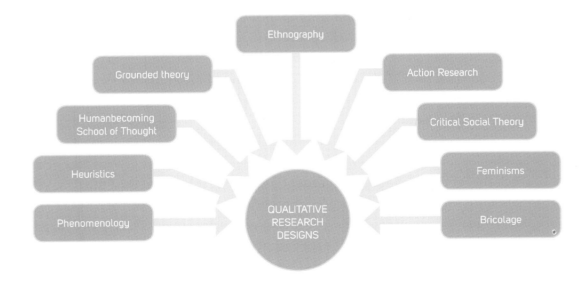

Phenomenology

Phenomenology as a research method can be traced back to the works of Franz Brentano (1838–1917), Carl Stumpf (1848–1936) and Edmond Husserl (1857–1938) in the late 19th century. Phenomenology as a scientific method of research emerged as an alternative to the traditional natural sciences commonly referred to as positive scientific methods or quantitative research, which was not concerned with researching the everyday world of human experience (Parse 2001). Since the initial work of Brentano, phenomenology, or what has been termed the phenomenological movement, has continued to develop. Two major pathways or streams of phenomenological research have developed over time: descriptive phenomenology and interpretive phenomenology. Although there are differences between the two approaches or pathways, some concepts are shared by both. These are intentionality, essences, life-world, intuiting and description of phenomena.

Intentionality is at the core of phenomenology. The term is used to refer to human consciousness or awareness. Phenomenology holds the belief that every act is an act of consciousness or an awareness of something, whether that be perceiving an object, recalling a memory, imagining an experience or anticipating a future event (Sokowloski 2000). For instance, one does not hear without hearing something, or hope without hoping for something or care without caring for something. 'Intentionality' should not be confused with 'intention', which is concerned with purpose and action, such as intending to buy a friend a present. Intentionality is at the heart of human experience as the act of creating meaning about what is being observed or experienced (Solomon 2001).

Essences are the essential structures of phenomena—what makes up a phenomenon. An essence is a basic unit of common understanding. For example, what is the essence or common understanding of caring? The nursing and midwifery literature often talk about the uniqueness of caring in these two disciplines. If you wanted to know what this uniqueness is all about you would be exploring the essence of caring as practised by nurses and midwives. One of the central aims of phenomenology, therefore, is to describe the essences or common understandings of phenomena as experienced by individuals and groups in everyday life.

Life-world denotes a world in which human beings live and through which they give expression and meaning to their personal existence—the world of lived experience. The inclusion of the word 'lived' denotes an experience that has been lived through. When we talk about lived-through experiences we are referring to experiences that have been reflected on in order to gain understanding of what occurred, for example, taking time to reflect on your clinical practice in order to learn from the experience.

Intuiting refers to the process of imaginative variation of the data—to look at the data in different ways—until a common understanding of the phenomenon emerges (Crotty 1998).

Description is a way of uncovering the essential nature or structure of phenomena. Within phenomenology description is considered the primary mode of communicating experiences of phenomena—'things'—as they occur in everyday life, for instance the experience of hoping, grieving, feeling loved, living with chronic pain, caring for another and so forth. The act of describing phenomena as experienced is fundamental to phenomenological enquiry.

Think about how you share your experience. More often than not it is by describing what has happened and what the experience was like for you. The same process is applied when you are undertaking phenomenological research.

In addition to the central concepts mentioned above, there is one further concept, the phenomenological attitude commonly referred to as 'bracketing'. Bracketing refers to the process by which the researcher reflects on their own personal assumptions, biases, beliefs and attitudes about the phenomenon or the focus of the study, and attempts to set them aside in order to reduce the possibility of allowing their own views and values to influence the findings of the study (Sokolowski 2000). Three elements are involved in phenomenological research: participant/s, the context or environment, and the researcher conducting the research.

Figure 5.2   Simple presentations of phenomenology and heuristic research designs

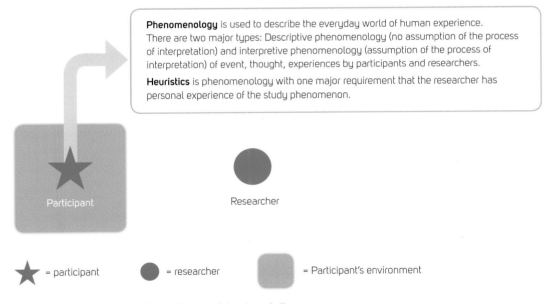

Phenomenology is used to describe the everyday world of human experience. There are two major types: Descriptive phenomenology (no assumption of the process of interpretation) and interpretive phenomenology (assumption of the process of interpretation) of event, thought, experiences by participants and researchers.

Heuristics is phenomenology with one major requirement that the researcher has personal experience of the study phenomenon.

Participant

Researcher

★ = participant   ● = researcher   ■ = Participant's environment

An arrow symbolises the data derived from participants and other sources.

Descriptive phenomenology

Description is the basis for all qualitative research. In-depth, rich, concrete description provides the foundation for qualitative enquiry (Patton 2002) through which the world of human experience is made visible. Descriptive phenomenology as a method of enquiry includes a range of approaches that have developed over time by researchers interested in seeking out new and innovative ways of researching human experience. Therefore, choosing a descriptive phenomenological approach is not a simple task of following one universally prescribed method but rather having to decide on one approach among many. Table 5.1 gives three examples of descriptive phenomenological designs.

Table 5.1   Three examples of descriptive phenomenology modifications

Amadeo Giorgi (1985)	Paul Colaizzi (1978)	Helen Streubert (1991)
• Read the entire description of the experience to get a sense of the whole. • Reread the description. • Identify the transition units of the experience. • Clarify and elaborate the meaning by relating them to each other and to the whole. • Reflect on the constituents in the concrete language of the subject. • Transformation of the concrete language into the language or concepts of science. • Integration and synthesis of the insights into a descriptive structure of the meaning of the experience.	• Description of the phenomenon of interest by the researcher. • Collection of subject's description of the phenomenon. • Read all the subject's descriptions of the phenomenon • Returning the original transcripts and extracted significant statements. • Trying to spell out the meaning of each significant statement. • Organising the aggregate formalised meanings into clusters or themes. • Writing an exhaustive description. • Returning to the subjects for validation of the description. • If new data are revealed during the validations, incorporating them into an exhaustive description.	• Explicating a personal description of the phenomenon of interest. • Bracketing the researcher's presuppositions. • Interviewing participants in unfamiliar settings. • Carefully reading the transcripts of the interview to obtain a general sense of the experience. • Reviewing the transcripts to uncover the essences. • Apprehending essential relationships. • Developing formalised descriptions of the phenomenon. • Returning to participants to validate descriptions. • Reviewing the relevant literature. • Distributing the findings to the nursing community.

As you read through these three designs you will notice that the processes involved differ. What is important is to make sure that whatever design you choose is appropriate to answer the research question and the chosen approach is consistent with the aims of your study.

Interpretive phenomenology

The development of an interpretive phenomenology is attributed to Paul Ricoeur (1976), Martin Heidegger (1962) and Hans Gadamer (1976). The rationale for such an approach to research is that to understand the ways human beings act, experience and find meaning in their everyday lives requires moving beyond description to interpretation. The interpretation of information or data is referred to as hermeneutics. Hermeneutics has its origin in biblical exegesis—the interpretation of biblical and historical texts (Bleicher 1980). Heidegger argued that hermeneutics is a fundamental element of human existence. Human beings are continually engaged in an ongoing process of interpretation in order to make meaningful sense of the world in which they live (Dreyfus 1991).

Interpretive phenomenology differs from descriptive phenomenology primarily in its adoption of the phenomenological attitude or the use of bracketing. In an interpretive phenomenological approach the use of bracketing is viewed as having limited value as human beings cannot be separated from the world in which they live. Therefore, it is not possible to take a purely objective stance, or separate ourselves from the world. People are sensate, meaning we experience our world from a subjective position. It is our interpretation of our experiences that creates meaning for us as human beings.

Within the realm of interpretive phenomenology there are a number of different approaches one can take depending on the focus of the research question. The works of Ricoeur, Gadamer and Heidegger are useful.

▸▸▸ TERMS, TIPS AND SKILLS

Phenomenological research is concerned with exploring the lived experience of everyday life.

5.1 RESEARCH DESIGNS FOR PHENOMENOLOGICAL STUDY

THINKING DEEPLY

Take a few moments to think about what research design you would choose if you were contemplating a phenomenological study. Think about the issue of concern you wish to explore then formulate a research question you wish to answer.

Once you have settled on a researchable question think about what would be the most appropriate design or approach in answering that question. Keep in mind that the focus of phenomenological enquiry is phenomena present in everyday experiences. Within the context of nursing and health care, questions may focus on caring for people with chronic pain, living with a chronic illness, being an advocate, giving birth, or coming to terms with dying.

In no more than one paragraph justify your choice of design in relation to the research question you wish to explore.

Heuristics

Heuristics is another form of phenomenological research. The aim of heuristic research is to explore a phenomenon through the personal experiences of the researcher and/or co-researchers. Heuristics has its origins in humanistic psychology with its emphasis on the primacy of human experience as a mode of discovery.

> The root meaning of the term heuristic comes from the Greek word heuriskein, meaning to discover or to find. It refers to a process of internal [personal] search through which one discovers the nature and meaning of experience and develops methods and procedures for further investigation and analysis. (Moustakas 1990, p. 9)

A fundamental requirement for undertaking heuristic enquiry is that the researcher must have a personal and intense experience of the phenomenon and a willingness to engage in such processes as introspective self-search, systematic enquiry and tacit knowing. Tacit knowing is defined as a process of 'giving birth to hunches and vague, formless insights' (Douglas & Moustakas 1985, p. 49) about the phenomena under investigation that surface in the course of the enquiry. In simple terms it can be said that the researchers are also the respondents. They become the participants. The processes involved in heuristic enquiry are:

- *initial engagement:* the beginning point where the researcher identifies the focus of enquiry
- *immersion:* the process of intense concentration involving self-dialogue, self-searching, pursuing intuitive clues and drawing from tacit knowledge
- *incubation:* a process of stepping back, taking a detached stance and being receptive to the emergence of new insights and understandings
- *illumination:* a point of new awareness and understanding
- *explication:* the process of describing or depicting core themes
- *creative synthesis:* the process of drawing together the core themes into a comprehensive description of the phenomenon being studied (Moustakas 1990).

The types of human experiences that you would focus on using this approach to research could include being a student nurse, feeling happy, feeling lonely, caring for another, or living on death row.

▶▶▶ TERMS, TIPS AND SKILLS

The aim of heuristic research is to explore a phenomenon through the personal experiences of the researcher and/or co-researchers.

The humanbecoming school of thought

The 'humanbecoming' school of thought has its origins in the human sciences (Parse 1998), in Martha Roger's (1970, 1980) science of unitary human beings, and in concepts from the body of existential-phenomenological thought, as described by a number of researchers (Heidegger 1962; Merleau-Ponty 1989; Sartre 1956). Parse synthesised concepts from these researchers into nine initial assumptions that were later collapsed into three pivotal assumptions. These three assumptions are philosophical tenets of the humanbecoming school of thought and have three main themes: meaning, rhythmicity and transcendence (Parse 1998), as follows:

1   *meaning:* humanbecoming or people freely choosing personal meaning in the intersubjective process of living value priorities
2   *rhythmicity:* humanbecoming or people co-creating rhythmical patterns of relating in mutual process with the universe or others
3   *transcendence:* humanbecoming or people co-transcending the multidimensional with the emerging possible. They can move beyond the 'now' moment and provide a unique personal path in an ongoing change (Cody 2010; Parse 1998, p. 29).

Three research methods have been further developed through the use of the humanbecoming school of thought in research. Comparisons between the three humanbecoming methods are presented in Table 5.2. The first two are basic research while the third is applied research:

1   The Parse research method is a phenomenological-hermeneutic method used to discover structures of universal lived experiences of an individual or a group.
2   The humanbecoming hermeneutic method focuses on interpretation and understanding of texts and art-forms from a humanbecoming perspective.
3   The qualitative descriptive pre-project-process-post-project method is used to explore what happens when humanbecoming is the framework guiding practice (Parse 2001).

Table 5.2   Three humanbecoming methods

THE HUMANBECOMING SCHOOL OF THOUGHT		
Basic research		**Applied research**
Purpose	To advance the science of humanbecoming school of thought		To evaluate the changes and effectiveness of health care when the humanbecoming theory guides practice
Contributions	New knowledge and understanding of humanly lived experiences to guide further research and practice		New knowledge and understanding of humanly lived experiences to guide further research and practice
Methods	Parse method	Humanbecoming Hermeneutic method	Descriptive qualitative pre-project-process-post-project method
Phenomena	Lived experiences (descriptions from participants)	Lived experiences (descriptions from published texts)	Change, satisfaction and effectiveness (descriptions from participants and documents)
Processes	Dialogical engagement Extraction-synthesis Heuristic interpretation	Discoursing Interpreting Understanding	Pre-project information gathered by evaluator Teaching-learning sessions on humanbecoming theory in practice Midway information gathered by evaluator Continue teaching-learning sessions Post-project information gathered by evaluator Analysis-synthesis of themes from each information source
Discover	The paradoxical living of the remembered, the now moment and the all-at-once	Emergent meanings	Thematic conceptualisations

Grounded theory

Grounded theory is a qualitative research method for generating a social theory through the study of basic social processes and social systems present in human interactions (Parse 2001). It is a systematic process of enquiry in which the researcher engages in a process of constant comparative analysis of data at each stage of the research process in order to generate theory about a particular phenomenon of concern. Data sources can include observation, fieldnotes, intensive interviews, review of documents, analysis of literature and research on the topic, and memo-writing.

The term 'grounded' refers to the fact that the emergent theory is grounded in or based on the actual data gathered by the researchers, who include Streubert Speziale and Rinaldi Carpenter (2007). The origins of grounded theory are attributed to Barney Glaser and

Anselm Strauss, two sociologists from the University of California. The initial works of Glaser and Strauss were influenced by two schools of thought—pragmatism and symbolic interactionism (Charmaz 2006; Glaser & Strauss 1967).

▶▶▶   TERMS, TIPS AND SKILLS

Grounded theory is a qualitative research method for generating a social theory through the study of the basic social processes and social systems present in human interactions.

The first school of thought, pragmatism, originated in the works of Charles Saunders Pierce (1839–1914) and was later modified and extended by William James (1976) and John Dewey (1929; see also McDermott 1981). The central focus of pragmatism (also referred to as the pragmatic method) was to 'bring intelligence to bear on the problems of moral and social life as an antidote to the often "unreflective and brutal" individualism' (McDermott 1981) pervading American life at that time.

The second school of thought, symbolic interactionism, which provides the theoretical framework for grounded theory (Fain 2004), has its origins in the works of George Herbert Mead and his student Herbert Blumer, two sociologists from the University of Chicago. The three assumptions underpinning symbolic interactionism stipulated by Blumer (1969) are:

- 'human beings act toward things on the basis of the meanings that these things have for them'
- 'the meaning of such things is derived from, and arises out of, the social interaction that one has with one's fellows'
- 'these meanings are handled in, and modified through, an interpretive process used by the person in dealing with the things he encounters' (p. 2).

The very nature of symbolic interactionism is a dynamic interactive process of personal engagement with others and the environment in the construction of understanding and meaning.

Since the original works of Glaser and Strauss (1967) in which the grounded theory method was developed, a number of modifications to the method have been proposed. The main contributors to the modifications have been Glaser (1992), Strauss and Corbin (1990) and Charmaz (1990). The modifications to the original grounded theory method are shown in Table 5.3.

Figure 5.3   Simple presentation of grounded theory research design

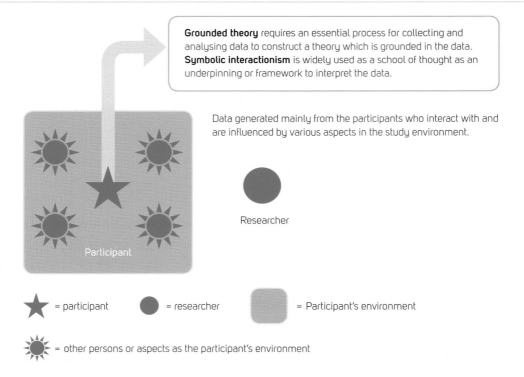

Grounded theory requires an essential process for collecting and analysing data to construct a theory which is grounded in the data. **Symbolic interactionism** is widely used as a school of thought as an underpinning or framework to interpret the data.

Data generated mainly from the participants who interact with and are influenced by various aspects in the study environment.

Researcher

Participant

★ = participant   ● = researcher   ▢ = Participant's environment

✷ = other persons or aspects as the participant's environment

An arrow symbolises the data derived from participants and other sources.

Table 5.3   Modifications to grounded theory

Theorist	Modification/refinements
Glaser and Strauss	The generation of theory without any particular commitment to specific kinds of data, lines of research or theoretical interests (Glaser & Strauss 1967).
Glaser	Continued to remain true to the original method developed by Glaser and Strauss (1967) but placed more emphasis on discovery, emergence of categories and strict adherence to each step of the method.
Strauss and Corbin	Moved towards verification with an emphasis on technical procedures and less emphasis on the constant comparative method.
Charmaz	Constructivist approach brings together traditional positivist/objectivist methods and post-positivist interpretive approaches to grounded theory research (Charmaz 2006).

Despite the various modifications to Glaser and Strauss's (1967) classic grounded theory method, processes that are generally considered essential are the following:

- Theoretical sampling means that decisions about whom to interview or what to observe next are determined by the state of theory generation, and that implies starting data analysis with the first interview, and writing down memos early.

- Constant comparative data analysis is the ongoing comparison between phenomena and contexts to make the theory strong.
- Theoretical sensitivity coding means that theoretical strong concepts are generated from the data to explain the phenomenon researched.
- Memo writing.
- Identification of a core category.
- The formulation of an explanatory theory (see also Chapters 8 and 11).

▶▶▶ TERMS, TIPS AND SKILLS

When choosing grounded theory as your research method it is important to remember that there have been a number of modifications to the original method which have resulted in different versions. Once you make a choice of a particular version for your study, it is important to remain true to that approach.

Ethnography

Ethnography has its origins in anthropology with its focus on the study of humans from evolutionary and social perspectives (New Webster's Encyclopaedia of Dictionaries 1990). Ethnography is defined by Fetterman (1989, p. 11) as 'the art and science of describing a group or culture' with particular attention on understanding the patterns and meanings of human behaviour such as belief systems, myths, rituals, symbols, customs, roles, events, social interactions and group interrelationships that form the basis of everyday life of a cultural group (McLeod 2001; Spradley 1980). At the core of an ethnographic study is 'to get at the implicit (back-stage) culture in addition to the explicit, public (front-stage) aspects of culture' (Germain 2001, p. 284) and to learn from the members that make up the cultural group.

Initially ethnographic studies were concerned with exploring traditional cultures about which little was known, such as tribal rituals, parenting behaviours in ancient civilisations, and patterns of communicating in different cultural groups. In contemporary society the focus of ethnography is on everyday social issues such as poverty, marginalised groups, homeless persons and organisational systems such as the health care system.

▶▶▶ TERMS, TIPS AND SKILLS

Ethnographic research is concerned with the art and science of describing patterns of living and human interaction of a group or culture.

Anthony Welch

Figure 5.4 Simple presentations of ethnography and ethnonursing

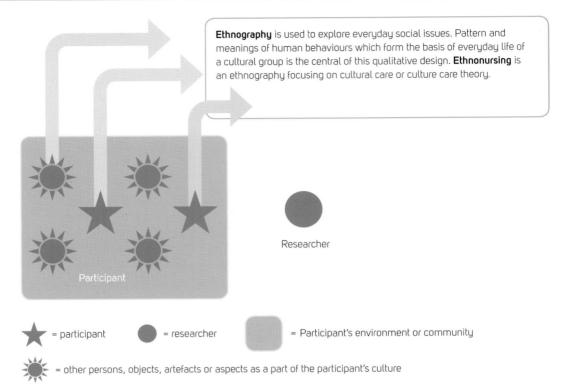

Ethnography is used to explore everyday social issues. Pattern and meanings of human behaviours which form the basis of everyday life of a cultural group is the central of this qualitative design. **Ethnonursing** is an ethnography focusing on cultural care or culture care theory.

Researcher

Participant

★ = participant   ● = researcher   ■ = Participant's environment or community

☀ = other persons, objects, artefacts or aspects as a part of the participant's culture

An arrow symbolises the data derived from participants and other sources.
These research designs gain data from different forms, modes and means.

Like other qualitative designs, a number of different approaches to ethnographic enquiry have evolved. These include classical ethnography, systematic ethnography, interpretive ethnography and critical ethnography (Muecke 1994).

Classical ethnography has as its central focus obtaining a complete description of all aspects of a cultural group: patterns of living of the people that make up a cultural group.

Systematic ethnography is concerned with 'defin[ing] the structure of culture, rather than [describing] a people and their social interaction, emotions, and materials' (Muecke 1994, p. 192).

Interpretive ethnography aims to 'discover the meanings of observed social interactions' (Muecke 1994, p. 193). The construction of meaning is the bedrock for human understanding. In order to understand human behaviour, therefore, it is necessary to discover the meaning behind what the person is doing (Muecke 1994).

Critical ethnography is the study of society that gives particular attention to uncovering social inequalities, oppression and injustices, with the aim of raising social awareness and instituting change (Patton 2002).

In addition to the contributions of Muecke, other ethnographic research approaches warrant mention—autoethnography and ethnonursing.

Autoethnography is concerned with the study of one's own culture through personal experience. The person's experience provides the conduit or means of exploring and gaining insights into the culture in which the person lives.

Ethnonursing as a research method was developed by Madeleine Leininger (1985, 1988). Its focus is on culture care patterns—care expressions and practices. The premises

Figure 5.5 Sunrise model

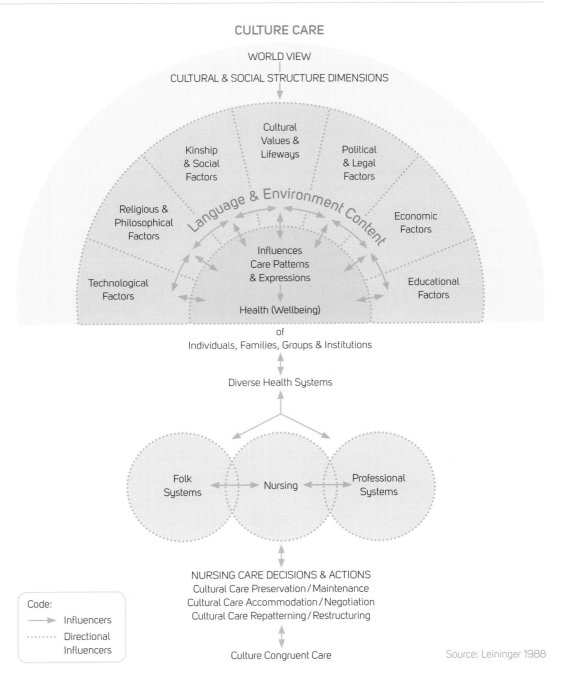

CULTURE CARE

WORLD VIEW
CULTURAL & SOCIAL STRUCTURE DIMENSIONS

Cultural
Values &
Lifeways

Kinship
& Social
Factors

Political
& Legal
Factors

Religious &
Philosophical
Factors

Language & Environment Content

Economic
Factors

Influences
Care Patterns
& Expressions

Technological
Factors

Educational
Factors

Health (Wellbeing)

of
Individuals, Families, Groups & Institutions

Diverse Health Systems

Folk
Systems

Nursing

Professional
Systems

NURSING CARE DECISIONS & ACTIONS
Cultural Care Preservation / Maintenance
Cultural Care Accommodation / Negotiation
Cultural Care Repatterning / Restructuring

Culture Congruent Care

Code:
⟶ Influencers
········· Directional
Influencers

Source: Leininger 1988

Anthony Welch

underpinning culture care theory are that care is fundamental to health and well-being, and the act of caring involves multiple universal and diverse elements. Therefore, in order to provide holistic humanistic culture care, elements that need to be considered include 'worldview, ethno-history, religious [philosophical and spiritual] orientation, kinship patterns, material cultural phenomena, the political, economic, legal, educational, technological, and physical environment, language, and folk and professional care practices' (Leininger 1991, p. 23). Leininger's Sunrise model was developed as a conceptual framework to depict the various dimensions of her culture care theory.

Critical social theory

Critical social theory focuses on uncovering social inequality and the reasons for social change. Critical theorists attempt to confront social injustices by critiquing the socio-political ideologies, conventional social structures and uncontested social beliefs that form the fabric of a society, shaping people's experiences, interactions with others and the way we view the world (Patton 2002).

The development of critical social theory can be traced to the seminal works of Karl Marx (1818–83). The fundamental issue for Marx was that those who hold economic hegemony (control) are able to shape the lives of those who do not (Crotty 1998). The issues of control, power, oppression, manipulation and social injustice implicit in Marxism have formed the foundation for much of contemporary critical social research. As a movement, critical social theory has its origins in the Institute for Social Research established in 1924 in Frankfurt, Prussia under the patronage of Felix Weil aided by Kurt Gerlach (Crotty 1998).

Figure 5.6 Simple presentations of critical social theory and feminism

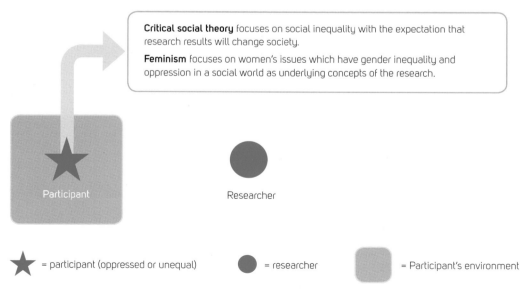

Critical social theory focuses on social inequality with the expectation that research results will change society.

Feminism focuses on women's issues which have gender inequality and oppression in a social world as underlying concepts of the research.

Participant

Researcher

= participant (oppressed or unequal)   = researcher   = Participant's environment

An arrow symbolises the data derived from participants and other sources.

Over time, critical social theory has become eclectic in orientation as a result of different ideological positions put forward by critical social theorists. Examples of different ideological approaches to critical social theory research are Communicative Reason by Jurgen Habermas, Paulo Freire's Pedagogy of the Oppressed, and Negative Dialectic by Theodor Adorno.

▶▶▶ TERMS, TIPS AND SKILLS

Critical social theory focuses on uncovering social inequality and the reasons for social change.

Feminism

Feminism is a term concerned with women's issues. At the centre of feminist thought is the recognition of women's experiences, beliefs, views, ways of being and ways of knowing as legitimate and authoritative sources of knowledge (Crotty 1998; Olesen 1994). Feminism is about raising awareness of gender inequality and oppression in the social world and exploring ways by which gender inequality can be rectified.

A range of feminisms within the feminist social movement have emerged in response to women's concerns about inequality and the desire to be free from male dominance. Examples of the various forms of feminism provided by Tong (1995) are given in Table 5.4.

Table 5.4   Forms of feminism

Category/type	Concerned with
Liberal feminism	Grounded in humanism, which privileges personal autonomy, self-fulfilment and sexual equality (Crotty 1998).
Marxist feminism	Women's oppression associated with 'the product of the political, social and economic structures associated with capitalism' (Tong 1995, p. 39).
Radical feminism	Taking a separatist stance from the dominant patriarchal system by creating 'woman defined systems, thought and culture' (Chinn & Wheeler 1985, p. 74).
Psychoanalytic feminism	Attributes women's oppression to the female psyche. Located in Freudian theory, the focus is on exploration of a non-patriarchal understanding of the Oedipus complex and/or pre-Oedipal relationship between mother and infant (Crotty 1998).
Socialist feminism	Represents 'a confluence of Marxist, radical and psychoanalytic streams of feminist thought' (Tong 1995, p. 173).
Existentialist feminism	Attributed to the work of Simone de Beauvoir, who illuminated the relationship between man and woman through Sartre's concepts of self and other. Man is denoted as Self and woman as Other. The Other, construed as a threat to Self, must be subjugated to a subordinate status/role.
Postmodern feminism	Draws on the works of Jacques Lacan (1901–81) and Jacques Derrida (1930–). The focus is on 'deconstruction [and] breaking down traditional antinomies such as reason/emotion, beautiful/ugly, self/other and conventional boundaries between established disciplines' (Crotty 1998, p. 168).

Anthony Welch

Action research

Action research has its origins in the work of J. L. Moreno, a physician who undertook community research with groups of prostitutes in Vienna during the early 1900s. The prostitutes were considered by Moreno as participants and co-researchers (McTaggart 1994). The term 'action research' as a mode of enquiry was coined by Kurt Lewin, who described a program of community research projects involving community groups in the USA to address post-Second World War social problems (Lewin 1946). Action research, as the name suggests, investigates an identified area or issue of concern to and by a group of interested people with the aim of generating solutions or interventions to bring about change. Action researchers go to the site of the problem and work with the people concerned as co-researchers. The processes for action research include a repeated cycle of enquiry, intervention and evaluation. Street and Robinson (1995) have developed a schematic representation for the conduct of action research based on Lewin's original model and their own experiences in working on nursing projects.

Figure 5.7   Simple presentation of action research

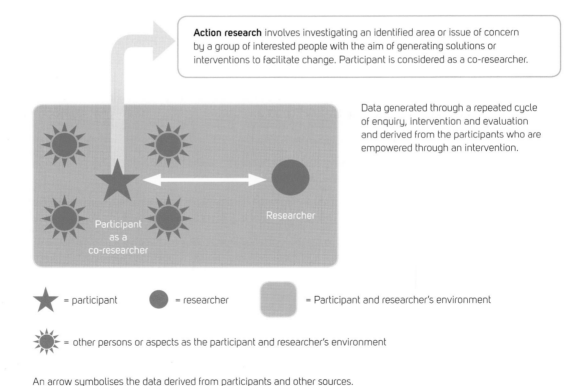

Action research involves investigating an identified area or issue of concern by a group of interested people with the aim of generating solutions or interventions to facilitate change. Participant is considered as a co-researcher.

Data generated through a repeated cycle of enquiry, intervention and evaluation and derived from the participants who are empowered through an intervention.

Participant as a co-researcher

Researcher

★ = participant   ● = researcher   ▮ = Participant and researcher's environment

✸ = other persons or aspects as the participant and researcher's environment

An arrow symbolises the data derived from participants and other sources.

From its original work by Lewin (1946), action research has witnessed a number of
modifications in response to different aims. Examples of the forms of action research and
specific aims are given in Table 5.5.

Table 5.5   Action research

Forms of action research	Foci/aims
Technical action research	Improvement of techniques and procedures through practitioner collaboration.
Practical action research	Improve existing practices and develop new ones.
Emancipatory action research	Take responsibility for actions that free the group from practice constraints through initiating change by transforming political, social and economic conditions (Taylor et al. 2007).

Bricolage

Bricolage has emerged over the past few decades in response to a perceived need by
researchers to move beyond adopting a singular philosophical position and its stipulated
method to embrace a broad sweep of philosophical perspectives and methodological
strategies from which to utilise the most appropriate methods for the collection and analysis
of data (McLeod 2001). The person using such an approach is described as the bricoleur,
a French word meaning 'someone who works with his hands, and uses [different] means
compared to those of the craftsman' (Weinstein & Weinstein 1991, p. 161). The idea of
researcher-as-bricoleur was introduced by Levi-Strauss (1966) to describe 'a person who
makes something new out of a range of materials that previously made up something
different' (Crotty 1998, p. 50). The bricoleur begins the enquiry by sifting through the
layers of assumed knowledge and perceptions to see the object of enquiry as it exists before
exploring its essential nature in a spirit of open receptiveness. The researcher-as-bricoleur
uses strategies or methods (whether or not they go against conventional approaches to
enquiry) deemed by the researcher as appropriate to ensure that the study is conducted in
the best possible manner. In other words, procedures for information-gathering and analysis
are not predetermined but are selected depending on which particular strategies will lead to
the most truthful, rich and informative findings.

Bricolage is an approach to research in which the researcher engages with a range of methods of data collection and analysis that do not fit with conventional approaches to enquiry.

The notion of researcher-as-bricoleur has not been without conjecture and criticism by adherents of traditional qualitative research methods. The main criticism is the apparent lack of a rigorous systematic research method. However, argument in defence of a bricolage approach cites the numerous modifications made over time to such qualitative research methods as phenomenology, grounded theory and ethnography, as previously discussed. It may well be that future developments in qualitative research see the researcher-as-bricoleur as a generally accepted approach to research.

RESEARCH AND EVIDENCE-BASED PRACTICE 5.1

5.1

REMOTE CARE

Mrs Morgan is a 55-year-old Aboriginal woman who has been admitted to hospital for management of chronic pain as a result of a long history of decubitus leg ulcers. Mrs Morgan lives in a remote community in north-west Queensland. Prior to hospitalisation Mrs Morgan has been treated by the flying doctor service, which has a scheduled monthly service to her community. On admission Mrs Morgan speaks of the difficulties in living daily with chronic pain. In talking with the nurse, Mrs Morgan speaks of many members of her community who have similar problems, especially chronic pain as a consequence of long-term illness. She also reveals that there is little assistance provided by her local community or the government in attempting to stem the increase in the number of individuals who are developing long-term illness. When questioned about her ability to self-manage her illness and chronic pain, Mrs Morgan informs the nurse that women have no authority in their community to make changes or even to suggest to the elders what changes would be appropriate in order to improve the health of the community. She states further that she would like to be involved in making a change in the way things are done to enhance both individuals' and the community's quality of life. The nurse reflects on what Mrs Morgan has shared with her and comes to realise she has no understanding of how this community is organised, including how members relate to each other, what are the important values of the group, and what processes are involved in making the community work together on a daily basis. At the end of the admission interview the nurse decides that there is a lot she does not know or understand about Mrs Morgan's and others' experience of pain, life in a remote Aboriginal community, the place of women in this society, how the social fabric of the community works, and what it means to be a nurse caring for this group of people.

From this case scenario think about what possible research studies could be conducted. Once you have listed the potential areas for research, what type of question would you ask?

In relation to the specific questions you have generated, identify the most appropriate research pathway or design to answer the research questions.

Summary

Qualitative research has emerged in the past six decades as a substantive and credible scientific mode of enquiry. Since its inception in the early 19th century with the birth of the phenomenological movement, a number of qualitative approaches to enquiry have been developed. Each has its unique philosophical frameworks, particular foci, and methods of data collection and analysis. Now we have a diverse range of research pathways from which to choose that fall under the umbrella of qualitative research. What becomes important is that the researcher—neophyte or experienced—is well informed about the various research pathways before selecting a particular approach to answer the research question. It requires considerable time and dedication to become familiar with both commonalities and differences in each approach. Qualitative research is an exciting enterprise, especially for health care professionals, who are in the privileged position of working with individuals, families and communities across the health–illness spectrum, and across the human life-cycle.

IMPLICATIONS FOR EVIDENCE-BASED NURSING AND MIDWIFERY

In recent times there has been considerable debate about how best to evaluate qualitative research in terms of its applicability to clinical practice. Because of the nature of qualitative research, which is concerned with exploring the lived world of people in their everyday situations, identifying outcomes that can be measured for their effectiveness has proved to be problematic. However, there have been developments in establishing guidelines to evaluate the usefulness of qualitative research to clinical practice. The Joanna Briggs Institute has adopted the FAME scale developed by Alan Pearson, which consists of four dimensions—Feasibility, Appropriateness, Meaningfulness and Effectiveness (JBI 2003). Janice Morse (2003) has developed a comprehensive evaluation framework in which she stipulates a number of evaluation criteria and their dimensions.

Qualitative research has much to offer the world of clinical practice, but in order to be accepted as a legitimate mode of enquiry by the scientific community, evidence of applicability to practice needs to be demonstrated. Qualitative researchers have taken on this challenge.

Practice exercise 5.1

a   Think of a topic or an issue of concern that you have a passionate interest in as a result of personal experience.

b   What would that be and why?

Practice exercise 5.2

Discuss how grounded theory could be a useful research method for investigating the following areas of clinical practice:

a   Performing an aseptic technique (How do we as nurses maintain asepsis on the unit in which we work?)

b   Pain management (How do we provide appropriate pain management for our patients?)

c   Clinical decision-making (How do we go about making clinical decisions?)

d   Providing culturally safe care (How do we provide culturally safe care?)

Practice exercise 5.3

a   Discuss the central concepts that underpin ethnographic research.

b   In what ways can ethnography be used in nursing and health care research? Identify an ethnographic study that has explored the culture of nursing and/or midwifery. What have you learnt about the culture of nursing and midwifery?

Practice exercise 5.4

a   What do you consider to be issues concerning inequality for nurses and midwives working in the current health care system?

b   What do you consider to be the basis for your assessment of the situation?

Practice exercise 5.5

a   What aspects of nursing could benefit by using a critical social theory or feminist research perspective?

b   Formulate a research question and rationale for your choice of a question for two of the approaches mentioned above.

Practice exercise 5.6

a   What do you consider are areas of nursing and midwifery practice that could benefit by undertaking an action research project?

b   Describe two areas in which action research would be appropriate in initiating change within your practice setting.

Practice exercise 5.7

a   What do you understand by the term qualitative research?

b   What are the main features or core elements of qualitative research?

c   What type of questions would be best suited to a qualitative research design?

d   When we talk about a philosophical position, what is meant?

e   What do you see as the relationship of qualitative research to nursing and midwifery?

f   What do you consider some of the useful ways in which qualitative research can contribute to advancing nursing and midwifery knowledge?

Further reading

Denzin, N. K., & Lincoln, Y. S. (eds). (1994). *Handbook of Qualitative Research*. Thousand Oaks, CA: Sage Publications.

Gadamer, H. G. (1976). The Universality of the Hermeneutical Problem. In L. E. Hahn (ed.), *The Philosophy of Hans-Georg Gadamer*. Chicago: Library of Living Philosophers vol. XX1V.

Heidegger, M. (1962). *Being and Time*. New York: Harper & Row.

Leininger, M. (1985). *Qualitative Research Methods in Nursing*. New York: Grune & Stratton.

Liamputtong, P. (2009). *Qualitative Research Methods*, 3rd edn. Melbourne: Oxford University Press.

Patton, M. Q. (2002). *Qualitative Research and Evaluation Methods*, 3rd edn. London: Sage Publications.

Ricoeur, P. (1976). *Interpretation Theory: Discourse and the Surplus of Meaning*. Fort Worth, TX: Texas Christian University Press.

Weblinks

<www.qualitative-research.net/index.php/fqs>

The Forum Qualitative Sozialforschung (Forum Qualitative Social Research) is a peer-reviewed multilingual online journal for qualitative research. You can gain access to the journal free of charge.

<www.humanbecoming.org>

The International Consortium of Parse Scholars focuses on a humanbecoming school of thought. This is an important qualitative approach which has been used in nursing research. It aims to contribute to human health and quality of life through research and practice.

<http://qhr.sagepub.com>

Sage publishes the *Qualitative Research Journal*, which can be useful for reviewing various published articles and discussion papers on various qualitative research issues.

Anthony Welch

The site of the *Grounded Theory Review*. This can be useful for readers who want to review the application of grounded theory in qualitative research.

References

Bleicher, J. (1980). *Contemporary Hermeneutics*. London: Routledge & Kegan Paul.

Blumer, H. (1969). *Symbolic Intervention, Perspective and Method*. Englewood Cliffs, NJ: Prentice Hall.

Charmaz, K. (1990). Discovering chronic illness: Using grounded theory. *Social Science & Medicine* 30, 1161–72.

Charmaz, K. (2006). *Constructing Grounded Theory: A Practical Guide Through Qualitative Analysis*. London: Sage Publications.

Chinn, P. L., & Wheeler, C. E. (1985). Feminism and nursing. *Nursing Outlook* 33(2), 74–7.

Cody, W. K. (2010). Parse's Humanbecoming school of thought. Retrieved 20 September 2010, from <www.humanbecoming.org/human-becoming.htm>

Colaizzi, P. (1978). Psychological research as the phenomenologist views it. In R. Valle & M. King (eds), *Existential Phenomenological Alternatives for Psychology*. New York: Oxford University Press.

Crotty, M. (1998). *The Foundations of Social Research: Meaning and Perspective in the Research Process*. Sydney: Allen & Unwin.

Dewey, J. (1929). *Experience and Nature*. La Salle: Open Court.

Dilthey, W. (1977). *Descriptive Psychology and Historical Understanding*. The Hague: Martinus Nijhoff.

Douglass, B., & Moustakas, C. (1985). Heuristic inquiry: The internal search to know. *Journal of Humanistic Psychology* 25, 39–55.

Dreyfus, H. L. (1991). *Being-in-the-World: A Commentary on Heidegger's Being and Time*. Cambridge, MA: Division 1, The MIT Press.

Ellis, C., & Bouchner, A. (eds). (1996). *Composing Ethnography: Alternative Forms of Qualitative Writing*. Thousand Oaks, CA: Sage Publications.

Fain, J. A. (2004). *Reading, Understanding, and Applying Nursing Research*, 2nd edn. Philadelphia: F. A. Davis Company.

Fetterman, D. M. (1989). *Ethnography: Step by Step*. Newbury Park, CA: Sage Publications.

Gadamer, H. G. (1976). The Universality of the Hermeneutical Problem. In L. E. Hahn (ed.), *The Philosophy of Hans-Georg Gadamer*. Chicago: Library of Living Philosophers vol. XX1V.

Germain, C. P. (2001). Ethnography. In P. Munhall (ed.), *Nursing Research. A Qualitative Perspective*, 3rd edn. Sudbury, MA: National League for Nursing.

Giorgi, A. (1970). *Psychology as a Human Science: A Phenomenologically Based Approach*. New York: Harper & Row.

Giorgi, A. (1985). *Phenomenology and Psychological Research*. Pittsburgh: Duquesne University Press.

Glaser, B. G. (1978). *Theoretical Sensitivity*. Mill Valley, CA: Sociology Press.

Glaser, B. G. (1992). *Emergence vs Forcing: Basics of Grounded Theory Analysis*. Mill Valley, CA: Sociology Press.

Glaser, B. G., & Strauss, A. L. (1967). *The Discovery of Grounded Theory: Strategies for Qualitative Research*. Mill Valley, CA: Sociology Press.

Grbich, C. (1999). *Qualitative Research in Health: An Introduction*. London: Thousand Oaks.

Heidegger, M. (1962). *Being and Time*. New York: Harper & Row.

Husserl, E. (1962). *Ideas: General Introduction to Pure Phenomenology*. New York: Macmillan.

James, W. (1976). *Essays in Radical Empiricism*. Cambridge MA: Harvard University Press.

JBI (Joanna Briggs Institute). (2003). *About the Institute*. Available at <www.joannabriggs.edu.au/about/history.php>

Kleinman, A. (1980). *Patients and Healers in the Context of Culture: An Exploration of the Borderland Between Anthropology, Medicine, and Psychiatry*. Berkeley, CA: University of California Press.

Leininger, M. (1978). *Transcultural Nursing: Concepts, Theories, and Practices*. New York: John Wiley & Sons.

Leininger, M. (1985). *Qualitative Research Methods in Nursing*. New York: Grune & Stratton.

Leininger, M. (1988). Leininger's theory of nursing: Cultural care diversity and universality. *Nursing Science Quarterly* 1(4), 152–60.

Leininger, M. (1991). The theory of culture care diversity and universality. In M. Leininger (ed.), *Culture Care Diversity and Universality: A Theory of Nursing* (pp. 5–68). New York: National League for Nursing Press.

Leininger, M. (2001). *Culture Care Delivery and Universality: A Theory of Nursing*. Boston: Jones & Bartlett.

Levi-Strauss, C. (1966). *The Savage Mind*. Chicago: University of Chicago Press.

Lewin, K. (1946). Action research and minority issues. *Journal of Social Issues* 2, 34–46.

Marx, K. (1961). *Selected Writings in Sociology and Social Philosophy*, 2nd edn, ed. T. B. Bottomore & M. Rubel. Harmondsworth: Penguin.

McDermott, J. J. (1981). *The Philosophy of John Dewey*. Chicago: University of Chicago Press.

McLeod, J. (2001). *Qualitative Research in Counselling and Psychotherapy*. London: Sage Publications.

McTaggart, R. (1994). Participatory action research: issues in theory and practice. *Educational Action Research* 2(3), 313–37.

Merleau-Ponty, M. (1962). *Phenomenology of Perception*, transl. C. Smith. New York: Humanities Press.

Merleau-Ponty, M. (1989). *Phenomenology of Perception*, ed. C. Smith, transl. J. O'Neill. Evanston, IL: Northwestern University Press.

Morse, J. M. (2003). A review committee's guide for evaluating qualitative proposals. *Qualitative Health Research* 13, 833–51.

Moustakas, C. E. (1990). *Heuristic Research: Design, Methodology, and Application*. Newbury Park, CA: Sage.

Muecke, M. A. (1994). *Critical Issues in Qualitative Methods*. California: Sage.

Natanson, M. (1973). *Edmund Husserl: Philosopher of Infinite Tasks*. Evanston, IL: Northwestern University Press.

New Webster's Encyclopedia of Dictionaries (1990). Melbourne: Budget Books.

Olesen, V. (1994). Feminism and models of qualitative research. In N. K. Denzin & Y. S. Lincoln (eds), *Handbook of Qualitative Research* (pp. 158–74). Thousand Oaks, CA: Sage Publications.

Parse, R. R. (1998). *The Humanbecoming School of Thought: A Perspective for Nurses and Other Health Professionals*. California: Sage.

Parse, R. R. (1999). *Illuminations: The Humanbecoming Theory in Practice and Research*. Sudbury, MA: Jones & Barlett.

Parse, R. R. (2001). *Qualitative Inquiry: The Path of Sciencing*. London: Jones & Bartlett Publishers.

Paterson, G. J., & Zderad, L. T. (1976). *Humanistic Nursing*. New York: Wiley.

Patton, M. Q. (2002). *Qualitative Research and Evaluation Methods*, 3rd edn. London: Sage Publications.

Polit, D. F., & Beck, C. T. (2004). *Nursing Research: Methods, Appraisal, and Utilization*, 7th edn. Philadelphia: Lippincott Williams & Wilkins.

Ricoeur, P. (1976). *Interpretation Theory: Discourse and the Surplus of Meaning*. Fort Worth, TX: Texas Christian University Press.

Ricoeur, P. (1981). *Hermeneutics and the Social Sciences*, ed. and transl. J. Thompson. Cambridge: Cambridge University Press.

Rogers, M. E. (1970). *An Introduction to the Theoretical Basis of Nursing*. Philadelphia: F. A. Davis.

Rogers, M. E. (1980). Nursing: A science of unitary man. In J. P. Riehl & C. Roy (eds), *Conceptual Models for Nursing Practice*. New York: Appleton-Century Crofts.

Sartre, J.-P. (1956). *Being and Nothingness: An Essay on Phenomenological Ontology*. New York: Philosophical Library.

Sokolowski, R. (2000). *Introduction to Phenomenology*. Cambridge: Cambridge University Press.

Solomon, R. C. (2001). *Phenomenology and Existentialism*. New York: Rowman & Littlefield.

Spradley, J. P. (1980). *Participant Observation*. New York: Holt, Rinehart & Winston.

Strauss, A., & Corbin, J. (1990). *Basics of Qualitative Research: Grounded Theory Procedures and Techniques*. Newbury Park, CA: Sage.

Strauss, A., & Corbin, J. (1998). *Basics of Qualitative Research: Techniques and Procedures for Developing Grounded Theory*, 2nd edn. Thousand Oaks, CA: Sage Publications.

Street, A. F., & Robinson, A. (1995). Advanced clinical roles: Investigating dilemmas and changing practice through action research. *Journal of Clinical Nursing* 10(3), 372–9.

Streubert, H. J. (1991). Phenomenological research as a theoretic initiative in community health nursing. *Public Health Nursing* 8(2), 119–23.

Streubert, H. J., & Carpenter, D. R. (1995). *Qualitative Research in Nursing: Advancing the Humanistic Imperative*. Pennsylvania: J. B. Lippincott Company.

Streubert Speziale, H. J., & Rinaldi Carpenter, D. R. (2007). *Qualitative Research in Nursing: Advancing the Humanistic Imperative*, 4th edn. Philadelphia: Lippincott, Williams & Wilkins.

Taylor, B., Kermode, S., & Roberts, K. (2007). *Research in Nursing and Health Care: Evidence for Practice*, 3rd edn. Australia: Thomson.

Tong, R. (1995). *Feminist Thought: A Comprehensive Introduction*. London: Routledge.

Van Kaam, A. (1966). *Existential Foundations of Psychology*. Pittsburgh: Duquesne University Press.

Van Manen, M. (1990). *Researching Lived Experience: Human Science for an Action Sensitive Pedagogy*. Albany, NY: State University of New York.

Weinstein, D., & Weinstein, M. A. (1991). Georg Simmel: Sociological flaneur bricoleur. *Theory, Culture and Society* 8, 151–68.

Winter, R., & Munn-Giddings, C. (2001). *A Handbook for Action Research in Health and Social Care*. London: Routledge.

CHAPTER 6

Quantitative Research Design

Sansnee Jirojwong and Karen Pepper

Chapter learning objectives

By the end of this chapter you will be able to:

▸ explain the definition of quantitative research

▸ understand the major underlying characteristics of quantitative research designs

▸ list and describe characteristics of major quantitative research designs

▸ explain terms frequently used in the design of quantitative research and apply the terms in a research scenario

▸ analyse the strengths and weaknesses of each quantitative research design

▸ discuss the implications of quantitative research for evidence-based nursing and midwifery.

KEY TERMS

Audit

Bias

Causality

Deductive hypothesis

Experimental research

Inductive hypothesis

Non-experimental research

Placebo effect

Quasi-experimental research

Reliability

Validity

Introduction

As professional health workers, nurses and midwives use and apply research in their daily work. For example, we wash our hands to reduce cross-infection from one patient to the other. Many studies have identified the cause (washing hands) and effect (reduction of cross-infection among patients) relationship through a number of observations and systematic investigations (Gould et al. 2007). In the 19th century, Ignaz Semmelweis (Rea & Upshur 2001) observed that medical students and obstetricians did not wash their hands properly after caring for women after birth, and this caused postpartum infection and deaths. Consequently, he ordered students and obstetricians to wash their hands before examining patients and this led to the reduction of postpartum infection (Rea & Upshur 2001). Florence Nightingale similarly observed that cleanliness reduced deaths among soldiers during the Crimean War (Meyer & Bishop 2007); later this led to strict rules of environmental cleanliness to reduce infection among patients.

Nurses are in a unique situation as they are frequently in contact with patients for longer periods than other health professionals. Nurses can observe events that potentially improve or worsen patients' health outcomes. These events can be systematically explored or tested to prove or disprove such observations. The use of honey to increase wound healing (Van der Weyden 2003) and having a pet to improve psychological health among people in residential care are examples of research initially based on observations by nurses (Krause-Parello 2008).

However, some nurses, midwives or students may wonder why they need to understand the details of how health research is done if they don't intend to carry out research themselves. The fact is that all health professionals must be able to understand and critically assess health research, as the knowledge base they use in their clinical practice is—or should be—based on evidence derived from research. Furthermore, as new research continually adds to this knowledge base health professionals must be able to judge whether such research results should be applied in their own daily work.

This chapter will help readers to understand the general concepts of quantitative health research and identify its strengths and weaknesses. Different quantitative research designs and their implications for nursing and midwifery care are described. When possible, we use research studies of hand washing and infection as illustrative examples of different quantitative research designs.

What is quantitative research?

The term 'research' is defined as 'an endeavour to discover new facts or collate old ones by scientific study of a subject. It is also a course of critical investigation' (Turner 1987, p. 940). The word 'quantitative' means 'measured or measurable by, or concerned with, quantity'

(p. 897). Quantitative research is a scientific and systematic enquiry used to investigate an event or phenomenon so that measurable and quantifiable information or data are collected to answer a research question (Polit & Hungler 1999).

RESEARCH AND EVIDENCE-BASED PRACTICE 6.1

6.1

IMPROVING HAND WASHING AMONG HEALTH WORKERS

Nurse managers of neonatal units have observed that not all nurses and medical doctors wash their hands between caring for babies. The managers want to know who regularly wash their hands and on what occasions. They have commenced a research process by identifying a problem that is likely to influence the infection rate among their patients. Evidence is needed to improve hand washing among health workers and to support the request for additional resources such as dispensing units of hand-washing gel.

▶▶▶ TERMS, TIPS AND SKILLS

A phenomenon is an abstract entity or concept under investigation in a study. In the case study, the phenomenon is irregularity of hand washing in health care workers' neonatal units.

Quantitative research is a scientific investigation method that can be used in different settings (health units, communities, geographical areas) and with various population groups (sick people, well people, people of different age or gender, and ethnic groups). A rigorous and controlled design is required to conduct quantitative research (LoBiondo-Wood & Haber 2006; Polit & Hungler 1999). Steps used in the research process need to be clearly defined and in detail and strictly adhered to. Researchers need to identify the study population and its representative samples, devise appropriate methods of measurement for the variables and create a good controlled research design. Logical and deductive reasoning are important to the development of quantitative research. Different steps in the investigation need to be logically linked together. Strengths, potential errors and weaknesses of every step including measurement, sampling, statistical analysis and generalisation need to be explored, and their impact on the study results has to be explained by researchers.

The overall philosophy of quantitative research is that knowledge and truth should withstand scrutiny and be upheld in different environments and population groups (Thompson 2003). The focus of quantitative research is concise, narrow and reductionist. Researchers should maintain objectivity, and not let value judgments influence the study. If this does not happen, bias occurs and can detrimentally affect the validity of the research.

Quantitative research aims to describe and examine relationships, and determine causality among variables. This method is useful for testing theories by testing the validity of the relationships that compose the theory. This is called the deductive hypothesis. Quantitative research incorporates logical deductive reasoning as the researcher examines phenomena in selected situations in order to make generalisations (Polit & Hungler 1999).

Quantitative research requires careful control. Researchers use techniques of control to identify and limit the phenomenon or problem to be researched. For example, they attempt to limit the effects of extraneous or outside variables not being studied. They also use measurement instruments to precisely measure the variables under investigation and produce numerical data. Statistical analyses can then be conducted to reduce and organise data, to describe groups and to identify differences between groups. Control of such aspects of the research provides findings that accurately represent the reality of the sample being studied, so the findings can be generalised. Generalisation involves the application of trends or general tendencies to a population that is identified by studying a sample of that population (see Chapter 8).

RESEARCH IN PRACTICE 6.1

6.1

BACTERIAL CONTAMINATION IN NEONATAL CARE

Iijima and Ohzeki (2006) explored bacterial contamination of the hands of nurses who provided basic neonatal care, and the efficacy of hand washing. They observed nurses' hand washing when they bottle-fed the babies and changed their nappies. They counted bacterial colonies on nurses' hands before and after hand washing, and after bottle-feeding and nappy change. The intention of this control (neonatal unit, in which one procedure—bottle feeding—is relatively 'clean', and the other procedure—nappy changing—is 'dirty') is to facilitate the more precise examination of the size of bacterial colonies when nurses contact and provide care to patients, and the effects of hand washing on these bacterial colonies. Results indicated that nurses will have increased bacteria count after providing care regardless whether it is a 'clean' or a 'dirty' procedure, and that hand washing reduced the bacteria count.

Question: Based on the above example, how did the researchers define hand washing?

(Answer: They observed nurses' hand washing when they bottle-fed the babies and changed nappies.)

Question: How was the efficacy of hand washing measured?

(Answer: They counted bacterial colonies on nurses' hands on four occasions: 1. before hand washing, 2. after hand washing, 3. after bottle-feeding, and 4. after nappy change.)

Question: How might the results of this research be applied to clinical practice?

(Answer: Hand washing is needed to reduce potential infection regardless of the procedures.)

Some concepts examined in research can be concrete and directly measurable, such as hand washing. Other concepts, such as intelligence, fear and pain, are abstract and only indirectly observable. Nevertheless, even abstract concepts can be measured with appropriate measurement tools such as psychological tests.

Conducting good quantitative research

During early stages of research, researchers need to consider a number of matters that potentially influence research, its credibility and results. Important issues will be discussed in the following sections. Understanding these will help researchers, nurses and midwives to grasp the strength and weakness of each research design and how it can affect the application of research findings.

Causality

We can observe cause-and-effect relationships in biological disciplines such as nursing and medicine, and in behavioural science disciplines such as sociology and psychology. In the biological disciplines, Susser (1973, 2001) and Friis and Sellers (2004) have proposed a set of principles to allow us to infer the causality of a disease. These principles are:

- *Association:* A strong link between the existence of a health effect and the suspected cause. For example, infection is reduced when all health care workers regularly wash their hands.
- *Consistency upon repetition:* The association between the cause and the health effect is identified by different researchers in different settings.
- *Specificity in causality:* The causal agent always predicts the occurrence of a disease. It should be noted that chronic diseases may have many causes and this should be taken into account when conducting research.
- *Time sequence:* A cause needs to come first, before the effect.
- *Plausibility:* The biological plausibility depends on current knowledge.
- *Coherence of explanation:* The relationship between the causal factor and its effect must not conflict with the biology of the disease or illness.
- *Experiment:* The expected effect should be produced to demonstrate the causality in either a natural environment or by introducing change to the causal factor.
- *Analogy:* An argument can be made for the proposed causality if similar causality is known. An example is the known reduction of infection in intensive care units when all health care workers wash their hands. It is therefore also highly probable that there will be a reduction of infection in surgical units if all health care workers regularly wash their hands (WHO 2009).

In order to identify causal relationships in the behavioural sciences, consistency can be applied to repetition, time sequence, coherence of explanation and experiment. In this case, the use of theoretical frameworks and literature to support suspected causal relationships may be needed because of the complexity of human behaviours. For example, health promotion theories including the Health Belief Model or Social Learning Theory have been applied to explore a causal relationship between a nursing intervention and improved adoption of patients' health promotion behaviours (Jirojwong & MacLennan 2003; Lim et al. 2008). Causes may be expressed within the propositions of a theory. Testing the accuracy of these theoretical statements indicates the usefulness of the theory. A cause that is not directly observable can be inferred from other similar phenomena.

Researchers need to identify and control potential risks that may occur during the research process and affect their ability to draw a cause-and-effect relationship. These are potential intrinsic and external risks to the causality (Polit & Beck 2004). A good plan drawn up during early stages of the research process will help reduce such risks.

RESEARCH IN PRACTICE 6.2

6.2 CONDUCTING A RESEARCH STUDY

We are going to conduct an experimental research project that aims to increase hand washing among nurses and medical practitioners who care for patients in medical and surgical wards in six Australian regional hospitals. A comprehensive in-service education program is designed and all nurses and medical practitioners are required to attend. Posters are strategically displayed to remind the health workers to wash their hands. Numerous hand-washing gel dispensers have been installed. We observed hand washing among all nurses and medical practitioners who met the selection criteria before the introduction of the program, and compared their hand washing three months after the program. During the planning of this research, we know that a certain percentage of nurses and medical practitioners may be against this research project as they think that the money should be spent on other things. This is one of the intrinsic factors that may influence our ability to assess whether there is causality between the comprehensive in-service education program (cause) and the increased hand washing (effect) among nurses.

We find that after the introduction of the program there is increased hand washing among nurses, but not medical practitioners. After collecting the data, we have found out that nurses who took part in the study are those who are keen to support the project.

Many questions have to be answered before drawing the conclusion that there is causality between the in-service education program (cause) and the increased hand washing (effect) among nurses. Some of these questions are:

- Who are included in the study (full-time, casual or agency nurses; enrolled nurses; shift or period of observation; length of observation)?
- Are the participants aware of the research?
- Who collected the data? Is the data collection process consistent across time periods (before and after the intervention) and for different persons who collect the data (research assistants)?

Sansnee Jirojwong and Karen Pepper

There are strategies that can be used to reduce the risks of causality. These include randomisation, homogeneity, matching and statistical control. The aim is to clearly demonstrate the effect of an independent variable on the dependent variable by ensuring that the intervention and control groups are as similar as possible at the outset of the study and by excluding the influence of potential extraneous variables.

Randomisation

Randomisation or random assignment of participants to study groups is used in a research project so that researchers can be certain that the variation of the dependent variable between groups is due to the intervention and not to existing differences in the participants. Randomisation ensures that all potential participants have the same chance of being included in the study. It also reduces the effect of unknown extraneous variables by distributing them across the study groups.

As an example, let us go back to the hand-washing study (Research in practice 6.2), but this time we will randomly select hospitals rather than individual health workers. We will study all staff that meet the selection criteria and that work in medical and surgical wards of the selected hospitals. The technique used is a simple random sampling (see Chapter 8). It will allow participants who have different characteristics and opinions on the project to have an equal chance of being included in the study. Transfer of information using hospitals as a sampling unit is less likely to occur than having individuals as a sampling unit. This randomisation also reduces selection bias.

Homogeneity

Homogeneity is a technique used when randomisation is not possible. Participants who have similar characteristics or similar extraneous variables are deliberately included as potential participants; that is, the group is homogeneous in those characteristics. For example, we may only include nurses and medical practitioners who are full-time or casual employees as participants in our project. This is to ensure similarity of extraneous variables such as access to in-service training and supervision. Their commitment and exposure to the intervention will also be similar. However, the use of homogeneity will limit the generalisation of the study results to other health worker groups. In this proposed project, the results will not be applied to agency nurses, enrolled nurses, visiting medical practitioners or locums, and students.

Matching

Matching is a technique used to match social demographic characteristics of individuals in the intervention and control groups. It also can be used when randomisation cannot be conducted. Researchers identify important extraneous characteristics that need to be controlled and match participants who have similar characteristics and systematically allocate them to a control group or an intervention group.

Statistical control

Statistical control is used in situations when it is difficult to study a particular group or randomisation. Researchers have participants from a range of social demographic characteristics and extraneous variables. After data are collected, a number of statistical methods such as multiple logistic regression analysis can be used to control the effect of extraneous variables when assessing a relationship between the independent variable (cause) and dependent variable (effect) (see also Chapters 2 and 12).

Validity

Researchers need to be certain that their research findings reflect the truth. Their credibility and dependability are reflected in the internal and external validity of the research findings. Internal validity is the methological rigour of a study, where any potential biases are minimised. It is also the ability to tell that the independent variable has actually made the difference or changed the dependent variable. External validity is the generalisability of the study findings to a wider population.

Let us consider our research project, which aims to explore hand washing among nurses and medical practitioners. In order to ensure that the findings reflect what truly happened, we have to consider several matters while conducting the study. These include the measurement tool we use, the accuracy of our observation records, a consistency of observations among those who collect the data, and ensuring that participants are included in the study without any prejudice. These are the kinds of things that influence the internal validity of the study.

Internal validity

The researchers' ability to control and explain the magnitude of potential threats to internal validity will influence the benefits of research results in clinical settings. A good example is the causal relationship between smoking and lung cancer. Early critiques analysed research on this link and used threats to studies' validity to dispute the claimed causality (Wingo et al. 1999). The threats to internal validity are history, maturation, testing, instrumentation, mortality or attrition, and selection bias.

History

History refers to an event that may have an effect on the dependent variable, either inside or outside the study setting or location. If there is an outbreak of SARS at the time when we assess hand washing after implementation, it is likely that all participants will increase their hand washing. This may influence the internal validity of the research in concluding whether the intervention is effective in improving hand washing. It will be difficult for the researchers to identify whether hand washing has increased because of the intervention or because of the SARS outbreak.

Maturation

Maturation can be physical, biological and developmental processes that a participant has experienced and that might influence the study directly and indirectly. For example, 'longitudinal' studies that collect data over a long period are likely to be influenced by the physical maturation of the participants.

Testing

The responses of participants who undertake the same test or a similar test may be influenced by the test itself. For example, we may observe the hand washing and monitor the change of knowledge and attitude towards hand washing by using the same test or measurement over time. Participants who complete the same test a few times may have a better score on knowledge and attitude because the test is repeated, not because of any actual change in their knowledge and attitude.

Instrumentation

Instrumentation for measuring the study variables can be a major threat to quantitative research if an inappropriate instrument is chosen. Using an inappropriate measurement will give results that do not reflect what the study variable intended to measure.

In a project that measures the amount of hand-washing gel used as a measurement of hand washing in hospital units, the internal validity of the study will be compromised, compared to direct observation of hand washing. Researchers need to be able to establish whether the gel is used for other purposes than hand washing, and the proportion of its different use. Chapter 10 discusses the characteristics of data collection instruments and their use in quantitative research.

Mortality

Mortality or attrition is the loss of participants between two or more points of the study, and includes drop-outs. Where possible, the characteristics of people who drop out need to be compared to those who remain in the study as the people who drop out may have an impact on the overall outcomes of the study.

Let us go back to our hand-washing project. A few participants who do not regularly wash their hands may have poor health behaviours compared to those who wash their hands regularly. They might be ill and taking time off work more often. They may not perceive the benefits of the study and may refuse to participate. Participants who are left in the study, who regularly wash their hands, may tend to have better health and good health promotion. The results of the study would be influenced by both the intervention and the characteristics of the participants.

Selection bias

Selection bias refers to bias introduced when selecting participants. Researchers may select a particular group that does not represent the whole study population. Recruitment methods should try to reach all potential participants to take part in the study. Self-selection that contributes to selection bias needs to be assessed or monitored. An example is the use of telephone interviews, which will exclude households with silent phone numbers or no landline phones. Similarly, personal observation studies of nurses during day shift will exclude nurses who mainly work during other shifts. Selection bias can influence the ability to draw conclusions or to allow generalisation of the study results to the population.

External validity

External validity is the same as 'generalisability', the ability to apply the results of the study to wider populations and locations. Matters that affect internal validity will also influence external validity. Internal validity applies to truth within the study. We can understand external validity by asking the question, 'To what extent can the results of this study be applied outside the study group and location?'

Three major threats to external validity are the interaction effect of selection, the reactive effects of being studied, and the interaction effect of testing (Schneider et al. 2007).

Interaction effect of selection

One or more factors that influence the validity of selection of the study sample, including the selection bias, mortality and maturation, can also affect the external validity.

Reactive effects of being studied

When participants' responses are distorted by their awareness that they are being observed (the Hawthorne effect), it will limit the researcher's ability to apply the results to wider populations.

Reactive or interaction effect of testing

Researchers also need to know the impact of testing and history on their study. The use of previous testing may influence the researcher's ability to generalise the study results to wider populations. For example, if a study is investigating changes in intelligence over time and requires participants to complete the same IQ test several times, their intelligence scores may increase over time simply because they have had so much practice with the test. Researchers need to be able to assess the impact of the frequency of completing the test on the study results.

Threats to validity can lead to type I and type II errors. A type I error occurs when researchers claim that there is a significant relationship between independent variable and independent variable when in fact there is no such relationship. A type II error involves claiming that there is no significant relationship between independent variable and independent variable when in fact a relationship does exist. One of the strategies to reduce the type II error is having a large enough sample size. (The section on hypothesis testing in Chapter 12 describes both errors in detail.)

Precision

Precision is another aspect of rigour in quantitative research. It refers to accuracy, order and the provision of full details. The statement of the research purpose and the detailed development of the study design need to be precise. The measurement or quantification of the study variables should be clearly defined and objectively measurable. For example, pain is a personal experience and can be influenced by various factors such as ethnicity and gender (Kim et al. 2004). One way to measure pain is to use drawings of facial expressions as a measurement tool (Royal College of Nursing 2009). Lin and Wang (2005) used this tool to measure pain among post-operative patients who received an intervention compared to pain among patients receiving routine care.

The research design

Before choosing a design

Before selecting a research design, it is important to review the purpose of the research. Researchers need to answer the following questions:

1   What is the purpose of the research? Is it to describe variables or groups within their environment, to examine relationships between two or more variables, or to examine causality?
2   Will a treatment or manipulation be used? How will the treatment be controlled by the researcher? How many groups of samples are included in the study? What is the type of sample selection?
3   How many times will variables be measured? Have extraneous variables been identified? If yes, will their information be collected? Will there be any strategy used to control for extraneous variables? What strategies are being used for comparison of variables or groups?

Choosing a research design

A research design is an overall plan with a general pattern that can be applied to many studies. It has defined structures within which the study is carried out (MacLennan 2009). Researchers use research questions, theoretical frameworks, literature reviews and clearly defined variables to devise a detailed research plan for data collection and data analysis. The research design needs to have specifications for enhancing the integrity of the study. A good quantitative research design should enable researchers to control or measure the environment of the study setting. Matters that influence validity, rigour or precision should be controlled or monitored. This is comparable to a detailed plan of a house, which will guide an owner, a builder and trade persons in building the house. The selected research design needs to guide data collection. Data can then answer the research question.

For example, researchers want to assess a relationship between the availability of hand-washing gel dispensing points close to patients (potential 'cause') and the regularity of hand washing among health workers ('outcome'). They could conduct a study into the proximity of dispensing points to patients. A number of hospitals could be included in the study and categorised to three groups according to different dispensing points. The first group of hospitals have dispensing points next to every patient bed. The second have dispensing points in procedure rooms and central working areas and the third have a single dispensing point in every room but not next to patient beds. The researchers would observe whether there is a relationship between the regularity of hand washing if the dispensing point is closer to the patient. A descriptive research design should allow researchers to collect data that meets the study's aim.

In a situation where there is a need to improve or increase the availability of hand-washing gel, researchers may want to assess whether or not this change will increase the regularity of hand washing among health care workers. In this scenario, there is an intervention, the introduction of new points for dispensers of gel. In order to meet the study aim, an experimental or quasi-experimental design has to be used.

The complexity of human behaviours will have impacts on the researchers' ability to demonstrate clearly the relationship between an independent variable and a dependent variable without the influence of extraneous variables. If a non-experimental study is conducted, researchers also still want to be sure that the information collected reflects the truth, not simply the fact that participants are aware of the research.

▶▶▶ TERMS, TIPS AND SKILLS

Variables are qualities, properties or characteristics of persons, things or situations that change or vary. In research, variables are characterised by degrees, amounts and differences. They are also concepts of various levels of abstraction concisely defined to facilitate their measurement or manipulation within a study (Burns & Grove 2009, p. 24).

There are three types of variables: independent, dependent and extraneous. A dependent variable is the outcome variable hypothesised to depend on or be caused by another variable, the independent variable. An independent variable is thought to cause or influence the dependent variable. In an experimental study that explores cause and effect between two or more variables, an independent variable is a 'cause' that is manipulated by researchers. An extraneous variable confounds the relationship between an independent variable and a dependent variable. Its effect on the study results needs to be controlled in the study design or by using statistical analysis.

Types of quantitative research designs

We use two major criteria in the categorisation of research designs. The first is the time when information is collected on the occurrence of the phenomenon being studied. The second is the degree to which the researchers manipulate an independent variable in order to explore whether or not there will be any change in the dependent variable. In this section we describe three major research designs: non-experimental design, quasi-experimental design and experimental design. Frequently used variations of each design will be described. There is a proliferation of research designs, and readers are advised to consult advanced research textbooks to explore the details of designs not included in this book.

We begin by describing fairly simple non-experimental research designs, then proceed to more complex experimental designs that require manipulation, control and comparison by researchers.

Non-experimental research designs

Non-experimental designs are used to describe a phenomenon in a more or less natural setting. There is no attempt to manipulate any study variable or to identify a cause-and-effect relationship between variables. No causation can be concluded from non-experimental research. Non-experimental research can be useful to describe a new phenomenon so that its data can be used to develop more complex future studies.

For example, early descriptive studies described patients with HIV and their characteristics such as gender, sexual partners and sexual relationships (Centers for Disease Control 1982; Kunanusont et al. 1988). Systematic and well-controlled non-experimental studies are useful in finding new health knowledge. Descriptive research design, trend design, comparative design and correlation design are frequently used non-experimental designs and are discussed below.

Descriptive research design

Descriptive studies are usually conducted when little is known about the phenomenon. Early studies of HIV/AIDS and SARS are descriptive studies that describe individuals who have the disease and their characteristics. The time, place and environment where the disease has occurred were systematically investigated (Centers for Disease Control 1982; Friis & Sellers 2004; Heymann & Rodier 2004; Kunanusont et al. 1988).

Researchers describe phenomena using descriptive statistics such as frequency, number and percentage. They use interviews, observation and questionnaires or checklists. Descriptive studies provide a knowledge base and a source of potential hypotheses to guide further correlational, quasi-experimental and experimental studies.

Descriptive study design aims to provide information (data) about the phenomena as they naturally happen. A descriptive study can involve observing one or many variables, but as there is no attempt to assess causality, the study variables are generally not defined as dependent or independent variables. Bias can be reduced by careful explanation of conceptual and operational definitions of the variables (Burns & Grove 2009), appropriate sample selection and size, valid and reliable measurement of the phenomena, and data collection procedures that achieve some environmental control.

Comparative design

Comparative design is used when the study aims to assess the differences between the study variables. An audit is a good example of a comparative design. Hospital or residential care audits have been used to monitor the quality of health services. Variables such as the actual length of hospital stay or waiting times are compared against the standard set by health departments. Bivariate statistical analysis such as a t-test can then be used to assess whether there is a significant difference between the actual data and the expected standard time period (see also Chapter 12).

Trend design

Trend design is used to assess changes of a phenomenon in the study population. Data are collected from different samples of potential participants at predetermined intervals. Changes are then assessed and presented as graphs, numbers and percentages. Bivariate statistical methods can be used to assess the difference of study phenomena across different groups and different times. Results can be generalised to a wider population.

For example, hospital units can be categorised into two groups according to the availability of hand-washing gel. The first group consists of the units with at least one gel dispenser available for every two patients. The second group consists of the hospital units with fewer dispensers. Researchers can randomly select samples from each group of hospital units. Study variables observed might include hand washing of each nurse and doctor, and attendance at in-service training programs. The trend of the regularity of hand washing against the other variables can be assessed.

Correlation study design

Correlation study design is used to assess a relationship between one or more independent variables and a dependent variable. When there is a change in an independent variable, researchers are interested to observe whether the dependent variable will also change consistently. If it appears that there is a relationship between the variables, the existence of a positive or negative correlation needs to be explored. A positive correlation exists if the changes of both the independent and dependent variable are in the same direction (Figure 6.1). In other words, an increased value of the independent variable is related to an increased value of the dependent variable, and vice versa. A negative correlation means that the change in the dependent variable is occurring in the opposite direction to that of the independent variable (Figure 6.2). In other words, an increased value of the independent variable is related to a decreased value of the dependent variable. The results of correlational research must be interpreted with caution. Correlation by itself does not prove that one variable causes the other; it merely shows that there is a relationship between the variables. When a correlational relationship is found between two variables, it is possible that Variable A has caused Variable B, or that Variable B has caused Variable A, or that a third variable has caused both A and B.

Figure 6.1 Positive correlation between independent and dependent variables

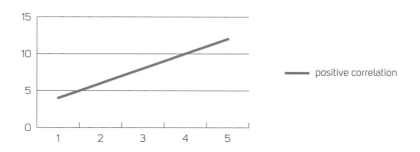

Figure 6.2 Negative correlation between independent and dependent variables

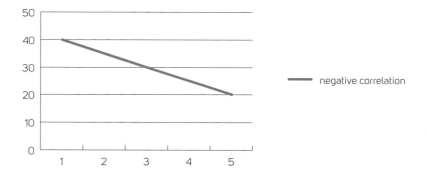

Quasi-experimental research designs

In both quasi-experimental research and experimental research, one or more independent variables are manipulated by the researcher to assess their causal relationship with a dependent variable. However, quasi-experimental research differs from true experimental design in that it lacks randomisation or control of extraneous variables. This lack of control can occur through the non-random selection of participants or study settings, and an inability to actively manipulate the intervention (Burns & Grove 2009, p. 252). This lack of randomisation or control means that researchers must be more cautious about inferring causal relationships between independent and dependent variables in quasi-experimental studies than they would in true experimental designs, as they cannot be sure that the outcomes they are observing are produced purely by manipulation of the independent variable rather than the effect of some inadequately controlled extraneous variable.

Specific quasi-experimental research designs and their characteristics will be described in the following section. The following symbols will be used to represent time of intervention and data collection.

O1 = Measurement of outcome (dependent variable) at Time 1
O2, O3, … On = Measurement of outcome variable at Time 1, 2, 3 to nth time
X = Intervention (independent variable).

Non-equivalent control group design

There is no randomisation in selecting either a control group or an intervention group. Reasons for absence of randomisation may include administrative or ethical implications of randomisation, or the potential for information relating to the intervention being transferred from one group to the other (LoBiondo-Wood & Haber 2006).

Table 6.1   Characteristics of non-equivalent control group design

Intervention group	O1 X O2
Control group	O1 O2

After-only non-equivalent control group design

No data are collected prior to an intervention. Data including the outcome variable (dependent variable) of both control and intervention groups are collected only after the intervention is introduced. If there is a difference between both groups in the outcome variable, researchers assume that this is caused by the intervention.

Table 6.2   Major characteristics of after-only non-equivalent control group design

Intervention group	X O1
Control group	O1

Pre-test-post-test design

Pre-test-post-test design is also called a one-group, before-after design (LoBiondo-Wood & Haber 2006). There is no randomisation or control group. Data are collected before and after the intervention. Changes of outcome or dependent variable are assumed to be caused by the intervention.

Table 6.3   Major characteristics of pre-test-post-test design

Intervention group	O1 X O2

Time series design

Compared to the pre-test-post-test design, a time series design allows researchers to monitor changes in the dependent variable over a long period. Data are collected a few times before and also after the intervention. This design is useful in assessing the influence of time on the outcome variable. Like the pre-test-post-test design, this design does not have randomisation and a control group.

Table 6.4   Major characteristics of time series design

Intervention group	O1	O2	O3	X	O4	O5	O6

Experimental design

Over the past few decades, scientific methods have been used to improve living standards. There have been interventions in clinical settings and communities to improve the health status of individuals and communities. Examples include immunisations to prevent infectious diseases and hand washing among staff in the postpartum ward to reduce postpartum infection (Beaglehole & Bonita 2004). The effectiveness of these and many other health interventions have been tested and proved by experimental research.

Experimental research involves manipulating one or more independent variables, and then observing subsequent changes in a dependent variable. In health research, this typically means introducing one or more health interventions and then observing the outcomes. It is a scientific method that provides level II evidence (see Table 1.1). Unlike quasi-experimental designs, both random assignment of interventions to subjects and the control of extraneous variables are present, so researchers can be more certain that any relationship they observe between independent and dependent variables is causal in nature.

The experimental design is the most powerful quantitative design in health research because it allows for rigorous control of variables. Threats to the validity of study results are controlled by randomisation, comparison groups and the active manipulation of the treatments or interventions by the researcher (Burns & Grove 2009, pp. 30, 252). Three main characteristics of experimental studies are (1) a controlled manipulation of at least one treatment variable (independent variable), (2) some of the subjects in the study receive the treatment or intervention (experimental group) and some do not (control group) and (3) random selection and assignment of subjects to treatment groups.

As an example, let's assume that we want to improve hand washing among all health care workers in long-term care units. A number of such units are selected for participation in the study, and each unit is randomly assigned to either an intervention or a control group. As an intervention in the selected units, we conduct an in-service program in order to increase the workers' awareness of the research issue, putting posters around the unit to prompt their hand washing and installing many dispensing points for hand-washing gel.

Units assigned to the control group receive no intervention program. We observe and measure hand washing in both groups of long-term care units both before the intervention and three months after it. Data collected from the intervention and control groups are then compared. If hand washing improves significantly more in the intervention group than in the control group, we are able to conclude that there is a cause-and-effect relationship between the intervention program and the improvement in hand washing observed.

True experimental design or randomised controlled (clinical) trial (RCT)

The true experimental design, often called randomised controlled (clinical) trial or RCT, provides level II evidence. It has the three major characteristics of an experiment: randomisation, control group and manipulation.

What does randomisation mean? The researcher randomly selects participants from the study population and assigns each participant randomly to either an intervention group or a control group. The intervention group then receives the intervention or treatment being tested by the experiment. The control group does not receive the intervention, but instead receives either a placebo treatment, an existing routine treatment or no treatment at all. These different treatments, which are actively manipulated by the researcher, constitute the independent variable of the experiment. Any differences in observed outcomes between the groups are likely to be caused by the manipulation, assuming that both the control group and the intervention group are similar in all aspects except the independent variable.

The following symbols are used to represent elements of the design: R represents randomisation to an intervention group, X represents the receipt of the intervention and O is the measurement of outcomes. The numbers 1, 2, 3 and so on represent the time data was collected (Polit & Hungler 1999).

Table 6.5   Major characteristics of true experimental design or randomised controlled trial

Group	Data collection		Data collection
	Before	Intervention	After
Intervention—Random selection (R)	O1	X	O2
Control—Random selection (R)	O1	No	O2

For example, White and others (2001) conducted an RCT to assess whether an alcohol-free, instant hand sanitiser containing surfactants, allantoin and benzalkonium chloride (SAB) could reduce illness-related absenteeism in elementary school students when regular soap-and-water hand washing was not readily available. The control group and the intervention group each had 16 classrooms randomly selected. The intervention group received SAB sanitiser to use, while the control group were given a similar-looking but inactive placebo. A double-blind strategy was used, so individual students did not know which of the two treatments they were using and the research assistants who collected data did not know what treatment each student was using. A comparison of outcomes showed that students using the SAB sanitiser were 33% less likely to be absent due to illness than those using the placebo.

Solomon four-group design

In experimental research, participants of both control and intervention groups are often required to undertake a pre-test which may by itself introduce change to the participants, and so may confound the effects of the intended independent variable on the dependent variable. The use of a Solomon four-group design (Table 6.6) will help identify the impact of the pre-test on the dependent variable. For example, consider a study on hand washing in which health care workers' existing knowledge about universal precautions is assessed by a test before an intervention is introduced, and its effects on hand washing is observed. Taking the test may in itself encourage them to improve their hand washing, so any change in subsequent hand-washing practices may owe as much to this pre-test as it does to the actual intervention. The Solomon four-group design is intended to account for such effects and increase the credibility of the study results.

Table 6.6   Major characteristics of the Solomon four-group design

Group	Data collection	
	Before	After
Intervention—with pre-test	O1	O2
Intervention—without pre-test		O2
Control—with pre-test	O1	O2
Control—without pre-test		O2

Factorial design

A factorial design is used when researchers want to manipulate two or more independent variables simultaneously. Multiple hypotheses can be tested at the same time. Each participant is randomly allocated to a group (Table 6.7).

As an example, consider a research project that aims to investigate patient recovery from surgery by providing two types of intervention: instruction in coping activities and information relating to the recovery from surgery. Table 6.7 shows the factorial design where participants in Group A will receive instruction in coping activities and a description of typical sensations experienced after surgery. Group B will receive instruction in coping activities and a description of typical events experienced after surgery. Group C will receive instruction in coping activities without any information relating to recovery from surgery. Group D will not receive instruction in coping activities but will receive information on the typical sensations experienced after surgery. Group E will not receive instruction in coping activities but receive information on the typical events experienced after surgery. Group F will not receive any type of intervention and serves as a control group (Johnson et al. 1978).

Table 6.7 Example of factorial design

		Instruction in coping activities	
		Receive	Not receive
Information given relating to recovery from surgery	Description of typical sensation	Group A	Group D
	Description of typical events	Group B	Group E
	No information	Group C	Group F

Crossover design

Crossover design is also known as counterbalanced design. Each participant will serve as participant in both intervention and control groups. They are randomly allocated to the sequence of receiving an intervention and being a control. This design will allow a participant to act as their own control and therefore reduce biases between the intervention and control conditions. The three criteria for experimental designs (randomisation, manipulation and control) are met.

Table 6.8 Major characteristics of crossover design

	Time 1	Time 2
Group 1 (randomly allocated)	Receives intervention treatment	Receives control treatment
Group 2 (randomly allocated to)	Receives control treatment	Receives intervention treatment

Researchers who conduct experimental research need to consider various practical matters such as cost and maintaining sufficient sample size throughout the study period. Timelines have to be adhered to, and strategies planned for participant recruitment and follow-up. If the study is expected to take a long time to complete, administrative and management issues need to be attended to at the beginning. These include having a protocol and manual for the project team (MacLennan 2009). Recently the CONSORT statement has been used to assess the quality of reports of randomised trials. It may be useful as a guide when designing an experimental study (Moher et al. 2001).

Other quantitative research designs

Quantitative research designs described in this chapter are not exhaustive. We will briefly present some frequently used epidemiological research designs.

Epidemiology

Epidemiology is the study of the frequency, distribution and determinants of health states and events in the community, and the evaluation of interventions aimed at improving health throughout the community. Epidemiological research may investigate the efficacy of an intervention, the cause of a health problem, or the magnitude of a health problem in the community. It does this by identifying health risk factors and relating them to health outcomes.

Historically, epidemiology was concerned with the patterns in the spread and population characteristics of acute-onset and short-latency problems such as infectious diseases. John Snow, the founder of epidemiology, was able to pinpoint the origin of an outbreak of cholera in London in 1854 by observing the geographic patterns in illness. He noted that the number of cases of cholera were greatest in an area of London supplied by one particular public water pump, and concluded that tainted water from this pump was the probable source of the outbreak. He confirmed this conclusion by having the pump disabled, and subsequently observing a rapid decrease in new cholera infections (Snow 1855). More recently, the increasing importance of chronic disease has seen epidemiologists turn to observing patterns of disease over longer periods in order to determine how and why these diseases develop.

Cohort study

Cohort study is used when participants are categorised according to the level of their exposure to risk factors, and then followed through a period of time to observe the occurrence of a disease. For example, a group of children who were exposed to sun were selected, and subsequently followed up to observe the development of melanocytic nevi later in their lives (Harrison et al. 2005).

Case control study

Case control study involves identifying existing groups of subjects who either have a disease or health condition ('cases') or don't have that condition ('controls'). The history of their previous exposure to risk factors is retrospectively collected from all participants. Comparison is made by the researchers about the difference in the proportions of people in each group who were previously exposed to risk factors. For example, English and others (1998) studied people with basal cell carcinoma, a form of skin cancer, and those without the disease. The timing and pattern of past sun exposure of both groups were then compared. This is an example of retrospective research, which involves the collection and analysis of data relating to past events. Researchers need to be aware of potential biases such as recall bias and the quality of record if information is collected retrospectively.

Cross-sectional design

Cross-sectional design aims to describe a phenomenon among a stratified study group that contains individuals who represent different stages of development, trends or patterns (Burns & Grove 2009). Data is collected from participants at a single point in time, then analysed in relation to the strata that the participants represent within the study group. An example is a study by Smith and Leggat (2005) that investigated needlestick and sharp injuries among nursing students of different years within their course, and found that third-year students suffered the highest rates of injury.

Longitudinal design

Longitudinal design (or a prospective study design) is used to follow up a group of participants whose data are collected at different times over a long period in order to assess temporal changes in the study variables. The term 'longitudinal design' may be used to describe a cohort study or an experimental study. An example is a longitudinal study by Karlsson and others (2000) assessing quality of life among patients before and after coronary artery bypass surgery.

Surveillance

Surveillance is the term applied to research when there is continuous analysis, interpretation and feedback of systematically collected data (Last 1995). Methods used to collect data emphasise practicality, uniformity and rapidity rather than accuracy and completeness. Information can be used to assess the trend of the studied variables according to time, place and persons. Change can be observed or anticipated and appropriate action (including investigative or control measures) can be taken (Last 1995, p. 163). An example is Australian food-borne disease surveillance (Food Standards Australia New Zealand 2010). The quality of data recording and reporting is a major problem when using the surveillance data.

Evaluation studies

Evaluation studies have a broader scope than traditional research designs (see details in Dunt 2009; Dykeman & Cruttenden 2009). In order to improve health outcomes, a health care team can introduce changes by implementing a program. Evaluation of this program can be conducted at the beginning of the program, at an early stage, at the end or throughout the course of the program. The scope of the intervention and its context need to be considered when deciding which research designs to use. The scope may include government policies and media campaigns. The context can be the underlying reasons for conducting an evaluation.

Use of quantitative research in nursing and midwifery

Experimental research provides the highest standard of evidence among the quantitative research techniques, and is usually the best way of determining whether a health intervention really works. However, well-planned and carefully conducted descriptive and epidemiological research can also provide useful data which later can be extended to quasi-experimental and experimental research. It also needs to be noted that because of practical or ethical constraints not all health issues can be explored or assessed by using experimental research.

▶ ▶ ▶   TERMS, TIPS AND SKILLS

A research team comprises doctors and registered nurses from medical and surgical units of a regional hospital who want to explore why nurses and medical practitioners do not wash their hands regularly. Each potential participant is asked to respond to a list of reasons that apply to them. They also are asked to respond to a series of questions about their personal characteristics including their highest qualification, work experience, gender and age. The research team does not want to assess a causal relationship between personal characteristics and their hand washing. This study does not have independent and dependent variables.

Although most quantitative health research is carried out by specialised health researchers, it is also possible for nurses and midwives working in clinical settings to observe health problems and initiate non-experimental quantitative research in order to investigate such problems and their treatment. The best practice guidelines for nurses and midwives are also based on a range of quantitative research studies.

▶ ▶ ▶   TERMS, TIPS AND SKILLS

In order to conduct an RCT, a large sample size is required. This is true when many extraneous variables are considered in order to assess a causal relationship between an independent and dependent variable. Results of non-experimental research designs are still useful in finding evidence that can be applied to health care services. Not all health issues need to be assessed using experimental research designs. Non-experimental designs that are well conducted and analysed can be as important and useful as experimental designs.

Summary

Quantitative research is considered to be a scientific and systematic investigation that provides evidence. The level of evidence varies according to the rigour, control, intervention and objectivity of researchers (Craig & Smyth 2007; NHMRC 2009). Researchers need to be aware of potential factors that can influence the validity of their study, and various strategies need to be planned and implemented at different stages of the research process. The use of the various quantitative research designs is determined by the research questions and purposes. It is important that researchers can identify the weaknesses and strengths of their own research so that the results can be useful in clinical settings and in the improvement of health outcomes of individuals and communities that is expected from this research.

IMPLICATIONS FOR EVIDENCE-BASED NURSING AND MIDWIFERY

Over the past few decades, the use of technology in health services has increased. New knowledge in health is discovered and made available to the public. Health consumers are encouraged and empowered to self-manage their health and illness. Health professionals and the general public demand health services that are evidence-based, and we as nurses and midwives have a responsibility to deliver evidence-based care.

Different types of research questions relating to intervention, diagnosis, prognosis, aetiology and screening are used to categorise research results to different levels of evidence (Table 1.1). There is a growing amount of nursing and midwifery research of various degrees of complexity and rigour. The particular contribution of quantitative research to this body of evidence lies in the precision inherent in its quantitative measurement and statistical analysis of health phenomena, and in the ability of experimental research designs to firmly demonstrate cause-and-effect relationships in health phenomena and provide proof that health interventions actually work as claimed.

▶▶▶ **PROBLEM SOLVING 6.1**

Bob and his team have conducted a research project that aims to assess whether or not giving instruction and printed health education materials relating to self-management of chest pain will reduce the proportion of patients who re-present to the ED with chest pain within six months.

Based on the information given, what is the type of research design the researchers are using? Identify the text to support your answer.

Practice exercise 6.1

From the following list, which one is likely to be the most precise measure of hand washing?

Direct observation

Self-report of hand washing

Measuring hand-washing product usage.

Practice exercise 6.2

Identify a research design from the following research objectives or research questions:

a   Will increasing the number of home visits by a midwife to women who have postpartum depression increase self-confidence in their ability to undertake their mothering role?

b   Patients with type 2 diabetes who receive health education from peers will better control their blood sugar level than patients with type 2 diabetes who receive health education from routine sources.

c   Two groups of women, women who have breast cancer and women who do not, were asked to recall their cigarette smoking and use of birth control in the past five years. Researchers want to find out whether cigarette smoking and use of birth control influence the development of breast cancer or not.

Answers to problem solving 6.1

Experimental design. However, the specific design cannot be identified (e.g. pre-test post-test or randomised controlled trial) because of the lack of information.

The text is, 'whether or not giving instruction and printed health education materials relating to self management of chest pain will reduce the proportion of patients...'

Answers to practice exercises

6.1

Direct observation

Health care workers may either under- or overreport their hand washing. Hand-washing products can be used for many activities which may or may not involve patient care (Haas & Larsen 2007).

6.2

a   Correlation design

b   Experimental design

c   Case-control study

Further reading

Craig, J. V., & Smyth, R. L. (2007). *Evidence-Based Practice Manual for Nurses*. Edinburgh: Churchill Livingstone.

Gordis, L. (2009). *Epidemiology*, 4th edn. Philadelphia: Elsevier/Saunders.

Howell, D. C. (2009). *Statistical Methods for Psychology*, 7th edn. Australia: Wadsworth, Cengage Learning.

Weblinks

ABC Health Report:

<www.abc.net.au/rn/healthreport/>

Centre for Applied Nursing Research:

<www.sswahs.nsw.gov.au/sswahs/canr>

Centre for Reviews and Dissemination, University of York:

<www.crd.york.ac.uk/crdweb>

Cochrane Collaboration:

<www.cochrane.org>

National Health and Medical Research Council (NHMRC):

<www.nhmrc.gov.au>

Joanna Briggs Institute:

<www.joannabriggs.edu.au/about/home.php>

References

Beaglehole, R., & Bonita, R. (2004). *Public Health at the Crossroads: Achievements and Prospects*. Cambridge: Cambridge University Press.

Burns, N., & Grove, S. K. (2009). *The Practice of Nursing Research: Appraisal, Synthesis, and Generation of Evidence*. St Louis, MI: Saunders Elsevier.

Centers for Disease Control. (1981). Pneumocystis pneumonia—Los Angeles. *Morbidity and Mortality Weekly Report* 30(21), 250–2.

Centers for Disease Control. (1982). A cluster of Kaposi's sarcoma and Pneumocystis carinii pneumonia among homosexual male residents of Los Angeles and Orange Counties, California. *Morbidity and Mortality Weekly Report* 31(23), 305–7.

Craig , J. V., & Smyth, R. L. (2007). *Evidence-Based Practice Manual for Nurses*. Edinburgh: Churchill Livingstone.

Dunt, D. (2009). Levels of project evaluation and evaluation study designs. In S. Jirojwong & P. Liamputtong (eds), *Population Health, Communities and Health Promotion* (pp. 267–83). Melbourne: Oxford University Press.

Dykeman, M., & Cruttenden, K. (2009). Frameworks of Project Evaluation. In S. Jirojwong & P. Liamputtong (eds), *Population Health, Communities and Health Promotion* (pp. 253–64). Melbourne: Oxford University Press.

English, D. R., Armstrong, B. K., & Kricker, A. (1998). Reproducibility of reported measurements of sun exposure in a case-control study. *Cancer Epidemiology, Biomarkers & Prevention* 7(10), 857–63.

Food Standards Australia New Zealand. (2010). *Monitoring and Surveillance*. Retrieved 2 October 2010, from <www.foodstandards.gov.au/scienceandeducation/monitoringandsurveillance>

Friis, R. H., & Sellers, T. A. (2004). *Epidemiology for Public Health Practice*. Sudbury, MA: Jones & Bartlett.

Gould, D. J., Chudleigh, J. H., Moralejo, D., & Drey, N. (2007). Interventions to improve hand hygiene compliance in patient care. *Cochrane Database Systematic Review* 18(2), CD005186.

Haas, J. P., & Larsen, E. L. (2007). Measurement of compliance with hand hygiene. *Journal of Hospital Infection* 66(6), 6–14.

Harrison, S. L., Buettner, P. G., & MacLennan, R. (2005). The North Queensland 'Sun-Safe Clothing' study: Design and baseline results of a randomized trial to determine the effectiveness of sun-protective clothing in preventing melanocytic nevi. *American Journal of Epidemiology* 161(6), 536–45.

Heymann, D. L., & Rodier, G. (2004). Global surveillance, national surveillance, and SARS: Emerging infectious diseases. *Medscape* 10 February 2004.

Iijima, S., & Ohzeki, T. (2006). Bacterial contamination on the hands of nursing staff in the most basic neonatal care. *Journal of Neonatal Nursing* 12(2), 53–5.

Jirojwong, S., & MacLennan, R. (2003). Health beliefs, perceived self-efficacy, and breast self-examination among Thai migrants in Brisbane. *Journal of Advanced Nursing* 41(3), 241–9.

Johnson, J. E., Rice, V. H., Fuller, S. S., & Endress, M. P. (1978). Sensory information, instruction in a coping strategy, and recovery from surgery. *Research in Nursing & Health* 1(1), 4–17.

Karlsson, I., Berglin, E., & Larsson, P. A. (2000). Sense of coherence: Quality of life before and after coronary artery bypass surgery—a longitudinal study. *Journal of Advanced Nursing* 31(6), 1383–92.

Kim, H., Neubert, J. K., San Miguel, A., Xu, K., Krishnaraju, R. K., Iadarola, M. J., Goldman, D., & Dionne, R. A. (2004). Genetic influence on variability in human acute experimental pain sensitivity associated with gender, ethnicity and psychological temperament. *Pain* 109(3), 488–96.

Krause-Parello, C. A. (2008). The mediating effect of pet attachment support between loneliness and general health in older females living in the community. *Journal of Community Health Nursing* 25(1), 1–14.

Kunanusont, C., Wangroonsarb, Y., Wattanasri, S., Kunasol, P., Wasi, C., & Limpakanjanarat, K. (1988). Surveillance of Acquired Immune Deficiency Syndrome in Thailand through July, 1987. Paper presented at the Regional Scientific meeting International Epidemiology Association, 24–30 January 1988, Pattaya, Thailand.

Last, J. M. (ed.). (1995). *A Dictionary of Epidemiology*. New York: Oxford University Press.

Lim, K., Waters, C. M., Froelicher, E. S., & Kayser-Jones, J. S. (2008). Conceptualizing physical activity behavior of older Korean-Americans: An integration of Korean culture and social cognitive theory. *Nursing Outlook* 56(6), 322–9.

Lin, L.-Y., & Wang, R.-H. (2005). Abdominal surgery, pain and anxiety: Preoperative nursing intervention. *Journal of Advanced Nursing* 51(3), 252–60.

LoBiondo-Wood, G., & Haber, J. (eds) (2006). *Nursing Research: Methods and Critical Appraisal for Evidence-Based Practice*. St Louis, MO: Mosby Elsevier.

MacLennan, R. (2009). Project planning: Projects and protocols. In S. Jirojwong & P. Liamputtong (eds), *Population Health, Communities and Health Promotion* (pp. 123–33). Melbourne: Oxford University Press.

Meyer, B. C., & Bishop, D. S. (2007). Florence Nightingale: Nineteenth century apostle of quality. *Journal of Management History* 13(3), 240–54.

Moher, D., Jones, A., Lepage L., & CONSORT Group (Consolidated Standards for Reporting of Trials). (2001). Use of the CONSORT statement and quality of reports of randomized trials: a comparative before-and-after evaluation. *JAMA* 285(15), 1992–5.

NHMRC (National Health and Medical Research Council). (2009). NHMRC levels of evidence and grades for recommendations for developers of guidelines. Retrieved 9 October 2010, from <www.nhmrc.gov.au/_files_nhmrc/file/guidelines/evidence_statement_form.pdf>

Polit, D. F., & Beck, C. T. (2004). *Nursing Research: Principles and Methods*. Philadelphia: Lippincott, Williams & Wilkins.

Polit, D. F., & Hungler, B. P. (1999). *Nursing Research: Principles and Methods*. Philadelphia: Lippincott.

Rea, E. & Upshur, R. (2001). Semmelweis revisited: The ethics of infection prevention among health care workers (Commentary). *Canadian Medical Association Journal* 164(10), 1447–8.

Royal College of Nursing, UK. (2009). *The Recognition and Assessment of Acute Pain in Children Clinical Practice Guidelines*. Update of full guideline. Retrieved 2 August 2010, from <www.rcn.org.uk/__data/assets/pdf_file/0004/269185/003542.pdf>

Smith, D. R., & Leggat, P. A. (2005). Needlestick and sharps injuries among nursing students. *Journal of Advanced Nursing* 51(5), 449–55.

Schneider, Z., Elliott, D., Whitehead, D., LoBiondo-wood, G., & Haber, J. (eds). (2007). *Nursing and Midwifery Research: Methods and Critical Appraisal for Evidence-based Practice*. Sydney: Mosby.

Snow, J. (1855). *On the Mode of Communication of Cholera*, 2nd edn. London: John Churchill.

Susser, M. (1973). *Causal Thinking in the Health Sciences*. New York: Oxford University Press.

Susser, M. (2001). Glossary: Causality in public health science. *Journal of Epidemiology and Community Health* 55, 376–8.

Thompson, M. (2003). *Teach Yourself Philosophy of Science*. Abingdon: Bookprint Ltd.

Turner, G. W. (ed.). (1987). *The Australian Concise Oxford Dictionary*. Melbourne: Oxford University Press.

Van der Weyden, E. (2003). The use of honey for the treatment of two patients with pressure ulcers. *British Journal of Community Nursing* 8(12), S14, S16–S18.

White, C. G., Shinder, F. S., Shinder, A. L., & Dyer, D. L. (2001). Reduction of illness absenteeism in elementary schools using an alcohol-free instant hand sanitizer. *Journal of School Nursing* 17(5), 258–65.

WHO (World Health Organization). (2009). WHO guidelines on hand hygiene in health care: A summary. First global patient safety challenge. Clean care is safer care. Retrieved 8 October 2010, from <www.whqlibdoc.who.int/hq/2009/WHO_IER_PSP_2009.07_eng.pdf>

Wingo, P. A., Ries, L. A. G., Giovino, G. A., Miller, D. S., Rosenberg, H. M., Shopland, D. R., Thun, M. J., & Edwards, B. K. (1999). Annual report to the nation on the status of cancer, 1973–1996, with a special section on lung cancer and tobacco smoking. *Journal of the National Cancer Institute* 91(8), 675–90.

CHAPTER 7

Mixed Methods Research

Janice Lewis

Chapter learning objectives

By the end of this chapter you will be able to:

▶ understand the purpose of mixed methods research

▶ identify the differences between quantitative and qualitative research

▶ describe different approaches to mixed methods research

▶ describe characteristics of mixed methods research designs

▶ discuss sampling techniques in mixed methods research

▶ explain approaches to analysing mixed methods data

▶ discuss issues of validity in mixed methods research

▶ identify the opportunities for mixed methods research in evidence-based nursing and midwifery.

Introduction

In previous chapters we have described aspects of quantitative and qualitative research designs, data collection approaches and analysis. Recent times, however, have seen the evolution throughout the social and behavioural sciences, as well as in nursing and midwifery, of an approach to research that Tashakkori and Teddlie (2003) have described as the third methodological movement. This approach, mixed methods research, is the subject of this chapter.

Mixed methods research is a term that has come to describe a class of research where the researcher mixes or combines qualitative and quantitative research methods in the same project. The other movements described in other chapters of this book are quantitatively oriented research and qualitatively oriented research. Mixed methods research represents a change in that the researchers are primarily interested in both narrative and numeric data and their analysis.

The use of mixed methods has a long history, with examples of research using this approach being identified throughout most of the 20th century and into the 21st. Mixed methods research as an identifiably different methodology, however, is fairly recent, emerging mostly since the late 1980s (Plano Clark & Cresswell 2008). Tashakkori and Teddlie (2003) recognise this recent development in methodology but suggest that the field of mixed methods research has now progressed beyond infancy into adolescence. Adolescence is a good description of the current position. Mixed methods as a research methodology is experiencing rapid growth as evidenced by the expanding body of literature and, advancing the field, the launch of several journals (e.g. the *Journal of Mixed Methods Research* and the *International Journal of Multiple Research Approaches*) and major conferences; for example, the Annual International Mixed Methods Conference will be in its sixth year in 2010. On the other hand, as with most adolescents, mixed methods research is still undergoing some difficulties with identity and differences of opinion.

Why conduct mixed methods research?

Following a review of the growing body of research using mixed methods, Greene and associates (1989) identified five purposes for conducting mixed methods research. These justifications have been quite influential and remain relevant today. These purposes are:

- Seeking convergence and corroboration of results from different methods that are studying the same phenomena. For example, in case studies several sources of data are used to describe a single case. This approach is frequently referred to as triangulation.
- Seeking to elaborate, augment or add clarification to results from one method with the results of another method. For example, interviews may be conducted to explain contradictory findings in the analysis of questionnaire data.

- Using the results from one method to inform or develop another method. For example, interviews or focus groups may be conducted before a questionnaire is developed.

- Using one method to discover new perceptions in an area of research enquiry leads to new perspectives and possible reframing of the research question. For example, interviews may be conducted with people who are known to have differing opinions so that the researcher can acquire an in-depth understanding of the issues before framing the research question and developing the research design.

- The results from one method are used to inform or develop another method. For example, direct observation methods may be used to access small populations and questionnaires may be used to access larger populations, both in the same research project.

There are other justifications for combining qualitative and quantitative research than those just listed. Bryman (2006a), for example, suggested 16 reasons for mixing research methods in the one study. Nevertheless, all the justifications offered reflect the underpinning notion that mixing methods offers a richer explanation than the sole use of quantitative or qualitative methods, drawing on the strengths of each approach and overcoming its weaknesses.

▶▶▶ TERMS, TIPS AND SKILLS

Mixing methods is thought to offer a richer explanation than the sole use of quantitative or qualitative methods.

Differences between quantitative and qualitative research methods

The possibilities of mixed methods are more clearly understood by considering the differences between quantitative and qualitative research methods. The strengths and weaknesses of the respective methods are worthy of reflection. The following tables have been adapted from Burke Johnson and Onwuegbuzie (2004).

Traditional quantitative and qualitative approaches to research have their strengths and weaknesses. One approach is not necessarily appropriate for addressing all research questions. Most mixed methods researchers (e.g. Plano Clark & Cresswell 2008; Tashakkori & Teddlie 2003) take the position that the research questions should drive the choice of research method. That is, the research method used should be the one that is thought to answer the question best. Not all researchers, however, agree with this position and argue that one approach is preferable and that mixing methods is not appropriate.

Janice Lewis

This debate is not yet resolved and although there is growing support for mixed methods research, the lack of universal acceptance reflects the immaturity of the methodology.

Table 7.1   Quantitative research

Strengths	Weaknesses
• testing and validating already constructed theories • hypotheses are constructed before the data are collected • may be replicated in different settings • may generalise findings to larger populations • the researcher can construct situations reducing confounding influences • the researcher can generate theory deductively • data collection may be relatively quick • produces numerical data • accommodates variation in researcher abilities • is useful for studying large numbers of people	• the categories or themes explaining the data generated by the researcher may not reflect the understanding of the subjects • underpinning theories may not be useful or reflect the subjects' understanding • hypothesis testing rather than hypothesis generation • knowledge produced may only be specific to local situations, context or individuals

Table 7.2   Qualitative research

Strengths	Weaknesses
• the data are based on the participants' categories of meaning • useful for studying a limited number of cases in depth • useful for describing complex phenomena • useful for research in areas about which there is limited prior research • study dynamic situations, exploring patterns of change • can identify contextual and setting factors that influence findings • can accommodate changes that occur during the study • can determine the course of the particular event • can generate theory inductively	• knowledge produced may not be generalisable to other populations or other settings • it is more difficult to test hypotheses and theories • data collection and analysis may be time-consuming • data collection and analysis is influenced by the researcher's abilities • results are more easily influenced by the researcher's personal biases

▶▶▶   TERMS, TIPS AND SKILLS

Quantitative and qualitative research methods have their strengths and weaknesses and one approach is not necessarily appropriate for addressing all research questions.

Views of mixed methods research

Incompatibility thesis

Much of the early debate about mixed methods research was based in what Bryman (2007, 2008) described as the paradigm argument. Schwandt (2001) defined a paradigm as a worldview or general perspective. In the research context, the word has come to mean the commitments, beliefs and values, methods and outlooks shared across a research discipline. Quantitative and qualitative research may be understood as belonging to particular and identifiably different paradigms. Quantitative research resides in the positivist paradigm, which takes the view that research must be value-free, with the researcher being independent of what is being researched. Objectivity is then the researcher's aim. Knowledge is arrived at by gathering facts that provide the basis for proving or disproving hypotheses. The aim of the research is to identify a single truth. Qualitative research, on the other hand, is considered to be in the constructivist paradigm, which views the researcher as inseparable from what is being researched. Research is bound by the values of the researcher and the notion of objectivity is rejected. Also rejected is the notion of a single reality. For those whose beliefs lie in the constructivist paradigm reality is multiple and is constructed by the observers.

> ▶▶▶   TERMS, TIPS AND SKILLS
>
> In the research context, paradigm has come to mean the commitments, beliefs and values, methods and outlooks shared across a research discipline.

Applying these worldviews to mixed methods research was seen to raise some insurmountable issues. For example, many saw it as impossible to be objective and subjective in the same piece of research. This has led to the view held by some that qualitative and quantitative research paradigms, including their associative methods, cannot and should not be mixed. This is the position that Howe (1988) labelled the incompatibility thesis where accommodation between paradigms is viewed as not being feasible because the two worldviews or paradigms are in opposition. Nevertheless, not all take that position and a growing body of literature continues to explore different views.

> ▶▶▶   TERMS, TIPS AND SKILLS
>
> The incompatibility thesis assumes that accommodation between paradigms is not feasible.

Pragmatism and mixed methods

For some researchers, the conflict between paradigms remains unresolved. Others (e.g. Creswell & Plano Clark 2007; Johnson & Onwuegbuzie 2004; Morgan 2007) have taken a different position, arguing that research should not be limited to the positivist or constructivist paradigms. They point out that there are other worldviews and one of them contends that pragmatism best fits mixed methods research.

▸▸▸   TERMS, TIPS AND SKILLS

Pragmatism has been proposed as a paradigm that best fits mixed methods research.

Pragmatism is a philosophical movement that began in the USA in the late 19th century. It aimed to find the middle ground between dogmatism and scepticism (Creswell 2003). Its focus was on rejecting traditional dualisms such as facts versus values or subjectivism versus objectivism, and finding workable solutions. Truth, meaning and knowledge were viewed as tentative in that they can and do change over time. Because of this, the emphasis is on practical theory and what works. By taking a pragmatic position researchers can reject the forced choice between methods based on paradigmatic position and in doing so also reject the incompatibility thesis. Thus for mixed methods researchers, the research question is more important than the paradigm that underlies the method.

Status of quantitative and qualitative elements

Another issue that emerged in the development of mixed methods research was debate about the way in which the methods would be used in the same study and whether or not one element of the research was more important than others. Morse (1991, 2003) took the position that mixed methods are possible but that paradigmatic positions must be kept clearly separate. She advanced the thinking on mixed methods research by suggesting that mixed methods studies could be designed in different ways. Quantitative and qualitative methods could be used at the same time or they could be used sequentially, with one method being used to plan the next. Morse also suggested that in a mixed methods study the quantitative and qualitative phases can have equal importance. When mixing methods the role of each method should be clearly expressed. In order to clarify the role of each method in this study, Morse developed a notation system. The elements of the system are summarised thus:

- use of the abbreviations QUAN for quantitative and QUAL for qualitative
- use of ✚ to indicate that data are collected simultaneously
- use of ➡ to indicate that data are collected sequentially
- use of UPPER CASE to denote that more priority is given to that orientation and use of lower case to denote a lesser role, thus indicating the relative weights of QUAL and QUAN.

▶▶▶   TERMS, TIPS AND SKILLS

Morse's notation system is used to describe how a mixed methods study is conducted.

The status of the quantitative and qualitative elements in mixed methods research continues to be a matter of debate. Decisions relating to priority (Morse 2003), weighting (Creswell & Plano Clark 2007) or dominance (Leech & Onwuegbuzie 2009) of the elements or phases of a mixed methods study are considered by many to be core considerations in mixed methods study designs.

Mixed methods as a continuum

Not all agree with Morse's position on the dichotomy between quantitative and qualitative research methods. Newman and colleagues (2003) argue that considering the comparative worth of the two approaches is pointless and suggest that quantitative and qualitative methods should be viewed as a continuum rather than a dichotomy (Figure 7.1).

Figure 7.1   The QUAL-MM-QUAN Continuum

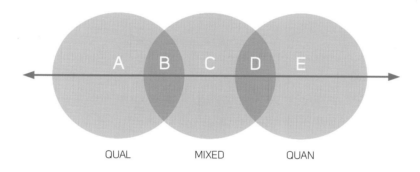

QUAL   MIXED   QUAN

Source: Adapted from Teddlie & Tashakkori 2009

In Figure 7.1 mixed methods research is represented by Zones B C and D. It is in Zone C that totally integrated mixed methods research occurs. This approach supports the notion of partially mixed methods and fully mixed methods proposed by some theorists such as Leech and Onwuegbuzie (2009). Nonetheless, the continuum approach suggests that the researcher can take a position at any point along the continuum. The choice of position will be driven by the optimal way in which to answer the research question.

Debates about methodological elements of mixed methods are ongoing. Over the last 15 years, however, there has been a dramatic increase in the published studies that use mixed methods and a growing number of textbooks focusing on mixed methods research (see e.g. Begman 2008; Creswell 1994, 1998, 2003; Creswell & Plano Clark 2007; Tashakkori & Teddlie 2003; Teddlie & Tashakkori 2009). Much of the debate relates to the best way to design a mixed methods study.

Mixed methods design

The ways in which researchers have combined quantitative and qualitative methods in any one study vary greatly. Bryman (2006b) investigated 232 published articles using mixed methods and identified 18 different ways of mixing methods. In order to provide some consistency, several authors have proposed typologies of mixed methods designs. Creswell and Plano Clark (2007) proposed four basic designs with a number of variants. Teddlie and Tashakkori (2009) suggested nine designs, while Leech and Onwuegbuzie (2009) proposed eight. The lack of clarity in mixed methods research designs is no doubt confusing and further reflects the evolutionary stage of the methodology. The research designs proposed by these authors address in various ways two underpinning design issues: the emphasis dimension and the time dimension. Decisions relating to these issues must be, as Maxwell and Loomis (2003) point out, clearly driven by the purpose of the study and the research question, by the questions that guide the study.

▶▶▶   TERMS, TIPS AND SKILLS

Mixed methods designs reflect emphasis and time dimensions.

Emphasis dimensions

These emerge from the notion that in the design of the study the status of the quantitative and qualitative elements should be identified. It now appears to be generally accepted that the quantitative or qualitative elements of a mixed methods study can have equal status or that one can be dominant.

Time dimensions

Time dimensions relate to when the phases of the mixed methods study are carried out. In a concurrent study, the quantitative and qualitative elements of the study are carried out at the same time. The interpretation of the findings of the research follows the integration of the findings from both elements. In the sequential mixed methods study one phase is carried out before the next and the first phase will inform or shape the second phase.

It is the various combinations of these two dimensions, time and emphasis, that generate the multiple research designs.

Concurrent mixed methods study design

Figure 7.2 illustrates a concurrent mixed methods study design. In this study the quantitative and qualitative data collection and data analysis are carried out in the same timeframe. Although there are two elements to the concurrent approach, it is a one-phase study. The interpretation of the research is when the results of the elements are combined. In the study design illustrated in Figure 7.2 the quantitative and qualitative elements are considered to have equal status (both are represented in upper case). Alternatively, one particular element could have been dominant (with one represented in upper case and one in lower case) if that was what the research question required. For this reason there are a number of possible variations on the concurrent design, depending on the emphasis of the methods. The purpose of this particular research design is to add to the explanation offered by one source of data by another source of data. It is based on the assumption that one method can add to the explanation offered by the other. This is often referred to as triangulation.

Figure 7.2 A concurrent mixed methods study design

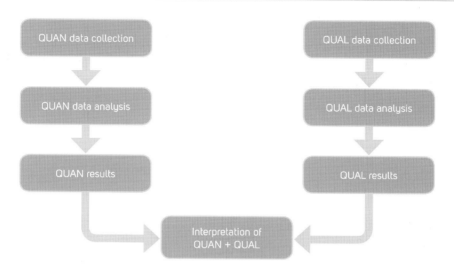

Concurrent mixed methods studies in nursing

The following examples of nursing research studies used concurrent mixed methods designs:

- Ream and others (2006) conducted an exploratory study to enable a detailed understanding of the phenomenon of fatigue in adolescents living with cancer. The researchers used a concurrent mixed methods design. The quantitative phase of the study was a life diary that used numerical rating across a number of items derived from previously developed scales. The qualitative phase of the study consisted of written responses to unstructured open-ended questions and semistructured in-depth interviews. The qualitative element was dominant in the study.

- Lehana and McNeil (2008) conducted a concurrent mixed methods study to determine how different parent groups (English-speaking and Spanish-speaking) understand medical care provided to their children and the procedural and research consent forms required by that care. The quantitative element of the research was a 36-item questionnaire requiring numerical responses, which measured comprehension or ability to read and understand health information. The questionnaire also collected demographic data. The qualitative element of the study was focus groups and individual interviews. The strength of the research was that the qualitative analysis enriched the quantitative results, hence strengthening the research. In the article reporting this study the status of the phases was not identified.

Sequential mixed methods study design

Figure 7.3 describes a generic sequential mixed methods design. Characteristic of this design is that there are two distinct phases that are conducted in separate timeframes. The first phase is used to develop and inform the second. Phase 1 can either be quantitative or qualitative, as can Phase 2. Similarly, Phase 1 or Phase 2 can be dominant or have equal status. For this reason there can be a number of variations of a sequential mixed methods study design, depending on decisions about sequence, timeframes and emphasis. The results of a study are normally in the interpretation of the data following the second phase. The dotted line connecting the results of Phase 1 indicates how results from both phases can influence the interpretation of the results of the study.

Figure 7.3   A sequential mixed methods research design

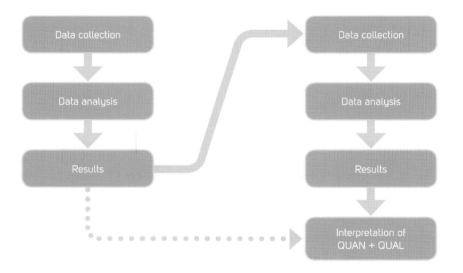

Sequential mixed methods in nursing

The following nursing research studies used sequential mixed methods designs:

*   Davila (2006) used a sequential mixed methods design to develop and evaluate an in-service program aimed at increasing nurses' knowledge and skills in responding to intimate partner violence. Phase 1 used interviews with nurses to identify their learning needs. The analysis of the qualitative data led to the development of an in-service

training program designed to meet the expressed needs of nursing staff for enhancing their intervention skills with the intimate partner. Phase 2 of the study was a one-group pre-test/post-test design to evaluate the effectiveness of the program. This phase used quantitative methods.

- In an Australian study, Farrell and Rose (2008) used a sequential mixed methods design to investigate whether personal digital assistants (PDAs) would enhance students' pharmacological and clinical contextual knowledge. In the first phase of the study, a quantitative phase, a quasi-experimental, non-equivalent experimental group design was used. Some student nurses were allocated to a clinical area with the use of PDAs and some were allocated to areas without the use of PDAs. Before the clinical placement both groups completed a questionnaire requiring numerical responses designed to assess pharmacological knowledge. Later both groups completed the same test on the completion of the clinical placement. The qualitative phase was also conducted on the completion of the clinical placement to explore issues related to the use of PDAs and the influence on students' pharmacological learning. Data were collected using focus group interviews.

Sampling techniques for mixed methods studies

In both quantitative and qualitative research, data are collected. Sampling techniques appropriate for each approach need to be considered. Qualitative sampling strategies normally employ purposive sampling techniques, whereas quantitative studies use probability sampling. See Table 7.3 for a brief overview of the essential differences between purposive and probability sampling.

Table 7.3   Purposive and probability sampling

	Purposive Sampling	Probability Sampling
Purpose	To generate a sample that will address research questions	To generate a sample that will address research questions
Generalisability	Form of generalisability (transferability)	Form of generalisability (external validity)
Selection of cases	Those that can best inform the research	Those that are collectively representative of the population
Sample size	Usually less than 30	Usually more than 50
Time of sample selection	Before and during study	Before study
Selection method	Expert judgment	Mathematical formula
Data	Narrative data	Numeric data

The researcher using mixed methods would follow the assumptions of the technique being used. See Chapter 8 for further discussion of sampling techniques.

Teddlie and Yu (2007) reviewed the literature for examples of mixed methods sampling techniques. They found that generally in concurrent mixed methods studies the sampling procedures occurred independently. Most of the reported literature appears to use only one research sample, with the purposive sample being drawn from the larger probability sample. There are nevertheless examples of studies that used two independent research samples. Sampling decisions were made according to the research question.

With sequential mixed methods studies sampling is determined by the research design and the related emphasis and sequence decisions. It was apparent, however, in most reported research that the results of Phase 1 influenced the sampling for Phase 2. Teddlie and Yu (2007), drawing on other authors and their own research, developed guidelines for mixed methods sampling:

- The sampling strategy should stem logically from the research question.
- The assumptions of the probability and purposive sampling techniques should be followed.
- The sampling strategy should generate quantitative and qualitative databases containing sufficient data to answer the research question and support the reported findings of the research.
- The sampling strategy must be ethical.
- The sampling strategy must be possible and realistic.
- The sampling strategy should be described in enough detail so that other researchers can assess the credibility of the research.

Analysis of mixed methods data

The analysis of quantitative and qualitative data is discussed elsewhere in this book (Chapters 11 and 12). In mixed methods research analysis offers some unique challenges. The way in which mixed methods studies may be differentiated from other studies is in the integration of the quantitative and qualitative elements. This integration may be in the design of the question, data collection and data analysis or at the point of interpretation or some combination of these. Most studies do not integrate data until the final interpretation of the findings (Bryman 2006b). The trend to date has been to treat the quantitative and qualitative data separately, thus avoiding integration of the data sets (Bazeley 2006). As Bazeley goes on to point out, the integration of data sets offers the possibility of enhanced understanding and more in-depth explanation of the data. With the integration of data sets, mixed methods research may likely realise its potential as a research methodology.

▶▶▶ TERMS, TIPS AND SKILLS

Integration of data sets is where quantitative and qualitative data sets are combined.

The integration of quantitative and qualitative data sets has proved challenging. In 1993 Caracelli and Greene identified four integration strategies for mixed methods analysis:

- Data transformation by numerically coding qualitative data (quantitising) or converting quantitative data into narrative (qualitising). Bazeley (2006) suggests that computer software offers considerable opportunities for such an approach, particularly in making qualitative data accessible for statistical analysis.
- Typology development where categories or themes are developed following the analysis of one data set is subsequently used as a framework for the analysis of the other.
- Extreme case analysis where a typical example is identified from the analysis of one data set is explored using data collected by alternative methods.
- Consolidated or merged data sets where both data types are jointly reviewed and consolidated into numerical codes or narratives for the purposes of further analysis.

Since that time, the development of approaches to the integration of mixed methods data sets has been slow. Integration of data sets before interpretation and discussion remains uncommon. Bazeley (2006) suggests that although a number of factors may have influenced this protracted development, the principal issue relates to the skills required to manage large data sets. In addition, if the integration of the data sets becomes too complex, this may place the satisfactory completion of the research at risk. The difficulty of the integration process is supported indirectly by Teddlie and Tashakkori (2009), who present a complex typology of mixed methods data analysis techniques related to the purpose of the research and the research design. The diversity of approaches and the skill mix needed by the researcher is intimidating, and as Bazeley (2006) points out it is for this reason that integration is frequently put in the 'too hard basket'. Nevertheless, approaches to integration of qualitative data sets is slowly developing, with Teddlie and Tashakkori (2009) suggesting that a datum is beginning to be considered as a transferable unit of information that can transition between quantitative and qualitative forms. It is likely that techniques for integrating quantitative and qualitative data sets will be the next step in the development of mixed methods research.

Janice Lewis

Issues of validity in mixed methods research

Issues of validity in mixed methods research are challenging because quantitative and qualitative research have different developmental pathways. While such issues in quantitative research have a long history, validity in qualitative research is less clearly understood. The way to address issues of validity in mixed methods is still evolving. Teddlie and Tashakkori (2009) report that at this stage there is no cohesive and comprehensive framework for establishing the validity of mixed methods studies. Onwuegbuzie and Johnson (2006) argue that because of the unique nature of mixed methods research a new nomenclature should be developed; they recommend that validity in mixed methods research should be thought of in terms of legitimation. Regardless of how validity is labelled, it is essential that the researcher establishes the credibility of mixed methods research. Drawing on Teddlie and Tashakkori (2009), the researcher needs to attend to several principles:

- establishing the suitability of the research design by clearly articulating the relationship between the research question and the methods of study
- ensuring that all the elements of the quantitative and qualitative components of the research design are conducted in a manner that demonstrates the established standards of research rigour required by each method
- demonstrating the relationship between the quantitative and qualitative elements of the study and how this relationship contributes to the findings of the study. In a concurrent mixed methods study this relates to how the findings of the concurrent elements are combined, and in a sequential mixed methods study to how the findings of Phase 1 inform Phase 2 and how the two phases inform the findings of the study.

▶▶▶ TERMS, TIPS AND SKILLS

Demonstrating the relationship between the quantitative and qualitative elements of the study is essential to establishing the credibility of the research.

The future of mixed methods research

The rapid growth of mixed methods suggests that the approach is offering something innovative to research. That narrative can be used to add meaning to numbers and numbers can be used to add precision to narrative is being recognised across many wide disciplines. A mixed methods approach draws on the strengths of both qualitative and quantitative methods and overcomes their weaknesses, and can conceivably be used to answer a broader and more complex range of research questions. In addition, a mixed methods approach can provide strong evidence through the convergence or corroboration of findings and can add insights and understandings that may be missed when only one method is used. In line with current trends, in the future mixed methods research is likely to make a considerable contribution as one of the methods available to study the complex phenomena that are of interest to nurses and midwives.

Mixed methods research still offers many challenges. The diversity of definitions, conceptualisations and nomenclature in addition to the confusing variety of research designs reflects the adolescent developmental stage of mixed methods as a research methodology. This lack of clarity can be confusing to students and researchers alike.

There are also some methodological issues which have yet to be resolved satisfactorily. The biggest challenge emerging relates to the way in which the quantitative and qualitative strands of the study are integrated. Generally understood methods for integration are yet to be forthcoming. This integration is nevertheless central to the concept of mixed methods research. A mixed methods study is not two separate studies that happen to be addressing the same issue in a different way; it is one study that uses different methods to address a clearly expressed research question. Developing protocols to the integration of these methods is essential if mixed methods research is to continue to develop.

On a more practical level, mixed methods research is frequently more complex and time-consuming, requiring high-level skills in the researcher. It can be difficult for a single researcher to carry out both phases of the study, especially when a concurrent design is being used. Having skills in both quantitative and qualitative methods could be particularly challenging for a student researcher.

Nevertheless, mixed methods is an exciting area of research and offers possibilities to explain the complexities of nursing practice in new ways. As Tashakkori and Teddlie (2003) say, 'Study what is of interest to you and what is of value to you, study it in different ways that you deem appropriate, utilise the results in a way that brings about positive consequences within your value system' (p. 21).

Summary

The strengths of both qualitative and quantitative research approaches have been combined in mixed methods research. The reasons for using mixed methods research are described in this chapter. Mixed methods constitute an important research approach because they are considered as a continuum embracing, on the one hand, the quantitative approach with its statistical rigour and its firm control by the researcher, and on the other, the qualitative approach, which is less rigorous in some ways but richer in others and driven to a great extent by the research participants. The chapter presents discussions relating to two major research designs: concurrent and sequential study designs, categorising both major research approaches according to the timeframe of the research. Research principles such as sampling techniques and data analysis have been discussed.

IMPLICATIONS FOR EVIDENCE-BASED NURSING AND MIDWIFERY

Evidence from empirical studies using mixed methods research is as important in health care services as studies that use a single approach. Mixed methods research is likely to be increasingly used by nurse/midwife researchers to explore health problems so that health services can be improved. Users and readers can use its principles to critique both quantitative research and qualitative research to identify the strengths and weaknesses of research publications. These may be challenging tasks but they are achievable by those who lack experience, in particular novice researchers or clinicians. Guidelines for synthesising evidence based on mixed methods research are not yet well developed.

Practice exercise 7.1

Jirojwong and colleagues (2007) explored identity and self-perception among young Muslim people in Queensland. A major aim of this research project was to explore the identity and self-perception of young Muslim people aged 9–19 years in three Queensland locations. They investigated social, cultural, political and structural environments, which influenced the identity and self-perception of young people and as described by them. Mixed methods research was used to collect quantitative and qualitative data from 117 youths. They took part in a group discussion and completed a short questionnaire. Social, cultural and political environments that influence the identity of young people were explored.

Based on the given information, was this a concurrent mixed methods design or sequential mixed methods design?

Practice exercise 7.2

A randomised control trial is to be conducted to evaluate the efficacy of a new style of motorised foam mattress in the prevention of pressure ulcers. This is to be a quantitative study. How might the collection of qualitative data enhance this research?

You are planning to answer the question: What are the health beliefs of patients who are hospitalised with myocardial infarction? Which quantitative and qualitative data would best answer this question?

Read: A. O'Cathain, J. Nicholl, F. Sampson, S. Walters, A. McDonnell & J. Munro (2004). Do different types of nurses give different triage decisions in NHS Direct? A mixed methods study. *Journal of Health Services Research & Policy* 9(4), 226–33.

What type(s) of mixed methods are being used?

What is the research design? Why was this design chosen?

How were the two phases of the study integrated?

A colleague suggests that quantitative and qualitative methods should not be used in the same study to answer the same research question. What is your response?

Answer to practice exercise 7.1

A concurrent mixed methods design.

Further reading

Andrew, S., & Halcombe, E. (eds). (2009). *Mixed Methods of Research for Nursing and Health Sciences.* Oxford: Blackwell.

Brannen, J. (2005). Mixing methods: The entry of qualitative and quantitative approaches into the research process. *International Journal of Social Research Methodology* 8(3), 173–84.

Burke Johnson, R., Onwuegbuzie, A., & Turner, A. (2007). Toward a definition of mixed methods research. *Journal of Mixed Methods Research* 1(2), 112–33.

Creswell, J. W., & Plano Clark, V. (2007). *Designing and Conducting Mixed Methods Research.* Thousand Oaks, CA: Sage Publications Inc.

Freshwater, D. (2007). Reading mixed methods research: Contexts for criticism. *Journal of Mixed Methods Research* 1(2), 134–46.

Giddings, L. (2006). Positivism dressed in drag? *Journal of Research in Nursing* 11(3), 195–203.

Morgan, D. (2007). Paradigms lost and the pragmatism regained: Methodological implications of combining qualitative and quantitative methods. *Journal of Mixed Methods Research* 1(1), 48–76.

Morse, J. (2005). Evolving trends in qualitative research: Advances in mixed-method design. *Qualitative Health Research* 15(5), 583.

Onwuegbuzie, A., & Leech, N. (2005). On becoming a pragmatic researcher: The importance of combining quantitative and qualitative research methodologies. *International Journal of Social Research Methodology* 8(5), 375–87.

Plano Clark, V., & Cresswell, J. (2008). *The Mixed Methods Reader.* Thousand Oaks, CA: Sage Publications.

Tashakkori, A., & Teddlie, C. (2003). *Handbook of Mixed Methods in Social and Behavioural Research.* Thousand Oaks, CA: Sage Publications Inc.

Teddlie, C., & Tashakkori, A. (2009). *Foundations of Mixed Methods Research: Approaches in the Social and Behavioural Sciences.* Thousand Oaks, CA: Sage Publications.

Weaver, K., & Olson, J. (2006). Understanding paradigms used for nursing research. *Journal of Advanced Nursing* 53(4), 459–69.

Wilkins, K., & Woodgate, R. (2008). Designing a mixed methods study in paediatric oncology nursing research. *Journal of Paediatric Oncology Nursing* 25(1), 24–33.

Weblinks

<http://videolectures.net/ssmt09_onwuegbuzie_mmr>
A video lecture by Tony Onwuegbuzie on Mixed Methods research. Recorded at the 2009 European Consortium for Political Research Summer School in Methods and Techniques in University of Ljubljana, Slovenia.

<http://mmr.sagepub.com>
The website for the *Journal of Mixed Methods Research.*

References

Bazeley, P. (2006). The contribution of computer software to integrating qualitative and quantitative data and analyses. *Research in the Schools* 13(1), 64–74.

Begman, M. (2008). *Advances in Mixed Methods Research.* London: Sage Publications.

Bryman, A. (2006a). Integrating quantitative and qualitative research. How is it done? *Qualitative Research* 6(1), 97–113.

Bryman, A. (2006b). Paradigm peace and implications for quality. *International Journal of Social Research Methodology* 9(2), 111–26.

Bryman, A. (2007). Barriers to integrating quantitative and qualitative research. *Journal of Mixed Methods Research* 1(1), 8–22.

Bryman, A. (2008). *Social Research Methods*, 3rd edn. Oxford: Oxford University Press.

Burke Johnson, R., & Onwuegbuzie, A. (2004). Mixed methods research: A research paradigm whose time has come. *Educational Researcher* 33(7), 14–26.

Caracelli, J., & Greene, J. (1993). Data analysis strategies for mixed method valuation designs. *Educational Evaluation and Policy Analysis* 15(2), 195–207.

Creswell, J. W. (1994). *Research Design. Qualitative and Quantitative Approaches.* Thousand Oaks, CA: Sage Publications.

Creswell, J. W. (1998). *Qualitative Inquiry and Research Design. Choosing Among Five Traditions.* Thousand Oaks, CA: Sage Publications.

Creswell, J. W. (2003). *Research Design. Qualitative, Quantitative, and Mixed Methods Approaches*, 2nd edn. Thousand Oaks, CA: Sage Publications.

Creswell, J. W., & Plano Clark, V. (2007). *Designing and Conducting Mixed Methods Research.* Thousand Oaks, CA: Sage Publications Inc.

Davila, Y. (2006). Increasing nurses' knowledge and skills for enhanced response to intimate partner violence. *Journal of Continuing Education in Nursing* 37(4), 171–7.

Farrell, M., & Rose, L. (2008). Use of mobile hand-held computers in clinical nursing education. *Journal of Nursing Education* 47(1), 13–19.

Greene, J., Caracelli, J., & Graham, W. (1989). Towards a conceptual framework for mixed method evaluation designs. *Educational Evaluation and Policy Analysis* 11(3), 255–74.

Howe, K. (1988). Against the quantitative-qualitative incompatibility thesis, or, dogmas die hard. *Educational Researcher* 17, 10–16.

Jirojwong S., H. D., Apellado H., & Ferdous, T. (2007). *The Nurturing Migrants Project: Outcomes and Achievements.* Report submitted to the Multicultural Affairs Queensland. Rockhampton: Central Queensland University.

Leech, N., & Onwuegbuzie, A. (2009). A typology of mixed methods research designs. *Qualitative Quantitative* 43, 265–75.

Lehana, C., & McNeil, J. (2008). Mixed methods exploration of parents' health information understanding. *Clinical Nursing Research* 17(2), 133–44.

Maxwell, J., & Loomis, D. (2003). Mixed methods design: An alternative approach. In A. Tashakkori & C. Teddlie (eds), *Handbook of Mixed Methods in Social and Behavioural Research* (pp. 241–72). Thousand Oaks, CA: Sage Publications.

Morgan, D. (2007). Paradigms lost and the pragmatism regained: Methodological implications of combining qualitative and quantitative methods. *Journal of Mixed Methods Research* 1(1), 48–76.

Morse, J. M. (1991). Approaches to qualitative-quantitative methodological triangulation. *Nursing Research* 40, 120–3.

Morse, J. M. (2003). Principles of mixed methods and multimethod research design. In Tashakkori & Teddlie (eds), *Handbook of Mixed Methods in Social and Behavioural Research* (pp. 189–208). Thousand Oaks, CA: Sage Pubications.

Newman, I., Ridenour, C., Newman, C., & DeMarco, G. (2003). A typology of research purposes and its relationship to mixed methods. In Tashakkori & Teddlie, *Handbook of Mixed Methods in Social and Behavioural Research.* Thousand Oaks, CA: Sage Pubications.

Onwuegbuzie, A., & Johnson, R. (2006). The validity issue in mixed research. *Research in the Schools* 13(1), 48–63.

Plano Clark, V., & Cresswell, J. (2008). *The Mixed Methods Reader.* Thousand Oaks CA: Sage Publications.

Ream, E., Gibson, F., Edwards, J., Seption, B., Mulhall, A., & Richardson, A. (2006). Experience of fatigue in adolescents living with cancer. *Cancer Nursing* 29(4), 317–26.

Schwandt, T. (2001). *Dictionary of Qualitative Enquiry*, 2nd edn. Thousand Oaks, CA: Sage Publications.

Tashakkori, A., & Teddlie, C. (2003). *Handbook of Mixed Methods in Social and Behavioural Research.* Thousand Oaks, CA: Sage Publications.

Teddlie, C., & Tashakkori, A. (2009). *Foundations of Mixed Methods Research. Approaches in the Social and Behavioural Sciences.* Thousand Oaks, CA: Sage Publications.

Teddlie, C., & Yu, F. (2007). Mixed methods sampling: A typology with examples. *Journal of Mixed Methods Research*, 1(1), 77–100.

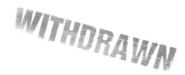

CHAPTER 8

Populations and Sampling

Maree Johnson and Sungwon Chang

Chapter learning objectives

By the end of this chapter you will be able to:

▸ understand the relationship between a sample and the target population

▸ distinguish probability and non-probability sampling approaches

▸ be aware of the meaning of generalisability within quantitative and qualitative sampling methods

▸ be familiar with sampling approaches for quantitative and qualitative research studies

▸ appreciate the importance of estimating sample size.

KEY TERMS

Cluster sampling

Convenience sampling

Population

Probability sampling

Purposive sampling

Random selection

Sample

Stratified random selection

Systematic sampling

Theoretical sampling

Introduction

In the previous chapters you have become familiar with some aspects of research. Sampling, or the selection of suitable persons to participate in a study, is often challenging and researchers consider this matter very carefully. Sampling has a major impact on the interpretation of the findings, length of the project and the overall costs. Selecting the right sample size and type of participants reduces time and costs for the investigator.

The importance of sampling

Often nursing and midwifery research involves studying a small number of cases (a sample) rather than an entire group (a population) in which the investigator is interested. This process of selecting a small number of cases from the population of interest is called sampling. The usual goal is to produce a representative sample (i.e. similar to the population in all characteristics except that there are fewer cases) in order to generalise the findings to the population from which the sample was drawn.

A population is defined as 'a complete set of persons or objects that possess some common characteristic of interest to the researcher' (Nieswiadomy 2008, p. 188). A sample is a subset of the population with the same characteristics as the original population.

The method of sampling should be considered in light of the research aims, questions or hypotheses, the interventions (if applicable) and the data collection methods. It is both effective and cost-efficient for researchers, with often limited funds, to accurately and appropriately define the sampling method to achieve the study aims.

There are two basic types of sampling method: probability sampling and non-probability sampling. In probability sampling each case from the population has an equal chance of being selected for the sample and the cases are chosen by a process known as random selection. In other words, in probability sampling the researcher identifies, in some way, all the cases in the population, and then allows random chance to determine which ones are to be included in the sample. Because the determination of the sample selection is directed by non-systematic and random rules, the researcher can assume that the characteristics of the sample approximate the characteristics of the total population. Probability sampling is sometimes called random sampling because of this random way of selecting cases to ensure a good representation of the whole population. A casual or haphazard sample does not qualify as a random sample. For example, just taking whoever is available does not constitute random sampling. In random sampling, all cases from the population must have an equal opportunity of being included in the study.

At this point we need to clarify the difference between target population and accessible population. In all research there is a desire to find an accurate listing of the entire population or target population of interest. However, this is usually not possible. Hence researchers tend to define a subset of the population or accessible population from which they can more readily sample. The listing of the accessible population from which the sample will be drawn is called the sampling frame. It is important to remember that the results of the research or generalisation from the research only apply to the accessible population and not to the target population. Any generalisations to the target population in research should be viewed as a provisional conclusion based on the experience and the wisdom of the researcher involved rather than on any logical or statistical necessity.

In non-probability sampling the researcher cannot ensure that each case in the population will be represented in the sample. Some cases may have little or no chance of being selected. As such, in non-probability sampling, researchers cannot claim representativeness and they are limited in their ability to generalise to the population. Non-probability samples may contain sources of bias not known or recognised by the researcher. As there is no assurance that each case has a chance of being included in the sample, it is difficult if not impossible to estimate the sampling error (i.e. the difference between the sample value and the population value) or to identify possible bias (i.e. a sample that is selected in a manner that is systematically different from the population).

Normal distribution and random sampling

Many characteristics studied in the biological, behavioural and clinical sciences reflect the shape of a bell curve, known more formally as a normal distribution. For example, the height of all Australian males would be normally distributed. There will inevitably be some men in the population who are tall and some who are short, while most will be around the 'average' height, sloping gradually in either direction towards the greater or the lesser heights (Figure 8.1).

By using random sampling, it is expected that more of the 'average' cases will be selected, as more of the 'average' exist in the population. Similarly, it is expected that a sample will also include fewer of those above and below the 'average' case as these cases are also represented in the population but in fewer numbers. The result is a sample that is representative of the population and also one that approximates a normal distribution. Furthermore, the central limit theorem (statistical concept) states that even if your population was not normally distributed, the distribution of the sample means will approximate a normal curve (bell curve) if the sample size is large enough (Munro 2005). This idea of a normally distributed sample is fundamental to many statistical analysis procedures used to generalise sample characteristics to the population.

The importance of probability sampling is in using a sample while also being able to make statements that are generalisable to the population. Furthermore, the use of probability sampling enables inferences to be made to the population with a level of precision that can be determined from statistical theory (Munro 2005).

All researchers recognise that no matter how hard a researcher tries, it is impossible to select a sample that perfectly represents the population. One way to express this lack of perfect fit between the sample and the population is by reporting the sampling error. Minimising sampling error, no more than 5%, is the goal of any sampling technique.

Figure 8.1   A distribution of participants selected through random sampling

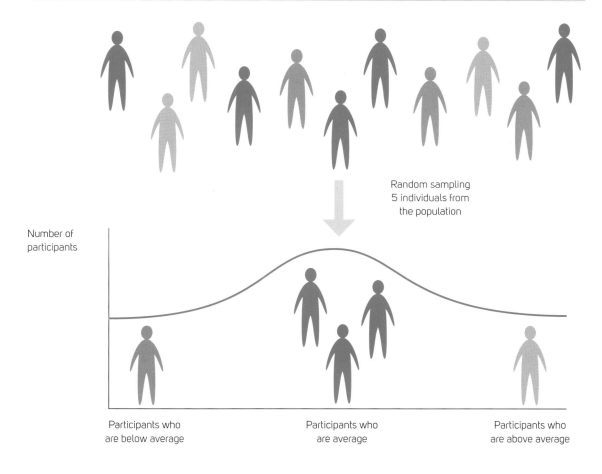

Source: Derived from the original figure from Edwards 2008, p. 12

These principles of generalisability also apply to qualitative studies (see also Chapter 4). In qualitative studies, Collingridge and Gantt (2008) suggest that the sample should reflect a 'well-defined rationale' or 'specific purpose' (p. 391). Like quantitative studies, a purposive sampling approach seeks to achieve the study's aims. However, Collingridge and Gantt suggest that qualitative research is seeking 'analytical generalisation' or whether the findings (themes or processes) defined from one study can be used in another context (p. 392). Qualitative sampling approaches are commonly understood as influenced by the methods— phenomenology, ethnography, grounded theory—of qualitative research (Hammersley &

Mairs 2004). One author proposes that the term 'case selection' rather than 'sampling' would be a more appropriate term for qualitative research (Chwalisz et al. 2008). Participant selection is also used.

RESEARCH IN PRACTICE 8.1

8.1

ELIGIBILITY CRITERIA

Eligibility criteria are used to define the characteristics of the study subjects the researcher is seeking (Hart 2006). These may include such attributes as category of nurse, type of presenting health problem of a patient, age of the person to participate in a study, or exposure to a particular situation. Inclusion and exclusion criteria are aspects of the eligibility criteria and are defined for a particular study.

In a study comparing two warming techniques for patients post-anaesthesia, 120 patients with mild or moderate hypothermia were systematically assigned to one of the two groups fulfilling the following criteria: 'The following selection criteria were used for all participants: having undergone general, orthopaedic, urological, vascular or gynaecological surgery; the procedure being greater than 20 minutes durations (excludes minor procedures); and having had a general, regional or epidural/spinal anaesthetic. All severely hypothermic patients (less than 35 degrees Celsius) were excluded from the study' (Stevens et al. 2000, p. 271).

Sampling approaches for quantitative studies

In quantitative studies both probability and non-probability approaches to sampling apply. Probability sampling approaches include simple random sampling, stratified random sampling, cluster sampling and systematic random sampling. Non-probability sampling approaches include convenience sampling, snowball sampling, purposive sampling and quota sampling.

Probability sampling approaches and procedures in quantitative studies

Simple random sampling

Simple random sampling is defined as an approach in which every case has the same opportunity to be selected for the study. The procedure involves obtaining a complete listing of cases in the population, allocating a number for each case, and generating a set of random numbers. Tools are available to generate random numbers such as add-on modules for Microsoft Excel™ or using a table of random numbers (see Appendix 8.1).

Table 8.1 outlines an example of random sampling using numbers. A nurse investigator needs to select, say, 10 study participants from an outpatient clinic that has 200 patient bookings per week. The nurse initially obtains a listing of all the health care record numbers of the patients attending during the defined period of one week. Every health care record number is then allocated a number from 1 to 200. Then, using either a random numbers table or random numbers generated by computer software, the following numbers are generated: 2, 3, 77, 85, 23, 45, 62, 99, 144, 192. The patients (health care record numbers) selected at random (using generated numbers) are requested to participate in the study.

Table 8.1   Selecting a random sample of 10 study participants from an outpatient listing of 200 patients

Health Care Record Number	Name	Numbers allocated by researcher
R6249	Frederick Topaz	1
P2278	Mary Jacobs	2*
Z4477	Amanda Chan	3*
T3395	Steven Jones	4
C2388	Samir Fernandez	5
...	...	...
D6785	Sophie Nyguen	200

*Patients selected using random numbers.

Stratified random sampling

This segments the population according to existing strata (category of nurse, qualifications, current place of work) that are relevant to the research study. The researcher obtains a listing of all cases within the relevant strata and then selects the sample from within the strata, so that the existing distribution within each stratum is retained. This method is used if each stratum (or group) contains distinctly different types of units or individuals from those in other strata. By using stratified sampling we can ensure that each distinct group within a population (or stratum) is fairly represented in a sample. As Lohr (2008) notes, for the sample to reflect the overall characteristics of the population, the researcher 'uses a stratified design with proportional allocation, in which the same proportion of population units is sampled in each stratum' (p. 107).

Cluster random sampling

Cluster random sampling is often used in studies where the entire population is being studied. It is commonly used to reduce the costs of the project by decreasing the geographic distribution of the sample (Neuman 2006). Here it is important that the clusters (or groups) are similar to one another or the sampling may contribute to a bias.

For example, we will assume there are 12 hospitals with operating rooms in Melbourne. Operating room nurses consist of registered nurses, nursing educators and nurse managers. We will randomly select four clusters (or hospitals), and all operating room nurses (i.e. registered nurses, nursing educators and clinical nurse managers) working in those selected four hospitals become our sample (Figure 8.2).

Maree Johnson and Sungwon Chang

Figure 8.2   Cluster sampling

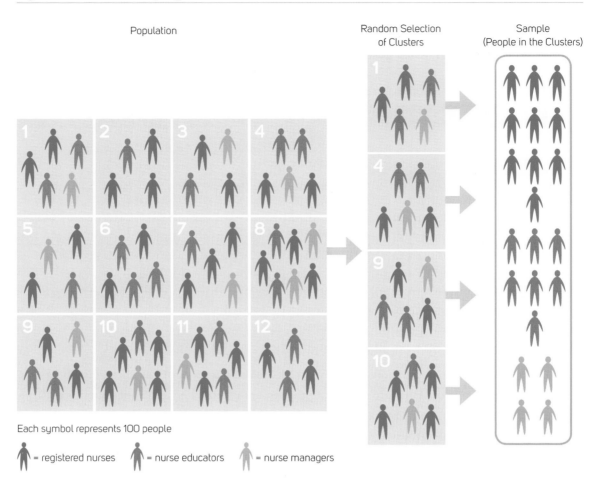

Population   Random Selection   Sample
                             of Clusters   (People in the Clusters)

Each symbol represents 100 people

👤 = registered nurses   👤 = nurse educators   👤 = nurse managers

Source: Derived from the original figure from Leedy & Ormrod 2005, p. 204

Systematic random sampling

This is an approach where the total number required is much smaller than the available population. For example, a researcher is seeking a total number of patients required (500 patients) from a listing of all patients who attended the outpatients clinic in 2008 (N = 5000). Since only 500 patients are required, every tenth patient (or having an interval width of 10; 5000/500 = 10) from the list is selected to result in the required 500 patients. For this method to be truly random the first selected patient in the list must be randomly selected (referred to as a random start). This is achieved by selecting a random number (from the random number table or by computer generation), in this example between 1 and 500 as the starting point (say, 44).

The relative merits of the various probability sampling approaches are outlined in Table 8.2.

Table 8.2   Summary of the advantages and disadvantages of the various types of probability sampling methods

Sampling method	When to use it	Advantages	Disadvantages
Simple random sampling	When the population is similar to one another on the research variable	No chance of introducing researcher bias as all units in the population have equal chance of being selected Does not require extensive prior knowledge of the population Ideal for statistical purposes	Requires an accurate list of the whole population, which is hard to achieve, especially in a large population Time-consuming
Stratified random sampling	When the population consists of different distinct groups that may influence the research outcome	Achieves an adequate representation of subgroups, which may not be achieved by simple random or systematic sampling	Required to know the characteristics of the target population in order that stratification can be achieved Time-consuming
Cluster sampling	When readily available sampling frame consists of clusters (or groups) as sampling units rather than individual units	Less expensive than simple random as it is easier to access units within a cluster than across a cluster	Larger sampling errors than simple or stratified
Systematic sampling	When the populations are similar on a research variable	Ensures a high degree of representativeness of the population Easier than simple random sampling as there is no need to use a randomisation process	Ordering of elements in sampling frame may create biases if the system interacts with some hidden pattern in the population Less random than simple random sampling

Sampling for surveys

Conducting a large survey requires particular attention to sampling procedures to ensure that an adequate sample is obtained. Three aspects of sampling ensure sampling adequacy: the sample frame (entire group of people or units with the characteristics or attribute under study), the sample size and the specific design of the sampling procedures. Crockett's guide comprehensively outlines considerations for surveys: the resources available (time, money and personnel), accuracy (standard error), the amount of detail needed in the results or number of subgroups, the proportion of the population with the attributes to be measured, the variability of the attributes in the target population, the non-response rate expected, and the sample design (Crockett 1989).

Sampling error refers to the variation of the sample mean from the population; the lower the sampling error, the less chance the responses received may not be reflective of the true answers of the entire population. Non-response rates are particularly important in estimating the sample size required. Wherever possible, the researcher should locate surveys carried out in similar populations to estimate the likely response rate. Response rates can vary within important subgroups—nurse managers may respond to surveys more frequently than clinical nurses, for instance. Response rates of 60% or more are recommended (Badger & Werrett 2005).

In many complex studies the use of several sampling strategies is required. For example, in the study of nurses' clinical skills, by Johnson and associates (2001), identified a sampling frame of nurses from the annual survey of the Nurses Registration Board of New South Wales (sampling frame), three types of sampling approaches were used:

> This database was accessed using a specially designed computer program and a series of sampling strategies—all nurses from some specialty groups; systematic sampling, or selecting every third nurse on the list of other specialty groups; and stratified random sampling from other groups—to result in a group of 11621 nurses being available to participate in the…study. (p. 48)

Random selection in experimental studies

Experimental studies or clinical trials use random selection and random assignment. These terms should not be used interchangeably. As noted above, random selection refers to the selection of a subset of cases from a listing of all cases using a random numbers table or computer number generation procedures. Random assignment or allocation refers to the assignment of a selected case (or patient) to a specific intervention group and is more fully described under designs (see Chapter 5).

> In a study of women's and midwives experiences of using perineal warm packs in the second stage of labour: '…a randomised controlled trial was undertaken. In the late second stage of labour, nulliparous women (N=717) giving birth were randomly allocated to having warm packs (n=360) applied to their perineum or standard care (n = 357).' (Dahlen et al. in press)

Non-probability sampling approaches in quantitative studies

The major non-probability sampling approaches include convenience sampling (also referred to as accidental), purposive sampling, network sampling, quota sampling and snowball sampling.

- *Convenience sampling* is an approach where the nurse researcher locates a sample that is 'convenient'. This sample may or may not be representative of the population. This approach is frequently used in nursing research and is appropriate when little is known about the topic.
- *Purposive sampling* is where the researcher recruits participants to the study based on some attribute that the researcher feels is appropriate. For example, a nurse researcher may wish to obtain information on decision-making in complex wound care. The researcher recruits nurses from the burns units and plastic surgery units because these wards would reflect complex wounds and the nursing management of such wounds.

- *Network sampling* is where the researcher knows a number of participants who could be involved in a study by virtue of their position.
- *Quota sampling* involves a process where nurse investigators wish to obtain a distribution on a particular characteristic that is important to the study. For example, a nurse investigator may wish to recruit patients with venous leg ulcers with a certain surface area (known to heal at differing rates). By having 10 patients with small wound surface areas (5–500 mm2), 10 patients with medium surface areas (501–2000 mm2), and 10 with large surface areas (2001–5000 mm2), a distribution of areas is included.

▶▶▶ TERMS, TIPS AND SKILLS

Quota sampling involves a process where nurse investigators wish to obtain a distribution on a particular characteristic (fill a quota) that is important to the study.

- *Snowball sampling* is the final approach and involves the identification of potential study participants through contact with key informants or other participants. This approach is often used where a condition or attribute is rare or sensitive in nature, where the best way to obtain a sample is by contacting an initial few cases and asking them about other potential participants. For example, in a study of adaptive behaviours of young women with multiple sclerosis, a researcher could contact the Multiple Sclerosis Society and ask if any initial members would be interested in participating. These initial study participants then recommend others known to them.

Sampling approaches for qualitative studies

There are a variety of sampling approaches suitable for qualitative research studies. In qualitative studies, information-rich study participants are being sought, and the researcher considers how that need for information influences their choice of sampling approach.

The most comprehensive listing was developed by Kuzel (1992), who also provided details of some issues to consider with the various approaches. The design of the qualitative study, in many cases, mandates a particular style of sampling. Table 8.3 gives an example of a qualitative design where a certain approach is applied.

▶▶▶ TERMS, TIPS AND SKILLS

To locate information-rich participants, consider which participants are most likely to describe the key study aspects: length of illness, experience with the context, intensity of symptoms.

A *convenience sample* is the simplest approach where those participants who meet the selection criteria and are available for inclusion in the study are included. This method is frequently used in studies conducted by nurses and midwives. As noted below, Kuzel (1992) suggests that this approach may reduce available depth of information and credibility (p. 38). Other writers confirm that this is a 'good place to start when little or no work has been done on a particular subject' (Shields & Twycross 2008, p. 37).

Purposive sampling is a common approach in qualitative studies and is defined as the selection of participants who fulfil a specific purpose consistent with a study's aims or purposes (Collingridge & Gantt 2008; Tuckett 2004). Miles and Huberman (1994) first described three types of information-rich cases in purposive samples as typical (average cases), deviant (extreme cases with unusual manifestations) and negative or disconfirming cases (cases that do not fit the pattern or rule) (Miles & Huberman 1994). The inclusion of a variety of participants enhances the depth of the text data available.

In *ethnography*, the focus on analysis of settings of interest to the researcher has created some confusion in relation to sampling in ethnographic studies. Wolf (2007) describes ethnography as concerned with studying cultures. The researcher seeks to become part of the cultural group in order to describe the cultural group norms, values and worldviews. A contemporary viewpoint proposed by Gobo (2008) is that sampling is relevant to ethnography and follows a two-step process, conceptualisation and selection of cases or observation units: 'The researcher clarifies the attributes of the topic that he or she intends to study; then, for each attribute he or she determines first the units of observation… second the setting(s) to be visited and then the set of cases (the sample)' (p. 98). Nurse ethnographers observe behaviours or activities between or by persons within a setting and are not observing a setting (such as a ward or hospital) as such.

In a study of how clinical nurses learn within a neonatal intensive care unit (NICU):

> An ethnographic approach was used…The context was a 20-bed NICU catering for infants with cardiac and surgical anomalies and complex medical conditions. Digital recordings of ward work between clinicians at the crib-side and recorded interviews with key informants from the different levels of nurse clinicians…The participants were 32 nurse clinicians, 14 medical registrars, 5 allied health workers, a nurse educator, a clinical nurse consultant, a nurse manager, 5 senior medical specialists and 1 administrative worker (57% of the unit population, constituting a mix of informants. (Hunter et al. 2008, pp. 657, 659)

Table 8.3 describes the various sampling approaches for qualitative studies and provides the reader with aspects or considerations for each of the methods and where such methods may be applied.

Theoretical sampling is related to research that generates grounded theory and is best described as a process by which findings from a small number of cases determine theoretically important aspects that direct the sampling or characteristics of the participants

Table 8.3 Sampling approaches for qualitative studies: considerations and designs

Approach	Aspects/Considerations	Designs
Convenience	Available participants	Phenomenology
Criterion	All participants meet some criterion †	Ethnography, grounded theory, phenomenology
Deviant case/atypical case	Seen as a subset of a purposive sample/theoretical sampling approach (Tuckett 2004)	Grounded theory, phenomenology
Discomfirming case/negative case	Seen as a subset of a purposive/theoretical sample Cases that do not fit the pattern	Grounded theory, phenomenology
Homogeneous	Focuses, reduces, simplifies: facilitates group interviewing †	Qualitative technique: content analysis, thematic analysis (Focus groups)
Intensity	Information rich cases that manifest the phenomenon intensely (but not extremely) †	Grounded theory, phenomenology
Maximum variation	A subset of a purposive sample/theoretical sampling Documents diverse variations and identifies important common patterns †	Grounded theory, phenomenology
Opportunistic	Taking advantage of the unexpected †	Grounded theory, phenomenology
Purposive	Participants that fulfil a specific purpose/criterion consistent with the study aims	Ethnography, phenomenology
Quota	Used in studies where there is a wide variation in the sample	Ethnography
Snowball or chain	Identifies participants of interest through informed persons who may include other participants	Grounded theory, phenomenology, ethnography
Theoretical	Small selection of cases then evolves into a theoretically driven sampling approach	Grounded theory
Typical case	A subset of a purposive sample or theoretical sample Highlights what is normal or average †	Grounded theory, phenomenology

Note: † Derived from the original table in Kuzel 1992, p. 38.

to be included in the study (Higginbottom 2006). Theoretical sampling is described as 'sequential, beginning with selective sampling and moving into theoretical sampling when concepts begin to emerge' (Draucker et al. 2007, p. 1138). The decision is made by the researcher as to when to move from selective to theoretical sampling. Writers in grounded theory propose that theoretical sampling should continue throughout the data collection period, suggesting that unlike other methods of sampling, theoretical sampling is continuous throughout this period. As Strauss and Corbin (1998) note, 'theoretical sampling becomes more specific with time…sampling is aimed at developing, densifying, and saturating…

categories' (p. 203). The selection of participants ceases only when 'codes are saturated (further information is redundant), elaborated upon, and fully integrated into the emerging theory' (Boychuk Duchscher & Morgan 2004).

In a study exploring the nature of nurses' practice with vulnerable and marginalised populations, Wilson and Neville (2008) note: 'The research with 38 indigenous Maori women aged between 24 and 65 years, inductively analysed interview data using constant comparative analysis, theoretical sampling and saturation of the core categories to generate a substantive grounded theory' (p. 165).

Phenomenology is concerned with studying a small group of persons experiencing a defined phenomenon. As data collection involves in-depth interviews and often repeated interviews, a small number of participants (5–25) who have all experienced the phenomenon of interest should form the sample (Creswell 2007). Purposive sampling is often used with this method.

Mixed methods sampling approaches

Given the proliferation of mixed methods studies within the nursing and midwifery literature, a brief discussion of sampling methods for mixed methods is appropriate. Several examples of sampling approaches that combine probability and purposeful sampling are presented.

Criterion sampling is defined as a kind of purposeful sampling approach in which cases are selected from a list of cases (perhaps derived from a large quantitative study) that represent a particular criterion (Sandelowski 2000), such as a high or low score on a particular scale.

> [In a study of women in Canberra, a] subgroup of women with high and low fatigue scores (as measured by the Postpartum Fatigue Scale (PFS) developed by Milligan and others (1997)) were further examined to determine their fatigue management strategies postnatally. These 54 cases were drawn from the original study sample of 504 women identified through the survey phase of the study. (Taylor & Johnson 2009)

Random purposeful sampling is an approach in which a subset of cases is randomly selected from a large pool. In this situation, cases are selected when meeting a specific criterion, but are so large in number, even within that criterion, that a random selection is made to deliver a more manageable set of cases and related text. Sandelowski (2000) gives the example of a study where participants have less pain (500 participants), similar pain (150 participants) or more pain (50 participants) on a standardised measure. Information-rich cases (typical, atypical, maximum variation, disconfirming) are still present, although the investigator can now reduce the number of cases selected to a manageable size (say 20) from each grouping.

Stratified purposeful sampling applies where a nurse researcher is seeking to select a subset of cases that vary on a collection of characteristics (rather than just one criterion) that are of importance to the phenomenon being studied (Sandelowski 2000). For example, in a large survey of patient-adverse incidents, there are incidents for patients that occur at varying times, and at varying locations, for varying types of adverse events. Incidents that represent the falls incidents in the morning for patients who are male and within the bathroom facilities may form one subset, while medication incidents in the afternoon for females occurring in the ward area may form another subset. Initial quantitative data of say 5000 cases with text data on the description of the incident would form the listing for selection. Then all cases would need to be coded into the three characteristics (type of incident, gender, location) and a subset selected within each of the groupings, or perhaps even a subset with only two characteristics would be chosen.

Bias in sampling

Bias is any influence or condition that distorts the data. It can happen in sampling when we generalise from the sample to the population. Among the conditions that lead to bias is when the accessible population is not a good representation of the target population. Non-responses may also cause bias, especially if the non-respondents differ from the respondents in some way on the characteristics of interest.

Sample size

After gaining some understanding of sampling, the next consideration is to determine an appropriate sample size. The size of the sample should be large enough to help answer research questions and to generalise the findings from your sample to the underlying population with a high degree of confidence. However, it should be small enough to be efficient and economical.

So how do you find the 'correct' sample size? There are a range of resources available to help you find the answer. There are tables that give approximate sample sizes for various situations as well as statistical programs to calculate sample size. There are also websites that can be used for calculating sample size (see Weblinks). But they all generally require some understanding of statistics, and the researcher needs to have decided on several key issues.

To start with, there is a slight difference in the information required to calculate a sample size for surveys (where the main purpose would be to estimate the population characteristics) to, say, clinical trials (where the main purpose is to test for differences between groups).

To make reliable estimates of population characteristics from your sample, the researcher needs to specify:

- an acceptable error rate involved in or making estimation of the population characteristics from the sample, usually referred to as level of precision or sampling error;
- an acceptable level of risk or confidence that the error rate will be larger than predicted. Another way to express it is an acceptable level of risk in selecting a 'bad' sample. It is sometimes expressed as a confidence level; and
- the amount of variability in the population on the characteristics of research interest.

For example, Table 8.4 shows approximate sample sizes for different population sizes at 5% level of precision and 95% confidence level. There are similar tables with a different combination of precision and confidence levels.

Table 8.4   Sample sizes based on the 95% confidence level and 5% level of precision for populations of 10 to 1 000 000

N	n	N	n	N	n	N	n
10	10	110	86	300	169	1 000	278
15	14	120	92	320	175	1 500	306
20	19	130	97	340	181	2 000	322
25	24	140	103	360	186	3 000	341
30	28	150	108	380	191	3 500	346
35	32	160	113	400	196	4 000	351
40	36	170	118	420	201	4 500	354
45	40	180	123	440	205	5 000	257
50	44	190	127	460	210	6 000	361
55	48	200	132	480	214	7 000	364
60	52	210	136	500	217	8 000	356
65	56	220	140	550	226	9 000	368
70	59	230	144	699	234	10 000	370
75	63	240	148	650	242	50 000	381
80	66	250	152	700	248	75 000	382
85	70	260	155	750	254	100 000	384
90	73	270	159	800	260	250 000	384
95	76	280	162	850	265	500 000	384
100	80	290	165	900	269	1 000 000	384

Source: Derived from original table by Krejecie & Morgan 1970, p. 608

Note: N stands for the size of the population; n stands for the size of the recommended sample.

In studies where the purpose is to detect an effect (e.g. difference between groups), the researcher needs the following information to calculate the sample size:

- the minimum size of meaningful clinical difference or an effect size
- the desired significance level
- the type of test to be used
- the population variability
- whether the analysis will involve one- or two-sided tests.

Estimating sample size is a complex area and more advanced readings are recommended. Explanations for the above terms as well as methods for calculating sample size can be found in general statistics books such as Bland (2000). Schlesselman (1982) describes a method used to calculate a sample size of case-control studies. For more specialised readings refer to Dattalo (2008).

As seen above, every situation is different and the sample size depends on the nature of the population as well as the type of statistical analysis expected to be used in the study. In general, the following situations require a larger sample size:

- If there is greater variability in population (i.e. there is more diversity in the characteristic of interest).
- If the population is diverse then you would need a larger number in the sample to ensure this diversity is represented.
- If the data analysis will take place on several subgroups, then a large enough sample size is required at the subgroup level.
- If a high level of precision is desired in making inference to the population from the sample you would require a larger sample size. Remember, the larger the sample size the smaller the sampling error (5% or less desired).
- When a less efficient sampling method has been used. For example, cluster sampling is less efficient in representing the population than proportional stratified sampling. Hence you would need a larger sample to generalise to the population with the same degree of confidence.
- If you expect that a low percentage of people will agree to participate in the study, then increase the sample size to ensure the final number in the study is adequate to answer the research question with adequate power.

Summary

Throughout this chapter we have explored both qualitative and quantitative sampling methods. Sampling is an essential part of the design of any research study and requires precise definition to ensure research questions are adequately addressed within the study. The selection of which sampling approach to take can be made using key criteria outlined in the tables provided for qualitative and quantitative sampling methods.

Finally, when a research study is published considerable detail of the sampling approach should be included so that other researchers can replicate the study. Attention to sampling within the design process can result in considerable cost and time savings for researchers.

IMPLICATIONS FOR EVIDENCE-BASED NURSING AND MIDWIFERY

Evidence-based practitioners are familiar with all the types of sampling approaches available. Contemporary perspectives on the selection and inclusion of studies into systematic reviews allow for both qualitative and quantitative studies to be considered. Randomised control trials (see Chapter 6) remain the best possible research evidence support for clinical interventions. Simple random sampling and probabilistic sampling are fundamental to RCTs.

Qualitative research also plays a vital role in shaping policy and an examination of the quality of any quantitative or qualitative study should include a review of the sampling methods used.

When using quantitative or qualitative designs the subtle nuances of the various sampling approaches should be carefully considered before undertaking any research study. Sampling is critical to ensuring that participants are representative of the population, or have experienced the phenomenon of interest, or represent key concepts in an evolving theory or a cultural context under consideration. Appropriate sampling approaches are responsive to the study aims, research questions or hypotheses and help to build sound nursing and midwifery knowledge.

▶▶▶ **PROBLEM SOLVING 8.1**

Bob and his team have conducted a research project that aims to assess whether or not giving instruction and printed health education materials on self-management of chest pain will reduce the proportion of patients who re-present to the emergency department with chest pain within six months. They list all 12 hospitals in their city and categorise each hospital using the following criteria: tertiary level of hospital (referral hospital) or non-referral hospital. Based on the reported number of chest pain events by the state health department and available resources, four hospitals will be included as study sites. One will be a referral hospital and three will be non-referral hospitals. They randomly picked four hospitals from the list they generated.

a   What is the sampling strategy they used?

b   Is a hospital a sampling unit, sampling frame or a sample?

c   Who/what is the sample?

d   Who/what is the population?

Practice exercise 8.1
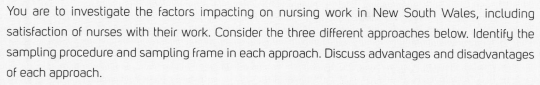

You are to investigate the factors impacting on nursing work in New South Wales, including satisfaction of nurses with their work. Consider the three different approaches below. Identify the sampling procedure and sampling frame in each approach. Discuss advantages and disadvantages of each approach.

- Take a random sample of 500 nurses from the list obtained from Nurses and Midwives Board NSW of all registered nurses.
- Take a random sample of 200 nurses from each area of practice as obtained from Nurses and Midwives Board NSW.
- Pick a random number K between 1 and 100. Starting with the kth nurse on the list from Nurses and Midwives Board NSW, select every 50th nurse on the list.

Practice exercise 8.2

For each of the sampling types below, decide first whether the type would be appropriate for quantitative or qualitative research or both, and second, whether the type represents probability or non-probability or both approaches. Present your answer as a table.

	Quantitative/qualitative/both	Probability/non-probability/both
1. Typical case		
2. Simple random sample		
3. Theoretical sampling		
4. Maximum variation case		
5. Deviation case		
6. Cluster random sample		
7. Systematic sample		
8. Purposive sample		
9. Convenience sample		

Practice exercise 8.3

Below are two fictitious studies outlining aspects of sampling:

Study a

A phenomenological study of women's lived experience of osteoarthritis was undertaken.

A purposive sample of 20 women with osteoarthritis was chosen based on the number of years of experiencing the disease, the range of medications taken including complementary medicines, and the use of other therapies. Typical and maximum variation cases were included to provide rich data.

Study b

A midwifery-initiated oral health screening tool and assessment process is to be trialled in the antenatal clinic at Christchurch Hospital. Women (200 in treatment group and 200 in the control group) will be randomly allocated to either the treatment group (women receive a set of oral health screening items and a free oral assessment by an oral hygienist) or the control group (women receive an oral health promotion brochure and a delayed treatment similar to the treatment group at a later stage in the study).

Answer the following for each of these studies:

i   What type of sampling approach was used?

ii   Was this approach appropriate for the study? If so, why? If not so, why?

iii Will the findings derived from this sample be likely to be generalisable to either the population or to other groups and why?

Practice exercise 8.4

Below is a fictitious study. Please suggest a sampling approach that you believe is appropriate.

The nurses' and midwives' registering authority of Western Australia has commissioned you to undertake a survey of all nurses and midwives to determine their beliefs about a national recruitment strategy for nurses not actively working in health care. Describe how you would ensure that all categories of nurses and midwives could be included in the study. Define the sampling frame and sampling plan or approach and say how you would proceed.

Answers to problem solving 8.1

a

stratified sampling method

b

sampling unit

c

patients who presented at the ED with chest pain at four hospitals

d

patients who presented at the ED with chest pain at 12 hospitals

Answers to practice exercises

8.1

The sampling procedure here is a simple random sampling. The population we wish to sample is nurses working in New South Wales. In this approach, we assume the sampling frame (the list of nurses from Nurses and Midwives Board [NMB] NSW) would be very close to the population (all nurses working in New South Wales) and the sampling units are the population units. The main advantage of this procedure is there is a high degree of representativeness in the sample, that is, the sampling frame should be similar to the population.

This is an example of stratified random sampling. This approach would be used if there is a belief that specific areas of nursing practice would affect work satisfaction (i.e. the topic of the study). The strata here are different areas of nursing practice. Hence the list obtained from the NMB will be prepared separately for each area of practice (emergency, medical/surgical, etc.). Stratified sampling ensures a high degree of representativeness. For the example here, all areas of practice will be represented in the final sample. The main disadvantage is that it is time-consuming.

This is an example of systematic sampling. The sampling frame is the same as for simple random sampling. The main advantage is you can achieve a high degree of representativeness without using a table of random numbers. The disadvantage is that it is less representative than a simple random sampling.

8.2

Type of sample	Quantitative	Qualitative	Both	Probability	Non-probability	Both
Typical case		X			X	
Simple random sample			X	X		
Theoretical sampling		X			X	
Maximum variation case		X			X	
Deviation case		X			X	
Cluster random sample	X			X		
Systematic sample (with random start)	X			X		
Purposive sample			X		X	
Convenience sample			X		X	

8.3a

i   Purposive sampling.

ii   Purposive sampling was appropriate as the researcher wished to include women experiencing the disease at differing stages, and using a range of therapies.

iii The findings (thematic understandings) may be generalisable to other groups of women with osteoarthritis who have similar characteristics.

8.3b

i   Simple random selection or allocation.

ii   The method is appropriate because the researcher wishes to ensure that every case has an equal chance of participating and that no bias is indirectly introduced by the researcher-selected patients, who are more likely to have a better response to the intervention.

iii The findings will be generalisable to similar populations with similar characteristics to this sample.

Appendix 8.1
A Random Numbers Table

Guide to using a random numbers table

A random numbers table is used to select random numbers. First, the researcher applies a number to each unit in the sampling frame. Next, consider the size of the accessible population in your sampling frame. If, for example, the population is 100 cases then only two-digit numbers (01–99) are considered. Determine the starting point randomly (i.e. close your eyes and randomly select anywhere in the table). Then start with the upper left-hand digits in the designated block and work downward through the numbers in the table.

In an example in Chapter 8, 'a nurse investigator needed to select, say 10 study participants from an outpatient clinic that has 200 patient bookings per week'. Hence we will need up to three-digit numbers less than 200. Say the starting point was column C, row 15 (612155). The first three-digit number is 612. As the population is 200, there is no one with a number allocation of 612 in your list. Hence this number is skipped. Then go to the next three-digit number <155> and there is a person with that number. Person 155 on the list is selected. Going down the list the next three-digit number is 36, also on the listing. Continue to select three-digit numbers until you have all 10 values between 001 and 200.

Maree Johnson and Sungwon Chang

Random numbers table

1	2	3	4	5	6	7	8	9	10
45280	67711	73860	2295	43548	46348	64506	83473	73456	30067
17913	23253	7231	55297	84542	70251	39680	4836	9368	48889
22185	10436	45684	39939	83733	25794	73051	57838	50361	72792
58097	2700	15777	29662	88005	12977	11504	42480	49552	54893
99091	53161	90950	51025	97359	31799	81596	32203	53825	42075
71724	8704	24322	4027	64911	55702	56770	53566	63179	34339
49293	75997	95887	62774	62111	37544	37803	90141	6568	30730
68779	70656	11909	14708	32867	78392	41816	98427	28594	91209
91614	75592	23658	79460	38612	8041	99755	77728	17249	98686
90546	78796	14045	8300	52093	94155	41412	52757	33471	45625
17854	65920	21722	80874	76860	42016	19990	59511	40948	23195
21058	56307	50562	94355	62975	83674	95019	87542	9972	42680
68720	39880	26399	40285	98628	50157	22126	53102	60175	65515
12109	36271	63784	28131	61647	34540	42421	92219	69383	64447
34135	70192	8904	45884	34944	14649	75533	92882	93950	90746
22790	77669	86474	13177	33067	73397	99291	74724	48425	764
31740	24263	46693	79401	7836	49089	25331	43489	89014	78997
86878	85405	16381	23454	28794	12772	60838	90082	75792	45221
24926	71261	5700	55498	6104	27726	15977	51225	18922	62715
60234	96291	35003	71983	61043	40748	1632	18981	20049	16845
3768	12572	39275	59166	99495	25390	823	74524	26862	69847
5500	33935	75188	51429	69588	15113	5095	61706	65315	27931
38871	86937	16181	1891	71319	36476	41007	80528	35407	44212
77324	45021	88814	57434	78133	89478	82001	4432	37139	65574
47416	61302	93087	44616	43144	74119	54634	59975	43953	92019
84801	22590	82664	28999	63438	86678	63843	58906	47157	82405
3363	40344	55961	35667	96550	87341	88410	85205	94818	65979
80933	7636	27526	94414	93750	69183	42884	95223	38207	62370
82606	98223	77928	38812	29603	30671	27467	37080	8241	21317
49898	69788	36676	36012	11445	11704	64043	80469	4632	58702
44557	85810	88610	6768	52293	15718	72329	2496	65111	77265
49493	97559	53361	12513	81942	73656	51630	91151	72588	54834
52698	87946	82201	25994	68056	15313	26658	19181	41612	47762
359	71520	58038	71924	30267	55239	53766	84742	91814	97155
43748	41353	95423	59770	93287	66179	74060	23858	74465	96087
35608	39217	1832	40544	50966	66584	46289	7173	24522	25590
10377	14909	54430	9309	18113	44816	38148	5036	30931	79806
26458	97618	84137	98023	56366	81337	79865	10840	80269	83069
67451	21522	85869	19385	92278	159	49957	564	47821	6972
66642	77065	92682	72388	33271	50620	51689	48484	76660	20454
70915	64247	31135	57029	5904	6163	58502	74928	52498	66383
76197	17449	1227	46752	36735	93346	96955	18518	89882	54229
81133	29199	2959	68115	46089	85610	67047	2900	35203	66988
84337	19586	89073	9772	21117	13640	36071	9568	96491	56566
22386	31999	24726	76256	48225	79201	86273	68315	14245	29862
80065	32403	87746	60638	68520	18317	95482	20249	81537	1427
17045	48021	28535	33876	58443	38408	57375	47357	3968	72992
37339	60579	37744	32808	13840	44153	13581	78737	83269	27063
70452	61243	62311	59107	76601	57634	99696	46953	31335	64852
67652	43085	16786	69124	48830	89678	3564	61906	59570	52034

Further reading

Bland, M. (2000). *An Introduction to Medical Statistics.* Oxford: Oxford University Press.

Creswell, J. W. (2007). *Qualitative Inquiry and Research Design: Choosing Among Five Approaches.* London: Sage Publications.

Dattalo, P. (2008). *Determining Sample Size: Balancing Power, Precision, and Practicality.* New York: Oxford University Press.

Lohr, S. L. (2008). Coverage and sampling. In J. Hox., E. De Leeuw & D. A. Dillman (eds), *The International Handbook of Survey Methodology* (pp. 97–112). New York: Lawrence Erlbaum Associates.

Neuman, W. L. (2006). *Social Research Methods: Qualitative and Quantitative Approaches,* 6th edn. Boston: Pearson/Allyn & Bacon.

Weblinks

A program that can be used for random selection and random assignment can be found on the following sites:

<www.randomizer.org>

<www.random.org>

Another site that provides a program for random assignment:

<www.graphpad.com/quickcalcs/randomize1.cfm>

Here is a sample size calculator for surveys:

<www.surveysystem.com/sscalc.htm>

The following two sites have a free G-Power Program to determine sample size needed:

<www.psycho.uni-duesseldorf.de/aap/projects/gpower/how_to_use_gpower.html>

<hedwig.mgh.harvard.edu/sample_size/size.html#ssize>

References

Badger, F., & Werrett, J. (2005). Room for improvement? Reporting response rates and recruitment in nursing research in the past decade: Methodological issues in nursing research. *Journal of Advanced Nursing* 51(5), 502–10.

Bland, M. (2000). *An Introduction to Medical Statistics*. Oxford: Oxford University Press.

Boychuk Duchscher, J. E., & Morgan, D. (2004). Grounded theory: Reflections on the emergence vs. forcing debate. *Journal of Advanced Nursing* 48(6), 605–12.

Chwalisz, K., Shah, S. R., & Hand, K. M. (2008). Facilitating rigorous qualitative research in rehabilitation psychology. *Rehabilitation Psychology* 53(3), 387–99.

Collingridge, D. S., & Gantt, E. E. (2008). The quality of qualitative research. *American Journal of Medical Quality* 23, 389.

Creswell, J. W. (2007). *Qualitative Inquiry and Research Design: Choosing Among Five Approaches.* London: Sage Publications.

Crockett, R. A. (1989). *An Introduction to Sample Surveys: A Users Guide.* Catalogue No. 12020.2. Canberra: Australian Bureau of Statistics.

Dahlen, G. H., Homer, C. S. E., Cooke, M., Upton, A. M., Nunn, R. A., & Brodrick, B. R. (in press). 'Soothing the ring of fire'. Australian women's and midwives' experiences of using perineal warm packs in the second stage of labour. *Midwifery.* Doi:10.106/j.midw.207.08.002.

Dattalo, P. (2008). *Determining Sample Size: Balancing Power, Precision, and Practicality.* New York: Oxford University Press.

Draucker, C. G., Marsolf, D. S., Ross, R., & Rusk, T. B. (2007). Theoretical sampling and category development in grounded theory. *Qualitative Health Research* 17(8), 1137–48.

Edwards, T. (2008). *Research Design and Statistics: A Bio-Behavioural Focus.* Sydney: McGraw-Hill Australia.

Gobo, G. (2008). *Doing Ethnography.* Los Angeles: Sage.

Hammersley P., & Mairs, H. (2004). Sampling methods. *Nurse Researcher* 12(1), 4–6.

Hart, M. (2006). Birthing a research project. *International Journal of Childbirth Education* 22(2), 31–4.

Higginbottom, G. (2006). Sampling issues in qualitative research. *Nurse Research* 12(1), 7–19.

Hunter, C. I., Spence, K., McKenna, K., & Iedema, R. (2008). Learning how we learn: An ethnographic study in neonatal intensive care unit. *Journal of Advanced Nursing* 62(6), 657–64.

Johnson, M., Marsden, J., Day, E., & Chang, S. (2001). Nursing skill assessment within populations: Scale developing and testing. *Contemporary Nurse* 10, 46–57.

Krejecie, R. V., & Morgan, D. W. (1970). Determining sample size for research activities. *Educational and Psychological Measurement* 30(3), 607–10.

Kuzel, A. J. (1992). Sampling in qualitative inquiry. In B. F. Crabtree & W. L. Miller (eds), *Doing Qualitative Research: Research Methods for Primary Care*, vol. 3 (pp. 31–44). Newbury Park, CA: Sage Publications.

Leedy, P. D., & Ormrod, J. E. (2005). *Practical Research: Planning and Design.* Upper Saddle River, NJ: Prentice Hall.

Lohr, S. L. (2008). Coverage and sampling. In J. Hox, E. De Leeuw & D. A. Dillman (eds), *The International Handbook of Survey*, (pp. 97–112). New York: Lawrence Erlbaum Associates.

Miles, M. B., & Huberman, A. (1984). *Qualitative Data Analysis. A Sourcebook of New Methods.* Beverly Hills, CA: Sage Publications.

Munro, B. H. (2005). *Statistical Methods for Health Care Research.* Philadelphia: Lippincott, Williams & Wilkins.

Neuman, W. L. (2006). *Social Research Methods: Qualitative and Quantitative Approaches*, 6th edn. Boston: Pearson/Allyn & Bacon.

Nieswiadomy, R. M. (2008). *Foundations of Nursing Research*, 5th edn. New Jersey: Pearson Education.

Safman, R. M., & Sobal, J. (2004). Qualitative sample extensiveness in health education research. *Health Education & Behaviour* 31, 9–21.

Sandelowski, M. (2000). Focus on research methods. Combining qualitative and quantitative sampling, data collection, and analysis techniques in mixed method studies. *Research in Nursing & Health* 23, 246–55.

Schlesselman, J. J. (1982). *Case-Control Studies: Design, Conduct, Analysis*. New York: Oxford University Press.

Shields, L., & Twycross, A. (2008). Sampling in quantitative research. *Paediatric Nursing* 20(5), 37.

Stevens, D., Johnson, M., & Langdon, R. (2000). Comparison of two warming interventions in surgical patients with mild and moderate hypothermia. *International Journal of Nursing Practice* 6, 268–75.

Strauss, A., & Corbin, J. (1998). *Basics of Qualitative Research. Techniques and Procedures for Developing Grounded Theory*. London: Sage Publications.

Taylor, J., & Johnson, M. (2009). How women manage fatigue after childbirth. *Midwifery* 26(3), 367–75.

Tuckett, A. G. (2004). Qualitative research sampling: The very real complexities. *Nurse Researcher* 12(1), 47–61.

Wilson, D., & Neville, S. (2008). Nursing their way not our way: Working with vulnerable and marginalised populations. *Contemporary Nurse* 27(2), 165–76.

Wolf, Z. R. (2007). Ethnography: The method. In P. L. Munhall (ed.), *Nursing Research: A Qualitative Perspective* (pp. 293–319), 4th edn. Boston: Jones & Bartlett Publishers.

CHAPTER 9

Data Collection: Qualitative Research

Anthony Welch and Sansnee Jirojwong

Chapter learning objectives

By the end of this chapter you will be able to:

▶ identify data collection methods used in qualitative research

▶ align data collection methods with different approaches to qualitative research

▶ discuss the use of triangulation as a means of data collection

▶ discuss the concepts of rigour and trustworthiness in relation to data collection methods in qualitative research.

KEY TERMS

Clarifying question

Closed-ended question

Focus group

Open-ended question

Participant observation

Probing question

Semistructured interview

Structured interview

Triangulation

Unstructured interview

Introduction

Fundamental to credible research—research that produces appropriate, accurate and reliable data—is the method/s by which data are collected. Research studies can be meticulously designed and rigorously carried out, but unless the method/s of data collection are consistent with the chosen research question and research design, and gathered in a competent and transparent manner, the findings of a study may be challenged for accuracy, completeness and therefore credibility. Qualitative research is no exception. This chapter introduces you to the various methods and processes of data collection used in qualitative research.

Data collection methods in qualitative research

Within the qualitative research paradigm there are various research designs that a researcher can use in search of new knowledge and understanding (see Chapter 5). Depending on the question being asked, the theoretical framework underpinning the study, the research design, the type of data and the method/s by which such data are collected vary. What is important is the interconnection of these three elements of research.

Figure 9.1 The interconnection of research design, type of data and data collection method

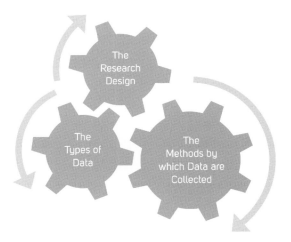

Preparing for the process of data collection

An essential aspect of any study is to ensure that the approach to data collection is consistent with the research question, the philosophical underpinnings of the research design, and the best approach by which 'rich' data can be accessed to answer the research question. This requires careful planning by the researcher. In planning the process of data collection for a particular qualitative study, three elements are of primary importance: a review of literature on the topic or phenomenon, participant selection and the methods by which data will be collected.

Figure 9.2   Key elements of the data collection process

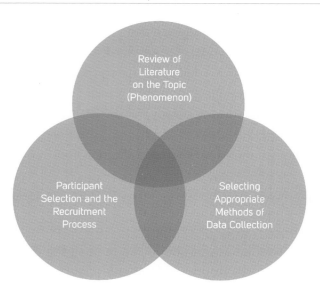

Review of the literature

An important component of the data collection process is to review what is already known about the topic to be investigated and to provide a context for the study. A review of literature is 'a systematic and rigorous exploration of the extant (existing) literature related to the concept(s) of interest' (Schneider et al. 2003) to the researcher. In some instances the review of literature may lead to refining the research question, clarifying the research design, altering the process(s) of participant selection and choosing strategies or modes for data collection.

In qualitative research, there is debate about the timing of a literature review. For instance, in phenomenological research, carrying out a literature review at the beginning of the study may lead to researcher bias. However, in grounded theory, a review of literature is made simultaneously with other modes of information-gathering such as interviews and participant observation.

Selecting participants

In qualitative research the process by which participants are selected is based on obtaining rich in-depth information of the research topic, the setting in which the study is to take place and who the participants are. Depending on the target group, different approaches to accessing participants can be used. Borbasi and others (2004, p. 134) have identified seven means by which participants can be accessed in qualitative research:

1   *Convenience sampling:* selection of participants based on availability
2   *Purposive sampling:* handpicking participants for a study

3   *Snowball sampling:* recruiting participants by asking those already in the study to identify others who would be suitable

4   *Extreme (deviant) sampling:* selection of participants who exemplify the phenomenon to be studied

5   *Intensity sampling:* selection of participants who can provide expert knowledge on the topic

6   *Maximum variety sampling:* selection of participants from different backgrounds who share a common experience such as happiness or being thankful

7   *Critical case sampling:* selection of participants who have been identified as a 'critical incident' while collecting data (modified from Borbasi et al. 2004, p. 143). (See also Chapter 8.)

Choosing a mode(s) for data collection

The choice of which mode(s) of data collection is to be used is important for the type of data to be collected. Each mode provides a particular form of data. Modes of data collection in qualitative research include individual, group and focus group interviews, dialogical engagement, observation, narrative descriptions, case studies, histories, field notes, audiovisual recordings, expressions of life/artistic representations and bricolage. Each of these methods provides unique avenues to accessing knowledge about an identified phenomenon or an issue of concern in the everyday world of human beings.

What is critical is ensuring that the right mode(s) is chosen for the type of study being undertaken and the type or form of information required to answer the research question. A brief description follows of the types or forms of data collection used in qualitative research.

Interviewing

Interviews are the most commonly used method of collecting data in qualitative research. Over time different interview methods have evolved as a means of eliciting particular forms of information. The various types of interviews can be perceived as 'on a continuum of structure ranging from highly structured to an unstructured' format (Taylor et al. 2007, p. 232). The use of a particular interview structure or format is determined by the purpose or aim of the study—the type of knowledge to be generated and the preferred means by which such information can be accessed. A number of terms have been assigned to particular types of interviews that have included 'unstructured' or 'informal conversational'; 'semi-structured', 'focused' or 'the general interview guide approach'; 'structured' or 'the standardized open-ended interview' (Patton 2002). However, the use of different terms to describe a particular approach can be problematic for the neophyte researcher. Clarification of the different terms assigned to a particular interview approach requires discussion.

▸▸▸   TERMS, TIPS AND SKILLS

The use of a particular type of interview format is determined by the purpose or aim of the study.

Figure 9.3   Frequently used types of interview

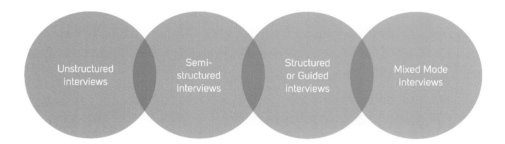

The unstructured interview

Unstructured interviews can be used in a variety of contexts to elicit in-depth knowledge of a particular topic or experience. The essential format of an unstructured interview involves either presenting a statement or posing a question and asking the participant to comment from their perspective. The initial statement or question is the central focus of the enquiry. Any additional questions asked by the researcher are generated from the participant's comments or descriptions for the purpose of clarification and/or elaboration to ensure that the information is accurate and a good understanding or comprehension of what the participant is saying is achieved. 'What might be rude to ask or be glossed over in friendly agreement in ordinary conversation—even with intimates—becomes grist for exploration' (Charmaz 2006, p. 26). The interview is not controlled by the researcher but moves with the flow of what the participant wishes to share about the topic under investigation. The term 'unstructured' is generic in nature—an interview approach that can be used in a range of qualitative research designs. Examples of research designs in which unstructured interviews usually form an important part of the information-gathering process include phenomenology, ethnography and grounded theory (see Chapter 5). However, unstructured interviews can be conducted in any qualitative research setting.

The phenomenological interview

The phenomenological interview is a relatively new term that owes its origins to the North American phenomenological movement of the middle to late 20th century. Rather than continuing the tradition of European phenomenology as originally presented in the works of Bretano and Husserl, in which phenomena were explored using the experiences of the researcher, phenomenology has been 'grafted' onto other philosophical movements such as humanism. The result for data collection has been the emergence of an approach to research that explores the life-world of others. The phenomenological interview has become the 'tool' for accessing the experiences lived by other human beings in the context of their everyday lives.

The goal of the phenomenological interview is to obtain a first-person description of a specified experience. Such an experience might focus on being ill, grieving the loss of a loved one or caring for a disabled child. The interview begins by asking the participant a question. The question is broadly stated to maximise the opportunity for the participant to respond in their own way by providing as full and rich a description of the phenomenon as possible. Such a question might be: What is your experience of being ill? Further questioning or comment by the researcher is concerned with seeking clarification about what the participant has described, or asking the participant to elaborate. An example of each type of question follows:

Clarifying question: You mentioned that being ill is a frustrating experience. Can you tell me what you mean by a frustrating experience?

Elaborating question: You mentioned you have been ill on a number of occasions. Can you tell me about those experiences?

What is essential in conducting a pheneomenological interview is to remain truthful to the subjective experiences of participants. The researcher does not deviate by asking questions of particular interest to themselves which are not directly related to the focus of the study, but moves with the flow of the participant's description of the phenomenon of enquiry. In other words 'all questions flow from the dialogue as it unfolds rather than having been predetermined in advance' (Pollio et al. 1997, p. 30). 'Why' questions are avoided because phenomenological enquiry is not concerned with causation. The introduction of a 'why' question has the potential to shift the focus of the discussion away from the actual experience of the phenomenon into unrelated areas that may ultimately compromise the findings.

▶▶▶ TERMS, TIPS AND SKILLS

In phenomenological enquiry 'why' questions are avoided because such enquiry is not concerned with causation.

Participants are viewed as co-researchers rather than research subjects (Giorgi 1989). The researcher is, in effect, a facilitator, assisting the participant to reflect on and provide the most comprehensive description of their experiences possible. Questions that facilitate an expanded discussion that contributes to achieving an information-rich, detailed description of participants' experiences could be:

'What was that experience like?'
'What was going through your mind at the time?'
'How did you feel when that occurred?'

In keeping with the principles of a rigorous and transparent approach to phenomenological research, two strategies or procedures have been identified to 'prevent, or at least miminize, the imposition of the researcher's presuppositions, and constructions on the data' (Crotty 1998, p. 83): the use of open-ended questions and the application of 'bracketing'. The only form of questioning throughout the interview process should be open-ended. To bracket is to attempt to acknowledge and set aside any pre-understandings of the phenomenon to be studied before data-gathering starts and to remain vigilant throughout the study to ensure that the data is not contaminated by the intrusion of the researcher's own agenda and bias.

Dialogical engagement

Dialogical engagement is a term coined by Dr Rosemarie Parse, the nurse theorist who developed the theory of humanbecoming (see Chapter 5). Dialogical engagement is defined by Parse (2001) 'as a true presence of the researcher [with the participant]' (p. 170). In contradistinction to the process of interviewing, in which the directional flow of conversation is guided by the researcher through the introduction of specific, often predetermined questions, dialogical engagement 'focuses on the phenomenon under study as it is described by the participant…the researcher stays in true presence with the participant without interjecting questions but may move the [dialogue] of the participant forward'.

The concept of dialogical engagement is a process of coming together (researcher with participant) (Parse 1998, p. 72). The dialogue with a participant commences with the researcher posing a question such as, What is it like to take life day by day? As the participant shares their experiences, the researcher moves with 'the rhythms of the sounds and silences [of the participant] as they describe the meaning of their experiences of the phenomenon under study' (Parse 1998, pp. 63–71). Throughout the dialogue the only verbalisation to be proffered by the researcher is to encourage the participant to expand their thoughts or to ask them to relate their comments to their experience of taking life day by day. Examples of such verbalisations are: 'Go on' or 'Please say more about your experience of…' (Parse 2001, p. 170).

Informal conversational interview

The informal conversational interview provides the researcher with 'maximum flexibility, spontaneity, and responsiveness to individual differences and situational changes' (Patton 2002, p. 343). The field of enquiry is regarded by the researcher as an open terrain for exploration. This form of information-gathering is sometimes referred to as unstructured or ethnographic interviewing. The term 'unstructured' is not to suggest that there is no intent or focus; on the contrary, although the interview is essentially a casual conversation, there is always 'a specific but implicit research agenda' (Fetterman 1989, p. 48). The researcher uses an informal approach as a means of accessing information.

Using an informal conversational interview approach, at the start of the study the researcher poses what Spradley and McCurdy (1972) term 'a grand tour question…designed to elicit a broad picture of the participant's…world, to map the cultural [or social] terrain' (p. 51). Such questions could be: Could you tell me about your family? or Can you show me around your nursing unit? Such an interview approach is most useful in ethnographic research.

As part of data collection the researcher engages in a sifting-searching process of enquiry because the open nature of the interview means that the information given by each participant will be peculiar to that person in content and delivery. Over a number of interviews with various participants a large amount of information is generated that requires synthesising and clarifying. One means by which this can be achieved is through repeat interviews. If repeat interviews are required with participants, the format and direction of the questions may change from the original interview as more specific information is sought. The use of predetermined questions in this later stage of clarifying information may be necessary in order to build on existing knowledge of what is being studied and to situate that knowledge within a context.

Conducting an unstructured or informal conversational interview appears on the surface not difficult. However, it requires great skill from the interviewer in several areas: interpersonal communication; the ability to ask probing and sensitive questions without intruding into the personal space of another; the ability to rapidly synthesise information on the spot and generate questions in a reflexive and timely manner; the ability to remain focused on the purpose of the study while moving with the flow of the conversation; and holding in abeyance personal biases and preconceived ideas.

Semi-structured interview

Semi-structured interviews are on a continuum between unstructured and structured interviews. They involve asking a certain number of predetermined open-ended questions about what is being researched without becoming prescriptive. Predetermined questions act as a guide to the interview, provide a systematic framework for exploring the topic, and enhance consistency in the process of data collection when more than one participant is involved (Patton 2002; Taylor et al. 2006). Additional questions may be asked by the researcher, but these are more of a probe to encourage participants to expand on what is being discussed. Using a semi-structured interview format assists the researcher to maintain a focus on the research topic and avoid deviating into areas not covered by the predetermined question guide.

At times during the interview the participant may wish to discuss a particular point or aspect of their experience that does not appear to the researcher to relate explicitly or directly to the focus of the study. In such situations the researcher respects the need of the participant to share such aspects of their experiences by providing a space within the interview for such a discussion. Such a discussion should not be dismissed by the researcher as irrelevant or simply a moment of 'wondering' on the part of the participant. What becomes important is for the researcher to ascertain whether there is a link or relationship between what is being discussed and the actual focus of the study. This can only be achieved by asking a question, such as: 'You have just described your feelings towards your wife. How do these feelings relate to the focus of this study, which is your experience of being ill?' If the researcher does not ask how the discussion relates to the focus of the study, important information may be dismissed by the researcher and so not included as study data.

Structured interview

Structured interviews are generally associated with quantitative research where specific, factual and objective data are required, the questions are closed-ended, and where the researcher has maximum control over the interview process. However, structured interviews can also be part of the data collection process in qualitative research.

The type of structured interview in qualitative research has been referred to by Patton (2002, p. 344) as 'the standardised open-ended interview'. The interview format involves asking a predetermined set of questions in a particular sequence (similar to an oral survey or questionnaire). The questions are designed in the form in which they will be asked during the interview. The main difference from a questionnaire is that the questions are open-ended, giving the participant the opportunity to respond in their own terms rather than being confined to restricted responses as with closed-ended questions. If any clarification is required by the researcher the actual clarifying question/s must be included in the interview transcript (Patton 2002). If more than one interview is conducted, the same fixed sequence of questions must apply. In conducting structured qualitative or standardised open-ended interviews 'the fundamental principle of qualitative interviewing [must apply, which] is to provide a framework within which respondents can express their own understanding in their own terms' (Patton 2002, p. 348).

A weakness of this approach is that the enquiry is limited to the predetermined line of questioning. Unanticipated information that might surface in the course of the interview cannot be pursued by the researcher.

Mixed mode interview: Combining different methods of data collection

Depending on the design to be used in qualitative research, the form of interviewing is generally clearly prescribed, as discussed above. However, the use of different modes or strategies for data collection within a specific interview process does not have to be limited to one form. Depending on the purpose of the interview, different modes of data collection can be used. For instance, you may decide to conduct the first part of an interview in an unstructured manner, and later use a more structured approach to ask the participant to comment on some specific questions that you had drafted before the interview, or you could reverse the process by asking those questions initially, and then provide an opportunity for the participant to share what is important to them about the topic (Patton 2002). Another approach could be to combine targeted or closed-ended questions with open-ended questions to elicit in-depth data on a specific area of interest to the researcher.

A further combination of interview strategies could include the initial interview being unstructured with a second follow-up interview being more structured, focusing on specific questions that have arisen from the analysis of the initial interview. These questions may be about seeking clarification, elaboration or making further enquiry about the context of the data provided by the participant. What is important is to ensure that whatever strategies are used by the researcher are consistent with the intent of the study and the interview.

Figure 9.4   Modes of interview other than one to one

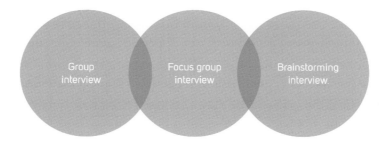

Group interview

Group interviews are another source of data collection in qualitative research. They can be used alone or in combination with other forms such as face-to-face interviews, participant observation or the administration of a questionnaire. The usual size of such groups is between six and eight members. Group interviews generally take two forms, focus groups or brainstorming groups, although there are various permutations to the way groups can be conducted.

Focus group interview

'A focus group is a collection of people working together on a particular research issue' (Taylor et al. 2006, p. 410). Focus groups are used in both quantitative and qualitative research for collection of data. Their main purpose is to provide a forum for group members, deliberately chosen, to 'concentrate their collective intelligence' (p. 410) in responding to a particular research question or area of investigation. Within the qualitative domain focus groups are about 'people talking together to share "life experiences, preferences, intentions, and behaviours"' (Fern 2001, p. 7). Focus groups provide 'the opportunity for multiple interactions not only between the interviewer and respondents but among all participants in the group' (Krueger 1994, p. 100). The format for conducting focus groups generally involves group members engaging in open discussion through the processes of attentive listening to other members' contributions, sharing their own insights, and responding to what is being discussed within the group.

Because of the number of people involved in focus group interviews, and the need to maximise exploration of a particular research topic, procedural rules and processes need to be clearly defined and stated before the interview begins. This can be done by seeking the opinions of the participants about what is important for them in sharing their experiences within a group setting and working with the group to achieve a consensus. Concerns that may be raised by participating group members could be concerned with whether what is discussed in the group will remain confidential, being comfortable about speaking honestly without feeling judged, respecting each member's contributions to the discussion and feeling safe in the 'expert hands' of the interviewer.

Competence in conducting focus group interviews is therefore an important consideration for credibility in data collection. Richard Krueger (1994), an expert in focus group interviewing, suggests that the person conducting the interviews should be more of a facilitator/moderator than an interviewer. For Krueger the term moderator 'highlights a specific function of the interviewer—that of moderating or guiding the discussion…where the conversation flows because of the nurturing of the [group by the] moderator' (p. 100).

Because of the complex nature of focus group interviews, it is recommended that two members of the research team are involved, allowing one person to focus on facilitating/moderating/managing the group while the other deals with the mechanics such as recording, videoing and note-taking, or attending to the needs of group members such as debriefing people who have decided to discontinue their involvement or supporting members who have left the group in a distraught manner (Patton 2002).

Brainstorming interview

If the intent is to canvass a broad sweep of ideas or attitudes about a particular topic in a free-flowing, creative and imaginative manner, brainstorming is an appropriate method of data collection. Such an approach to enquiry requires participants to be spontaneous and unrestricted in their responses to questions posed by the researcher-facilitator or to comments and questions from members of the group. The use of materials such as a whiteboard, computer or butcher's paper may be used to track the discussion and collate and synthesise the shared information.

Other modes of conducting interviews

In addition to forms of face-to-face interviews there are other means by which interviews can be conducted. These include telephone and internet (Skype) interviews.

Telephone interview

Telephone interviews are one alternative to face-to-face interviews; they are a less time-consuming means of data collection. The type of interviews conducted by telephone can range from structured to unstructured depending on the type of data required for the study. What is important is to ensure that the researcher is able to obtain an accurate account of the participant's responses. This means listening attentively to what the person is saying, and being attuned to the tonal changes in voice and expression such as nuances, inflections, emphases and pauses in conversation, each of which provides a context for what the person is communicating. Because of the absence of visual contact with the person, audiotaping of the interview is recommended. If this is not possible, note-taking during and immediately after the interview by the researcher is required in order to minimise data loss. Tape-recording the researcher's account and insights of the interview would enhance the quality of data collected.

Internet interview (Skype)

The use of Skype to conduct interviews is another alternative to face-to-face interviewing. The advantage of this approach over telephone interviewing is visual contact between participant and researcher—an important element in conducting in-depth conversational interviews. However, allowances need to be made for time delay and image distortion, which can be very disruptive to the flow of conversation and subsequent quality of data. The choice of Skype as a method of data collection should be based on the quality of data.

Tape-recorded and audiovisual recording of interviews

The preferred means of recording interviews for the purpose of research is by audiotaping and audiovisual recording. The tape-recorded interview gives the researcher the opportunity to listen to the recordings. What can be picked up through this process is the person's pauses, nuances such as emphasis on important points, and the general sense of what is being described. These are important considerations in capturing the participant's story of their experience. Audiovisual recording of interviews provides an additional source of information to that of the tape-recorded interview. It is most useful in situations where the researcher is attempting to gain as full as possible a 'picture' of the interview discussion or when non-verbal cues are required for the analysis process (Taylor et al. 2006). Audiovisual recording also provides the researcher with an opportunity to revisit the interview as a learning tool for refining of interviewing skills, especially for researchers who are new to qualitative research.

Observation

Observational methods of data collection are used in both quantitative and qualitative research. When the intent of the data collection process is to gain as complete a picture as possible of what is being studied, observation is often used. Observation as a method of data collection in qualitative research has its origins in anthropology. The practice of observation within anthropology has in more recent times been used in ethnography, ethnonursing and grounded theory. The purpose of observation is 'to seek detailed knowledge of the multiple dimensions of life within the studied milieu [natural setting] and to understand members' taken-for-granted assumptions [meanings] and rules' (Charmaz 2006, p. 21) from the perspective of those being observed.

Choosing a form of observation for a study

Observation can take a number of forms, as presented in Figure 9.5.

Figure 9.5   Different forms of observations

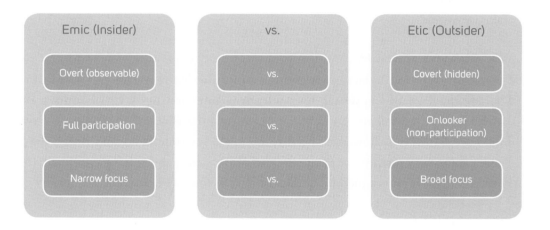

▶▶▶   TERMS, TIPS AND SKILLS

The purpose of observation within these research approaches is 'to seek detailed knowledge of the multiple dimensions of life within the studied milieu [natural setting] and to understand members' taken-for-granted assumptions [meanings] and rules'.

Depending on the type of data the researcher requires for the study, the form(s) of observation will differ. The form(s) selected by the researcher are crucial to the aims of the study and the quality of data required.

Emic versus etic view

The word 'emic' refers to an insider's perspective or point of view. 'An emic perspective compels the recognition and acceptance of multiple realities…which is crucial to an understanding of why people think and act in the different ways they do' (Fetterman 1989, p. 31). An emic perspective focuses on a particular social or cultural situation.

The companion term 'etic' refers to an outsider's perspective or point of view. A point of professional distance from the actual setting provides an objective perspective. An etic perspective allows a comparison between similar situations or cultures.

There has been considerable debate about the value of each approach, but the general consensus is that other perspectives are integral to an understanding of the setting as each perspective contributes different forms of knowledge.

Overt versus covert observation

The use of overt and covert forms of observation have been used in qualitative research as methods of data collection. Overt observation requires full disclosure to the participants that they are being observed for the purpose of research. Covert observation is the non-disclosure to participants that they are to be observed as part of the study. Considerable debate has taken place over the years about the value of both forms of observation. Informing participants that their behaviour will be observed may lead to the participants not behaving in their normal everyday manner, resulting in distortion of what is observed. On the other hand, covert observation captures the natural everyday behaviour of participants. However, not disclosing the researcher's intent to observe participant behaviour has been considered to be ethically wrong (Patton 2002). There is a global move to outlaw research that engages in such apparently deceptive practices.

Full participation versus the onlooker

Full participation requires immersion in the research setting. Ideally the researcher lives and works in the community under study for a period of time during which they become part of the community, internalising social norms, beliefs, attitudes and ritualistic behaviours. Where possible the researcher feels, thinks and acts as one of the group (Patton 2002). Through this process of immersion the researcher is able to gain insights and understanding of the cultural/social setting and way of life of the group or community. At the other end of the continuum the researcher adopts the position of an onlooker—someone who assumes a position of detached observer in order to gain an objective view of what is going on. The choice of what position the researcher wishes to take depends on the type of data being sought.

Anthony Welch and Sansnee Jirojwong

Narrow versus broad focus

Observation can be narrow or broad in focus. Depending on the aim of the study, the researcher may choose to come from either angle. In general, however, the researcher first takes a broad look at what is occurring in the research setting, noting down observations in order to gain an overview of what is taking place, such as the way members interact with each other. Once the researcher has developed a broad sense of what is going on they may decide to hone in on a particular aspect in order to have an in-depth understanding. Both forms of observation complement each other and therefore are usually used in combination.

Field notes

Field notes are an essential means of data collection, especially in situations of observation such as an ethnographic study. The purpose of field notes is to document all that the researcher observes during the enquiry. Field notes are descriptions of what has taken place and what is considered by the researcher to be important information for future reference during the process of analysis. It is primarily descriptive in nature, without interpretation. What is described may include the context of the event or situation, the interactions that take place, what is actually said, the researcher's own feelings, thoughts and reactions to what has taken place, and insights gleaned through researcher reflections (Patton 2002).

Narrative method

Narrative research has its origins in the human sciences. Its purpose is to gain insight into human stories or life events, with an emphasis on capturing the whole event or experience of the person or group of people (Parse 2001). During an interview narratives are captured in the participant's own language. The interview is conducted in such a way as to encourage the participant to describe the sequence of events that make up the whole story. The central assumption of narrative enquiry is that 'stories about life events shed light on the meanings of human experience' (Parse 2001, p. 43).

Case study method

A case study approach occurs in both qualitative and quantitative studies. The focus of a case study is on a particular phenomenon or issue of concern in a particular person, a number of persons, groups or institutions over time. Methods for undertaking a case study along with data collection vary depending on the focus and parameters of the research. Case study research draws on a range of information sources that may include interviews, observation, records, historical documents and statements by others in order to assemble a comprehensive bank of data and to contextualise the information (Patton 2002). The data can be both quantitative and qualitative in nature.

Historical method

Historical research is concerned with exploring a particular event or events and trends over time. The validity of historical research relies on the truthfulness or legitimacy of the information sources. Information sources have been categorised as primary—the original source(s) of data, and secondary—sources once removed from the primary source (Schafer 1980). Data collection therefore may involve oral history, archival documents, government reports, artworks and photography, to name a few.

The arts as a mode of data collection

Within the domain of qualitative research, in particular phenomenology, the arts are recognised as an avenue for data collection in advancing knowledge of the human condition—the affairs of the everyday world of human beings. The arts (referred to as 'expressions of life' by Dilthey [1977]) include but are not limited to literary works, which in turn include but are not limited to poetry, painting, music and drama. These art forms have been part of human experience throughout recorded history. Each of them has been a vehicle through which human experience has been expressed in personally significant ways (Dilthey 1977).

Figure 9.6 Different art forms as sources of data

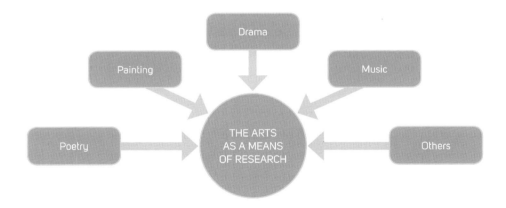

Poetry is concerned with how humans seek meaning in experience (Knights 1995). It is a mode of expression through which personal hopes and dreams, amid the uncertainties and confusions of life, are rendered intelligible. Knights (1995) suggests that poetry is a form of praxis: finding a way to speak the things a person needs to say through reflective action. Freire (1972) describes such action as critical self-insertion into the reality of one's own situation, opening up the potential for insight and personal transformation. Human experience expressed in verse is a potent means of sharing one's personal world with others.

Painting as an 'expression of life' can be traced back to the cave dwellings of our Palaeolithic ancestors living between 30 000 and 8000 BCE. Down the millennia painting has remained a major vehicle of expression through which the everyday world of human beings is portrayed. Panzine (1955, p. 9) suggests that 'Art follows life as the shadow follows the body'. Painting has the power to overcome distance and time and to engage the viewer in a dialogue with the 'author-painting' as if they were contemporary partners with (the viewer) (Gadamer 1997, pp. 545–6).

Music reaches beyond word in evoking and expressing the tones, rhythms and patterns of human existence as lived in the everyday world of humans. Music has the ability to evoke and reveal human experience that otherwise would remain silent. Music is human beings' oldest form of expression, older than word or art (Menuhin & Davis 1979). Throughout history human beings have woven the tonal world of music into the fabric of everyday life marked by experiences of birth, joy, hope, sadness, suffering and loss.

> For most of history, music has been elevated to the highest place in society…It was [and continues to be] the essential ingredient of public ceremony and celebration. It served occasions of grief. It was [and is] there for public and private fun. It marked the days. People's lives revolved [and continue to revolve] around it. (Blackwood 1991, p. 12)

Langer (1953) posits that the tonal world of music bears a close resemblance to the ebb and flow of human feelings—a tonal analogue of emotive life (p. 27). In other words, music is a mode of thought—a way of thinking in tones (Ferguson 1982, p. 1).

Drama in the form of theatrical performance can also be included as an expression of life. Drama is both representation and illumination of life themes—love, hope, despair, tragedy. It provides a space in which the presumed and familiar can be challenged, creating a renewal of perception and awareness (Cox & Theilgaard 1994). Drama invites one to engage with the perspectival world—a world of multiple perspectives. Poole (1972) crystallises such a conception in stating: 'We are all conscious that there is only one world, but we are also quite sure that we all see it differently, we all interpret it differently, and we all attribute differing meanings to it at various times' (p. 89).

Expressions of life—poetry, painting, music and drama—are potent media for explicating human experiences that cannot be illuminated through everyday language. Dewey (1958) supports such a belief: 'In the end works of art are the only media of communication between man and man that can occur in a world of gulfs and walls that limit community of experience' (p. 105).

As expressions of life, the arts have a significant part to play in expanding understanding of the world of human beings. In research the arts have the potential to contribute to the development of new knowledge. The use of the arts is now recognised as an important source of data collection within qualitative research. Data collection using the arts can take many forms. These may be used as an adjunct to an interview where the participant is asked to share an art form that best conveys their experience of the phenomenon under study. This approach can be very useful when a participant has difficulty expressing what they wish to communicate or in situations where language is a barrier. Participants may wish to engage in an artistic expression to convey their experience such as dance, singing, drawing, or making a montage (Taylor et al. 2006). Researchers may decide to use art forms such as painting or music as a vehicle for asking participants to share their thoughts and feelings about the subject matter. The arts as symbolic representations of a person's experience can be a potent source of research data.

RESEARCH IN PRACTICE 9.1

9.1

SELF-MANAGEMENT OF GESTATIONAL DIABETES

Jirojwong and others (2008) explored Southeast Asian migrant women's responses and experiences of having gestational diabetes. A qualitative study was used and aimed to describe how Cambodian, Laotian, Thai and Vietnamese women use information from health professionals to self-manage their illness during pregnancy. Nineteen women participated in the study, recruited at two major hospitals in Sydney. An individual face-to-face interview was conducted at a place nominated by participants. The following broad questions were used:

- When you were told that you had high blood sugar, what was your feeling? Why did you feel that way?
- How do you feel now?
- What have you done to make you change or not change your feelings?
- In your opinion, what is the effect of having high blood sugar on your own health and the health of your baby? Give examples. (REASSURE CONFIDENTIALITY)
- In your opinion, what are the causes of your high blood sugar? There is no right or wrong answer.
- What do you think are the effects of having high blood sugar on your own health in 10 or 15 years? Give examples. (REASSURE CONFIDENTIALITY)
- What do you think are the effects of having high blood sugar on your baby's health in 10 or 15 years? Give examples. (REASSURE CONFIDENTIALITY)

An interview was about one hour and audio-recorded. Later it was transcribed verbatim. Field notes and diary were used to record observation information. Data were analysed using content analysis to identify themes and categories (Miles & Huberman 1994). The steps described by Miles and Huberman were used.

Source: Modified from Jirojwong et al. 2008

Bricolage

Bricolage is an approach to enquiry (see Chapter 5) that uses a broad sweep of data collection methods. The bricoleur is not restricted to one stipulated approach but selects the most appropriate methods for obtaining data (McLeod 2001). Such an approach begins with the researcher engaging in a process of open receptiveness without predetermining what avenues will be required. In other words, procedures other than the initial method of data collection are not established before the enquiry but are selected depending on what particular strategies will lead to the most truthful, rich and informative data. Openness and creativity are at the core of data collection. The researcher interacts with each new piece of information, after which a decision is made about what further data is needed and what is the best way to obtain it. The methods of data-gathering are not ad hoc but a discerning, carefully thought out process.

▶▶▶ TERMS, TIPS AND SKILLS

Bricolage is an approach to enquiry that uses a broad sweep of data collection methods.

Triangulation in data collection

Triangulation is a process of using two or more methods for either data collection or data analysis in order to strengthen a study. The rationale for the use of triangulation has been put forward by Denzin (1978, p. 28): 'Because each method reveals different aspects of empirical reality, multiple methods …must be employed. This is termed triangulation. I… offer as a final methodological rule the principle that multiple methods should be used in every investigation.'

Types of triangulation that come under the umbrella of methodological triangulation include data triangulation, investigator triangulation and theoretical triangulation. For the purpose of this chapter the focus is on data triangulation.

Figure 9.7   Three major types of triangulation

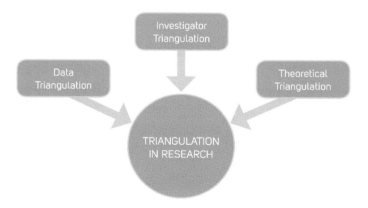

Data triangulation is concerned with the use of more than one method of data collection in one research study (Begley 1996). Within the domain of qualitative research there are a number of different approaches to this.

As outlined above, data triangulation can take a range of forms depending on the type of data sources required to answer the research question. Different combinations are often used; for example, in grounded theory data are collected from interviews (face-to-face and focus groups), observation and the researcher's field notes. In ethnographic research data are collected from interviews, observation, field notes, artefacts and the researcher's diary about their personal experiences of being immersed within a setting or culture. In phenomenological research face-to-face focus group interviews and the arts can be used in combination. Case studies often draw on a range of information sources. Contemporary documents (Bergen & While 2000) are also used.

Data triangulation also includes obtaining data from individuals, groups, communities, documents, artistic expressions, photographs and diaristic accounts of participants' experiences to name a few. An example could be that if you as the researcher wanted to explore the experience of caring for a dying person at home, you might consider not only interviewing the primary carer, but also the person being cared for. You might even expand the study to include the community nurse who is also involved in the care of the person, as well as family members who live in the house.

Data collection in a mixed method research study is collected from both the quantitative and qualitative domains, for example, the use of questionnaires followed by in-depth interviews or vice versa.

In using triangulation as a process for data collection it is important to ensure that selected data collection methods are appropriate for answering the research question.

Rigour and trustworthiness

The term 'rigour' refers to 'the strictness in judgement and conduct that must be used to ensure that the successive steps in a project have been set out clearly and undertaken with scrupulous attention to detail, so that the results/findings/insights can be "trusted"' (Taylor et al. 2006). The concept of rigour in qualitative research can be traced back to the works of Guba and Lincoln (1981), who believed that the terms 'validity' and 'reliability' denoting rigour in quantitative research were not the appropriate language to reflect the philosophical 'fit' in determining rigour in qualitative research. The term 'trustworthiness' was introduced by Lincoln and Guba (1986) to express the central nature of rigour in qualitative enquiry. 'Trustworthiness of the data is tied directly to the trustworthiness of the person who collects and analyses the data—and his or her demonstrated competence...[in] building a "track record" for quality work' (Patton 2002).

▶▶▶ TERMS, TIPS AND SKILLS

In using triangulation as a process for data collection it is important to ensure that the selected data collection methods are appropriate for answering the research question.

▶▶▶   TERMS, TIPS AND SKILLS

'Rigour' refers to 'the strictness in judgment and conduct that must be used to ensure that the successive steps in a project have been set out clearly and undertaken with scrupulous attention to detail, so that the results/findings/insights can be "trusted"' (Taylor et al. 2006).

In order to achieve trustworthiness in data collection in qualitative research, a number of key elements need to be demonstrated: researcher competence; transparency of the research process—the decision trail; and congruence between the selected philosophical and methodological approaches for a particular study.

Quality of research data is dependent on researcher competence. Three aspects are of particular importance here: having an informed understanding of the philosophical underpinnings of the theoretical framework to be used for the study, being able to discern the appropriate data collection strategies, and being appropriately skilled in the use of the selected data collection methods.

Beginning the process of data collection without having a solid grasp of the theoretical framework or ontology (underlying values and beliefs) informing the study has the potential to compromise the study's integrity. Each theoretical framework within qualitative research has its own underlying values and beliefs about how a study should be conducted. Failure to have such an understanding before commencement of a study inevitably leads to errors in the focus of the data collection process(es). An example would be choosing a phenomenological approach to enquiry to explore the phenomenon of everyday lived experience of women when the intent of the researcher is to explore the experiences of social inequality for women. The former is about the lived experience of women whereas the latter is concerned with the social inequality of women.

In addition to theoretical competence, the researcher also needs to be able to select the appropriate data-gathering methods for the study. The methods of data collection need to be consistent with the theoretical framework underpinning the study.

Transparency in the decision-making processes of the researcher is fundamental to credibility. This can be achieved by the researcher maintaining ongoing documentation of the decision trail (audit trail) concerning data collection and analysis throughout the course of the study. In terms of data collection, any issues in the process need to be carefully documented.

A final and critical point is researcher competence in the use of data collection methods. The range of data collection methods in qualitative research can provide significant challenges to the new researcher or even to the advanced researcher who is not familiar with the processes involved in the selected data collection methods. It is therefore incumbent on the researcher to acquire the necessary competence to ensure the collection of quality data. Failure to do so has the potential to compromise the integrity of the study.

▶▶▶ TERMS, TIPS AND SKILLS

Transparency of the decision-making processes of the researcher is fundamental to achieving credibility.

Summary

The need for researchers undertaking qualitative research to demonstrate a competent, transparent and rigorous approach to data collection is essential for conducting credible research. There is a broad range of means by which data can be collected for a study. At times the array of data collection methods can be overwhelming for the beginning researcher. What becomes important is to ensure that the methods chosen are consistent with the intent or aim of the study, the research question(s) and the research design. If each of these components 'fit' with each other, you are on the path to conducting a study that will be credible in the eyes of the research community.

IMPLICATIONS FOR EVIDENCE-BASED NURSING AND MIDWIFERY

Qualitative research has the potential to make a significant contribution to evidence-based practice by providing in-depth information about the perceptions, expectations and experiences of health care consumers concerning the quality of health care they have received. Qualitative research complements quantitative research in providing a different source of knowledge about quality care and how the outcomes of health care can be evaluated.

▶▶▶ PROBLEM SOLVING 9.1

Ann and her team conducted a research project that aims to explore the meaning of chest pain and the decision process patients used before presenting at the hospital emergency department. Major issues explored include social support and help-seeking behaviours of the patients. The team will interview respondents at their own homes. In addition to an interview schedule with open-ended questions, what else do you think could be data collection tools?

Practice exercise 9.1

You have been invited to join a research team to conduct a study about pain management practices in your facility. The purpose or aim of the proposed study is to identify the ways in which nurses provide pain relief for patients with chronic pain. You are asked by the head of the research team to explore the most effective means of data collection and to give a reason for your choice(s).

Practice exercise 9.2

Think of a research topic that you would like to investigate.

What is the topic or area you wish to investigate?

What is the question you wish to explore?

What type of information do you believe will assist you to answer your reseach question?

What form of data collection methods do you consider would be appropriate to answer the research question?

What forms of information-gathering would be inappropriate and why?

Practice exercise 9.3

1   In what research designs would you use the following interview formats: unstructured, semi-structured and focus groups? Give a reason for your decision.

2   What are the strengths and weaknesses of collecting data through the following observational processes: emic versus etic, full participation versus onlooker, covert versus overt?

3   Describe three forms of trialgulation used in research.

4   What are the strengths of using triangulation in research studies?

Answer to problem solving 9.1

Ann and her team may want to have a list of observations that they may have to make, for example, photographs of family that can be used as a starting point to explore the issues surrounding social support. Respondents may be asked to keep a diary about sources of help that they use when they have concern about their health and how they feel during the day when they are well. Using a combination of sources of data will help triangulate the data from an interview.

Further reading

Berg, B. L. (2007). *Qualitative Research Methods for the Social Sciences.* Boston: Pearson.

Burgess, R. G. (1987). *In the Field: An Introduction to Field Research.* London: Allen & Unwin.

Pelto, P., & Pelto, G. (1978). *Anthropological Research: The Structure of Inquiry.* Cambridge: Cambridge University Press.

Weblinks

<http://qhr.sagepub.com>

Sage publishes *Qualitative Research Journal*, which can be useful for reviewing various published articles and discussion papers on various qualitative research issues.

<www.srcd.org>

The Society for Research in Child Development which has a number of useful issues relating to research among children.

References

Begley, C. (1996). Using triangulation in nursing research. *Journal of Advanced Nursing* 24(1), 122–8.

Bergen, A., & While, A. (2000). A case for case studies: Exploring the use of case study design in community nursing research. *Journal of Advanced Nursing* 31, 926–34.

Blackwood, A. (1991). *Music of the World*. Oxford: Facts on File.

Borbasi, S., Jackson, D., & Langford, R. W. (2004). *Navigating the Maze of Nursing Research: An Interactive Learning Adventure*. Sydney: Mosby.

Charmaz, K. (2006). *Constructing Grounded Theory: A Practical Guide Through Qualitative Analysis*. London: Sage Publications.

Cox, M., & Theilgaard, A. (1994). *Shakespeare as Prompter: The Amending Imagination and the Therapeutic Process*. London: Jessica Kingsley.

Crotty, M. (1998). *The Foundations of Social Research: Meaning and Perspective in the Research Process*. Sydney: Allen & Unwin.

Denzin, N. K. (1978). *The Research Act: A Theoretical Introduction to Sociological Methods*, 2nd edn. New York: McGraw-Hill.

Dewey, J. (1958). *Art as Experience*. New York: Capricorn Books.

Dilthey, W. (1977). *Descriptive Psychology and Historical Understanding*, transl. R. M. Zaner & K. L. Heiges. The Hague: Martinus Nijhoff.

Dilthey, W. (1989). *Introduction to the Human Sciences*, transl. R. J. Bentanzos. Detroit: Wayne State University Press.

Ferguson, D. (1982). *A History of Musical Thought*. Westport, CN: Greenwood.

Fern, E. F. (2001). *Advanced Focus Group Research*. London: Sage.

Fetterman, D. M. (1989). *Ethnography: Step by Step*. Newbury Park, CA: Sage.

Freire, P. (1972). *Cultural Action for Freedom*. Harmondsworth: Penguin.

Gadamer, H. G. (1997). The philosophy of Hans-Georg Gadamer in L. E. Hahn (ed.). *The Library of Living Philosophers*, vol. xxiv. Illinois: Open Court.

Giorgi, A. (1989). Some theoretical and practical issues regarding the psychological phenomenological method. *Saybrook Review* 7, 71–85.

Guba, E., & Lincoln, Y. (1981). *Effective Evaluation*. San Francisco: Jossey-Bass.

Jirojwong, S., Schmied, V., Hannah, D., & Johnson, M. (2008). Health literacy and self management of gestational diabetic: a study among Vietnamese, Cambodian, Thai and Laotian women in Sydney. Research proposal submitted to College of Health and Science, Sydney: Unversity of Western Sydney.

Knights, B. (1995). *The Listening Reader: Fiction and Poetry for Counsellors and Psychotherapists*. Pennsylvania: Jessica Kingsley.

Krueger, R. A. (1994). *Focus Group Interviews: A Practical Guide for Applied Research*, 2nd edn. Southern Oaks, CA: Sage.

Langer, S. K. (1953). *Feeling and Form: A Theory of Art Development from Philosophy in a New Key*. London: Routledge & Kegan Paul.

Lincoln, Y. S., & Guba, E. G. (1985). *Naturalistic Inquiry*. Beverly Hills, CA: Sage Publications.

McLeod, J. (2001). *Qualitative Research in Counselling and Psychotherapy*. London: Sage.

Menuhin, Y., & Davis, C. (1979). *The Music of Man*. Toronto: Methuen.

Miles, B. M., & Huberman, A. M. (1994). Introduction: Three approaches to qualitative data analysis. In B. M. Miles & A. M. Huberman (eds), *An Expanded Sourcebook: Qualitative Data Analysis* (pp. 8–12). London: Sage Publications.

Panzine, A. (1955). In W. Boeck & J. Sabartes (eds), *Picasso*. New York: Harry N. Abrahams.

Parse, R. R. (1998). *The Human Becoming School of Thought: A Perspective for Nurses and Other Health Professionals*. California: Sage.

Parse, R. (2001). *Qualitative Inquiry: The Path of Sciencing*. Boston: National League for Nursing.

Patton, M. (2002). *Qualitative Research and Evaluation Methods*, 3rd edn. Thousand Oaks, CA: Sage Publications.

Pollio, H., Tracy, H., & Thompson, C. (1997). *The Phenomenology of Everyday Life*. Cambridge: Cambridge University Press.

Poole, R. (1972). *Towards Deep Subjectivity*. London: Allen Lane.

Schafer, R. J. (1980). *A Guide to Historical Method*. Homewood IL: Dorsey Press.

Schneider, Z., Elliot, D., LoBiondo-Wood, G., & Haber, J. (2003). *Nursing Research: Methods, Critical Appraisal, and Utilization*, 2nd edn. Sydney: Mosby.

Spradley, J. P., & McCurdy, D. W. (1972). *The Cultural Experience: Ethnography in Complex Society*. Chicago: Science Research Associates.

Taylor, B., Kermode, S., & Roberts, K. (2006). *Research in Nursing and Health Care: Evidence for Practice*, 3rd edn. Australia: Thomson.

CHAPTER 10

Data Collection: Quantitative Research

Jan Taylor and Jamie Ranse

Chapter learning objectives

By the end of this chapter you will be able to:

▸ analyse the usefulness of different data collection methods

▸ create a simple questionnaire

▸ choose an existing instrument or scale to be used in research

▸ judge the validity and reliability of a scale or instrument

▸ describe the use of a personal digital assistant to collect research data.

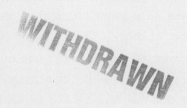

Introduction

Most of us have provided information to various organisations for their research purposes. Some of us complete a satisfaction form before we check out from a hotel. Every five years, we complete a census form conducted by the Australian Government. We may be approached at an airport or a supermarket by a research assistant who is collecting information for marketing purposes. Information about our use of cancer screening is stored by the Department of Health and Ageing and then analysed and used to report to the wider public. Particular attention to the methods used in data collection ensures the quality of research. This chapter will explore various methods used to collect data in quantitative research.

Data collection methods

Surveys

A survey is a system for collecting self-report information. Surveys can be divided into two broad categories: questionnaires and interviews.

Questionnaires

Questionnaires are one of the most commonly used data collection methods in nursing and midwifery research. They can be used to measure knowledge, behaviours and perceptions as well as gathering factual information about respondents (Nieswiadomy 2008). Questionnaires contain different types of questions including closed-ended, open-ended, checklist and rating scales. General characteristics of each type of question will be briefly described and examples of the questions are presented in Box 10.1.

Types of questions

The following types of questions may be used in a questionnaire:

- *Closed-ended question:* Respondents choose an answer from a given set of alternatives. The dichotomous question (yes/no, male/female) is one example. When using closed-ended questions, the alternatives need to cover all the possible answers or be collectively exhaustive and mutually exclusive, that is, with no overlap between the categories. When unsure that all possible alternatives are covered, the researcher can have an additional category of 'other'.
- *Open-ended question:* An open-ended question allows respondents to answer the question in their own words with sufficient space provided for the answer.
- *Checklist:* A checklist is a list of behaviours, characteristics or information in which the researcher is interested. The participants select possible answers from

the list. Some questions allow more than one response. For example, Jirojwong and MacLennan (2004) explored what actions rural Australians take when they are seriously sick. A list of five options ranging from doing nothing to going to a hospital was presented to respondents, who could choose more than one answer.

- *Rating scale:* A rating scale is more useful when the behaviour or characteristic requires precise measurement rather than merely being present or not. Examples of rating scales include the Likert scale, visual analogue and semantic differential.

  - The Likert scale is used to measure attitudes and beliefs. Respondents indicate their position on a continuum ranging from strongly agree to strongly disagree. In the classic Likert scale the number of possible responses ranges from five to seven.

BOX 10.1
EXAMPLES OF QUESTIONS

Fixed response

Closed-ended questions: the dichotomous question (yes/no) is one example.

'Do you usually speak English at home?'
1.   Yes, I usually speak English at home
2.   No, another language (Please specify) _____

The question is collectively exhaustive and mutually exclusive.

'During the last week, approximately how many hours of sleep have you usually been getting each night?' (Please circle one number only).
1.   0–4 hours
2.   5–6 hours
3.   7–8 hours
4.   More than 8 hours

The use of 'other' category.

'How are you feeding your baby at present?' (Please circle one number only).
1.   Breastfeeding only
2.   Breastfeeding plus some formula
3.   Formula only
4.   Other (Please specify) _____

Jan Taylor and Jamie Ranse

BOX 10.1

Open-ended questions allow respondents to answer the question in their own words.

'Overall, what do you think is contributing to and/or causing the fatigue you have experienced in the past week?' _____

_____

Checklists

A checklist is a list of information in which the researcher is interested. The participant checks the appropriate answer.

'What method/s of pain relief have you been using in the past 24 hours?'

(Please circle ALL that apply; you may circle more than one).

1.   Tablets such as panadol (or similar drug)
2.   Injections of Pethidine (or similar drug)
3.   Patient Controlled Analgesia (PCA)
4.   Other. (Please specify) _____
5.   None, I have not required any analgesia

Rating scale questions

Likert Scale: Creedy et al. (2008) examined midwives' breastfeeding knowledge. One of the tools they used was the Newborn Feeding Ability Questionnaire. This questionnaire contained 21 questions with a five-point Likert scale. Question 1 is set out below.

A normal full-term infant is born with instinctive reflex ability to breastfeed effectively.

1 strongly disagree, 2 disagree, 3 not sure, 4 agree, 5 strongly agree.

Visual Analogue Scale

Here pain is ranked on a VAS scale with 0 representing no pain and 10 representing the worst pain possible.

No Pain   Worst Pain Possible

0   10

Semantic differential scale: Norman (2001) used a semantic differential scale to test nursing students' attitudes towards drug-using patients. One of the questions is set out below.

Smart   Stupid

1   2   3   4   5   6   7

- A Visual Analogue Scale (VAS) is a straight line, 100 mm in length, with anchors representing the extremes of the particular concept being measured. Participants record the intensity of their feelings by placing a cross on the line and scores are calculated by measuring from the lowest extreme point to this cross. The VAS is used to measure concepts such as pain and anxiety.
- The semantic differential scale asks respondents to indicate their position or attitude to a concept using two adjectives at opposite ends of a continuum. The number of positions on the scale ranges from five to nine.

Administering a questionnaire

Questionnaires can be administered by various methods including the post, the internet and via an interview. Researchers need to carefully choose the most appropriate method to reach the target study group and design the questionnaire to maximise the response rate as a low response rate will introduce bias and reduce the power of the study.

Postal questionnaires

It is recommended that you search the literature and databases for an existing questionnaire that you could use. If you cannot locate a suitable one you can develop your own. Producing a questionnaire from the beginning is a complex task and beyond the scope of this chapter, but we will cover some basic principles.

Before starting

Write down the study goals and only develop questions that directly relate to the goals, not just because the information would be interesting. Locate some examples of questionnaires or specific items by searching databases identified in Weblinks at the end of this chapter. Alternatively, approach a researcher who has used a questionnaire and ask for a copy. Researchers usually respond positively to this request. You may locate two or three questionnaires and assess their applicability to your research. You may want to assess their layout, their language and their ease to complete. Compare them and make a note of the features you like for future reference. Now, decide on the information you need to answer the research goals (demographic, outcome and/or explanatory variables). The next step is to develop the questions that will ensure you have the information you need.

When developing the questions, consider the following:

- Use simple everyday language.
- Keep your intended respondents in mind. Will they understand the wording?
- Develop one or more questions for each variable you have identified.
- Check that each question only deals with one matter. For example 'I am confident in assessing and swabbing infected wounds' should be 'I am confident in assessing infected wounds' and 'I am confident in swabbing infected wounds'.

- Make sure there are no leading questions or double negatives. For example, 'Don't you think the government should fund home births?'
- Clear and unambiguous instructions for completing the questions.
- Each different type of question should have instructions on how to complete it.

When sequencing the questions:

- Group questions together logically.
- Sequence all the questions related to each variable/topic together.
- Precede each new topic with a descriptive statement to alert the respondent to the change in topic. An example is 'Now I am interested in how you…'
- Start with demographic questions such as age, education.
- Place sensitive questions towards the end of the questionnaire when respondents may be more comfortable in answering them.
- Questions asking for personal details such as income may also be better placed towards the end of the questionnaire.

Formatting the questionnaire

It is important to consider the appearance of a questionnaire as this may influence the response rate. Suggestions for formatting include:

- Use an easy-to-read font with a 10–12 point size.
- Ensure there is enough space between questions.
- Make sure the instructions for completing questions, the questions and the spaces for responses are on the same page.
- Leave a space for general comments at the end of the questionnaire.
- Aim to keep the questionnaire as short as possible. Longer questionnaires are usually associated with a poorer response rate (Kitchenham & Pfleeger 2002).

Pilot-testing is critical and may entail more than one testing. First, ask experts in both the content area and questionnaire design to review your questionnaire and then revise it. Second, pilot-test with a group of between 60 and 100 persons with similar characteristics to those who will participate in your study. Take the opportunity to seek information on the clarity of the instructions, wording of questions, general layout, as well as completion time. Revise the questionnaire with the suggestions from experts and the responses from participants.

Finally, give your questionnaire a short, meaningful title, and include a covering letter outlining the purpose of the research, who you are, your contact details and why the respondents' participation will be valuable, instructions for returning the questionnaire and expected return date. Mail your questionnaire together with a reply-paid envelope to the potential participants (Houser 2008; Nieswiadomy 2008).

Advantages and disadvantages

A postal questionnaire is a very cost-effective way of collecting data from large numbers of participants who may be spread across a wide geographic area. They allow anonymity, which can encourage participation when sensitive topics are being explored. A significant problem of surveys is the low response rates. Response rates of 25% to 30% for mailed questionnaires are common. A response rate lower than 50% places the representativeness of the sample in question (Burns 2000). Another disadvantage of questionnaires is their inability to clarify questions and probe responses. This may result in missed questions or inaccurate responses. Finally, questionnaires may not be appropriate for some groups such as participants from culturally and linguistically diverse backgrounds. Careful attention to detail and an understanding of the processes involved in developing a questionnaire are of immense value to the novice researcher. While developing questionnaires can be complex, Thom (2007) argues that simple self-designed questionnaires can be used to quickly and effectively collect information to inform nursing and midwifery practice.

Internet questionnaires

The internet has increasingly become a well-recognised tool for use in everyday activities. In 2001, approximately 35% of Australians households had internet access. In 2006, this figure had almost doubled to approximately 63% (Australian Bureau of Statistics 2007). In the health care environment, adequate access to the internet is accepted as a necessity. With an increase in internet availability and access to nurses and midwives, research using the internet is increasing. However, it is important to consider the participants' experience, researcher implications and general advantages and disadvantages of this approach.

The experience of potential participants may directly reflect the success of the research project. They are commonly notified via email of an invitation to participate in an internet-based research project. The initial email invitation should be motivational and easy to read (Dillman et al. 1998). A hyperlink will direct the participant to a unique, specifically designed survey. Occasionally, the internet survey site may be password-protected, to prevent non-invitees from completing the survey. If this is the case, the original email should contain a username and password. While online surveys can be developed and distributed with ease, institutions and associations should be strategic in the number distributed as oversaturation of research may result in decreased participation.

Social networking websites such as Facebook and MySpace are increasing in popularity and provide access to potential research participants. These Web 2.0 applications are interactive and have the capacity to generate internet-based polls, surveys and other data collection methods. Additionally, these social networking sites commonly allow users to select networks or groups with whom they wish to be affiliated. The Royal College of Nursing Australia is one example of the growing number of organisations that have a group on Facebook, which users can join. These methods of participant recruitment may be of particular interest to social researchers.

When contemplating an internet-based survey, a number of matters should be considered, such as the use of hybrid approaches, strategies to increase responses, design principles and protection of participants.

Some participant populations may not have regular access to the internet and prefer a traditional mail survey approach. In these circumstances, the researcher should consider a hybrid approach, where participants receive a paper copy of the survey and are provided with an internet site where they can choose either (Duffy 2002). Various stand-alone software packages exist that will assist the researcher in designing and collating their survey. There are software programs that combine data collected from online and postal surveys. An example is the Remark software packages. The Remark OMR (optical mark recognition) software scans and collates paper-based surveys, while the Remark Web Survey assists with developing, distributing and collating online surveys.

Various strategies can be applied to increase the response rate of online surveys, such as pre-notification of the survey, personalising messages, using simple formatting and strategically reminding participants (Morris et al. 2004).

Morris and colleagues explored trends in nursing education. The researchers emailed deans of schools of nursing and midwifery to complete an online survey. It was on the second email to non-responders that most participants completed the survey.

The design principles outlined in Box 10.2 need to be considered when using the internet. They will assist in promoting a user-friendly survey and enhance a favourable response rate. Many internet-based survey tools are available, including SurveyMonkey (www.surveymonkey.com). Depending on the survey tool, the input from the participant may be delivered to the researcher in varying appearances. The researchers may receive an email of individual responses, or alternatively they may access an internet site that contains a contemporaneous collation of the responses.

BOX 10.2

INTERNET-BASED SURVEY DESIGN PRINCIPLES

- Have a motivational introductory screen.
- Focus on ease of reading.
- Start with an easy question.
- Use a similar format to that of a paper-based survey.
- Keep questions to one screen and avoid the need to scroll.
- Allow participants to skip questions and return at a later time.
- Avoid advanced and/or specialist programming.
- Be cautious when using problematic question types, such as open-ended and 'tick all that apply'.

Source: Adapted from Dillman et al. 1998

An important part of an online design is testing the environment or piloting (Duffy 2002). Having someone who has previously designed an internet survey may assist novice researchers in designing, building and testing the survey appropriately.

Data collected should be stored on a password-protected individual computer, rather than on public-accessible computers (Duffy 2002). The researcher should establish their survey on their institution's server in preference to a free online survey site such as the SurveyMonkey. Storage data on free online survey internet sites may have some level of accessibility to others than the researchers. Some human research ethics committees may prefer that researchers do not use free online surveys. Anonymity and confidentiality, security, self-determination and authenticity, full disclosure, and fair treatment of participants' data entry need to be considered (Im & Chee 2002).

Advantages and disadvantages

An internet survey is cheaper than telephone and postal surveys as it does not require postage or a hard copy of a survey form (Duffy 2002; Stewart 2003). The main costs associated with online surveys are incurred at the beginning of the data collection process, with the establishment and uploading of the survey. Some internet sites offer free surveys, which may suffice the novice researcher with a small budget and sample size. Cost savings occur during data collection and data entry. The researcher will usually receive responses in a usable format such as an Excel spreadsheet. Further, the time lag between distributing an internet survey and the researcher receiving it back is shorter than other types of survey. One month is a reasonable time for the distribution and collection of the web information (Stewart 2003).

It is important to know the response rate. Depending on the distribution strategy of internet surveys, a response rate may be difficult to ascertain, particularly surveys accessible to all internet users. In internet-based surveys for specific populations, such as a workplace, all employees should be included so that the denominator is known. Response rates in the literature from internet surveys have been less than those from traditional methods.

The potential population's characteristics that may affect their accessibility to an internet survey have to be considered (Courtney & Craven 2005). On the other hand, internet surveys may provide access to populations that are otherwise difficult to reach (Ahern 2005). Internet surveys may be useful for research across continents or with geographically diverse populations.

In summary, the internet provides a rapid approach to designing, developing and delivering a survey. Questionnaires can be distributed and the responses can be collected in a timely manner. Although researchers have an initial cost outlay in the design stage, this method reduces the cost of production of hard copy of the questionnaire, postage and data entry.

Interviews

Structured interviews

Structured interviews use an interview schedule to collect data and can be administered face to face or over the telephone. Participants respond to a set of questions where the questions and the possible answers are predetermined, similar to a questionnaire. The structured interview is most appropriate when you are collecting factual data from participants in a study.

Participants need to know what is required of them when taking part in the study. Interviews should be scheduled at a time suitable for both the interviewer and the interviewee, and they should know the length of time required of them. An interview should be carried out in a quiet private area so the interviewee is able to speak freely without being overheard. Choosing an area where the interviewee feels comfortable is also essential (White 2003).

Matters to consider include developing questions, pilot-testing the interview schedule, training interviewers and recording responses. Developing interview questions is similar to the process of designing a questionnaire. Questions are generally closed-ended with a range of possible predetermined responses (Polit & Beck 2008). The interview schedule has to be piloted using participants with similar characteristics to those who will be included in the study. Problems with the questions, the sequence of questions and the proposed method of recording the responses are assessed during this pilot stage.

To ensure consistency in interviewing, the interviewer has to ask the same questions in the same sequence using the same manner and tone of voice. If more than one interviewer is collecting data, they need to be trained and a protocol needs to be drawn up (MacLennan 2009) so that the same set of procedures is followed with each participant. Training includes having the interviewers rehearse the interview and the use of role play, with each interviewer playing the part of the interviewer as well as the interviewee (Nieswiadomy 2008). Data from interviews is recorded on data collection sheets, tape-recorded or videotaped with the participants' consent.

White (2003) used the following process to explore the extent to which 40 Australian intensive care nurses from seven metropolitan intensive care units considered brain death a meaningful concept of death.

The structured one-hour interview consisted of 38 items which had been previously reviewed for their applicability for the study by an expert panel. Interviews were conducted adjacent to the participant's place of work and were audiotaped with their consent. Responses were also entered into a record of interview sheet. Interviewer reliability was determined by having an observer present during the early interviews (White 2003).

Advantages and disadvantages

This type of data collection allows the interviewer to clarify any questions that are unclear. Researchers can control who participates as it is clear who is being interviewed—unlike mailed questionnaires where someone other than the intended participant may complete it (Polit & Beck 2008). However, structured interviews are costly in time and money. Other expenses such as travel and venue hire add to the costs. In summary, while costly, structured interviews are more personal, gain a higher response rate and result in fewer missing responses.

Telephone interviewing

With the increasing coverage of the Australian population with fixed telephone lines and mobile phones (Nielsen Media Research 2001), telephone interviews are a viable method for use in clinical research.

Participants need to understand their commitment, which includes timing of calls, number of calls needed to complete the study, estimated length of time of each call, and the types of questions. Participants should have access to a toll-free number should they wish to reschedule a call, ask questions or raise concerns. This information is usually provided during the consent process (Musselwhite et al. 2007).

Telephone interviews are generally not designed to last longer than 20 minutes. They are best suited to research with a specific focus rather than a general topic. Computer-assisted telephone interviewing (CATI) has made the process of telephone interviewing easier and quicker. CATI is a software program that allows the questions to be displayed on a computer screen (Polit & Beck 2008) and the interviewer codes the respondent's answers directly into the computer file. It facilitates data collection and improves the quality of data as there is less opportunity for data entry errors. The technique is suitable for large surveys.

Advantages and disadvantages

Telephone interviews are less costly than face-to-face interviews. The data can be collected quickly and easily across states and time zones, giving access to populations that are otherwise hard to reach. They provide a degree of anonymity that may encourage participation in research where sensitive topics are being explored, such as illicit drug use. However, it may be more difficult to ensure a representative sample as only potential respondents with telephones can be reached. Whether or not this is a problem depends on the purpose of your study. When a potential respondent is not available, call-backs may be time-consuming.

In summary, telephone interviewing is most useful in research with a specific focus, but it may be more difficult to obtain a representative sample. Telephone interactions have the potential to be impersonal, so it is important to build rapport with the interviewee (Smith 2005).

Structured observation

Structured observation uses a non-participatory approach and the term is used to indicate that a researcher or an observer only gathers data without interfering with any study variables or research participants' activities. The researcher collects data on specific behaviours, actions and events by visual observation (Polit & Beck 2008). It is used when there is prior knowledge of the particular behaviour, for example nurses' and midwives' hand-washing practices. Data collection tools such as checklists are used to identify and quantify the behaviour.

There are two types of non-participant observations. Non-participant observation (overt) involves observation by the researcher with the full knowledge of the participant. The participant is aware of being observed, knows what will be observed and who will observe them. Non-participant observation (covert) involves observation where the participant is not aware that they are being observed (Nieswiadomy 2008) (see also Chapter 9, Overt versus covert observation). There are a few situations when this observation would be considered ethical, so the researcher needs to justify the need for concealment when seeking ethical approval for this data collection method (Elliot & Schneider 2007).

A number of steps are needed when using non-participant observation. They include identifying who and what is to be observed and having clear and objective definitions of the behaviour, action or event. As before, the categories for observation need to cover all the possible behaviours (collectively exhaustive) as well as ensuring no overlap between the categories (mutually exclusive). The categories then form the basis for constructing the data collection instrument (Polit & Beck 2008). Researchers need to check whether or not an existing checklist or rating scale is available. The process of locating and choosing an existing scale is covered in the following section.

In structured observation the researcher is aiming for objectivity. However, total objectivity is not possible because the process of observing is susceptible to bias. The observers' knowledge, experiences and values all contribute to how events may be interpreted and recorded. Researchers need to be mindful of the tendency to rate a participant's observed behaviour more highly because of a positive overall impression of that participant (the Halo effect). The use of a structured data collection tool may reduce these subjective elements of observation.

Participants may change their behaviour when they know they are being observed (the Hawthorne effect). Nieswiadomy (2008) suggests that although people initially change their behaviour if they know they are being observed, over time they revert to their usual behaviour. Aiming to make observation as unobtrusive as possible is one way to manage this problem. If there is more than one observer, training is essential (see also the 'Structured interview' section above). Interrater reliability, that is, the degree to which two or more observers allocate the same score to an observation, is essential.

Video-recording and audio-recording methods can be used where the events are too rapid or too complex for pen and paper. The data can be collected at the time of the action or event and then analysed later. These methods permit the researcher to play and replay the data, ensuring accuracy of coding and analysis (Kermode & Roberts 2007a).

Gerdtz and Bucknall (2001) used structured observation to describe triage nurses' decision-making in an adult emergency department in an Australian tertiary hospital. A single observer collected data using a 20-item instrument adapted for the study. Before use, the reliability of the instrument was tested using two independent observers who recorded 10 occasions of triage with 94.6% agreement. The authors acknowledged that the Hawthorne effect may have influenced the results but argue that the observed behaviours reflect what the nurses believed were their best performance.

Advantages and disadvantages

Structured observational methods collect data about what participants do rather than relying on their verbal accounts of their own behaviour, which may or may not be accurate (Kermode & Roberts 2007a). It is very useful when it is difficult for participants to give answers or to give reliable answers—for example pre-verbal children and older persons with impaired communication skills (Polit & Beck 2008).

It is challenging to be both a researcher and a midwife or nurse, particularly if an event that places an individual at risk occurs during observation. In these circumstances the welfare of the individual takes precedence and the researcher's role is abandoned for the clinician's role. Observing in the clinical setting is time-consuming as time is required for the behaviours or events to occur. Ensuring sufficient participants may also be difficult as many people do not want to be observed. The use of audio- and video-recording methods can be expensive as they require specialist equipment (Kermode & Roberts 2007b). In summary, structured observation is a useful data collection method for nursing and midwifery research. The structured observation needs checklists and this is not suitable where there is limited understanding of the topic.

Table 10.1 summarises the advantages and disadvantages of various data collection methods in terms of time, cost, response rate and access to potential respondents.

A range of instruments can be used to collect quantitative data. We will explore issues relating to the use of existing instruments or scales, the personal digital assistant (PDA), personal computers and laptops.

Table 10.1   Advantages and disadvantages of different data collection methods

	Questionnaires		Interview		
	Mail	Internet	Face-to-face	Telephone	Observation
Cost	Provides large amounts of structured data at a relatively low cost	Cheaper in comparison to traditional methods

Main cost occurs during the development phase | More costly than mailed questionnaires | Less costly than face-to-face interviews

More costly than mailed questionnaires | Can be costly if the behaviours to be observed occur infrequently |
| **Time** | Additional time required for sending reminders and repeat questionnaires to non-responders | Decreased data collection period as there is no lag time for postal delivery | More time-consuming | Allows data to be collected quickly and relatively easily

Call-backs may be time-consuming | Immersion in the field requires considerable time commitment |
| **Response** | Typically low response rates | Harder to track accurate response rates

May not accurately represent the desired population | Higher response than mailed questionnaires | More difficult to get a representative sample | More difficult to get a representative sample |
| **Accessibility** | Provides access to populations spread over a wide geographic area

Those who respond to the survey may be different from those who did not, thus biasing the findings | Provides access to hard-to-reach populations

Provides access to larger number of potential participants

Assumes potential participants have access to the internet | | Provides access to hard-to-reach populations | Provides access to populations who are not able to answer questions: pre-verbal children and older persons with impaired communication skills |
| **Other** | Allows anonymity, which can encourage participation when sensitive topics are being explored

Less suitable for some groups (e.g. participants from culturally and linguistically diverse backgrounds) | Anonymity of participants is easier to maintain

Some online surveys lack flexibility and have limitations in the number and type of data entry fields that are available | Permits clarification of questions | Allows anonymity, which can encourage participation when sensitive topics are being explored

Lack of visual cues may inhibit flow of interview | The presence of the observer may influence the situation |

Choosing an existing instrument or scale

A psychometric scale is a set of written questions or statements designed to measure a particular concept, for example, anxiety or self-esteem. The questions or statements in the scale are called items (Macnee & McCabe 2008). A number of ways can be used to locate a validated scale. A review of the literature on the topic may identify an already existing scale. Another source is a compendium of research tools. These texts summarise the characteristics of scales that have been used in nursing and midwifery research including the name, the variables measured, the population, reliability and validity data and where to access the scale. The book *Instruments for Clinical Health-Care Research* (Frank-Stromborg & Olsen 2004) contains reviews of clinical scales that measure concepts such as body image, fatigue and sleep.

Data collection tools

Another source of research tools is the Mental Measurement Yearbook available via the Ovid interface. This database covers more than 4000 commercially available tests in categories such as personality and sensory motor assessment. The Health and Psychosocial Instruments (HAPI) database is also available via OVID. HAPI contains a variety of measurement instruments in various formats including questionnaires, interview schedules, scales and checklists. Many scales are copyrighted and the researcher will need to obtain written permission to use the tool. Some cases will involve a cost. As previously stated, developers of these research instruments are generally delighted but they may stipulate that the scale is not to be altered in any way. Some scales, such as the Edinburgh Postnatal Depression Scale, are available in the public domain and permission to use is not required.

There are a number of factors that should be considered when selecting a scale for use. It is essential to ensure that the scale you use measures what you want to measure in your study. For example, if you want to measure resilience it is essential that the instrument you choose measures resilience, not some other concept like coping. Selecting a reliable and valid scale is also important. Frank-Stromborg and Olsen (2004) argue that there is a strong relationship between the amount of psychometric information provided by the developer and the quality of a scale. Where the commonly expected measures of reliability and validity are missing it should be assumed that the quality of the scale is not supported. Understanding what are the most appropriate measures for demonstrating quality and how to interpret these statistics will be covered in the next section. The feasibility of using the scale also needs to be assessed. If you were interested in measuring fatigue in a group of women undergoing chemotherapy for metastatic breast cancer, a brief and simple instrument to measure their fatigue is required, so that it does not contribute to the fatigue the women experience. Some scales are costly to purchase and require particular expertise in scoring or administering. Unless you have access to these resources and expertise, it may be easier to choose another scale. In some scales the wording may not be relevant for the current population and substitution of some words may be necessary, for example, substituting 'nappy' for 'diaper' in a scale originally developed in the USA, for use with Australian parents. In summary, many factors should be considered when evaluating a scale, and whether or not the scale is the most appropriate for the study often calls for judgment (Frank-Stromborg & Olsen 2004).

Quality of existing tools

Quality is an important consideration when selecting a scale for use in research. Frank-Stromborg and Olsen (2004) describe a good scale as valid and reliable. It measures what it is supposed to measure (validity) and it measures the concept consistently across settings and groups of participants (reliability).

Reliability is the degree of consistency or dependability with which a scale measures a concept (Polit & Beck 2008). Three types of reliability will be considered: equivalence, homogeneity and stability.

Equivalence involves comparing the degree to which two raters measuring the same event obtain the same results (Burns & Grove 2009). This is also referred to as interrater reliability. Exploring interrater reliability is an essential step if the researcher intends to use an observational scale. Cohen's kappa statistic is used to examine the agreement between two raters observing the same event simultaneously and rating it independently. The value of Cohen's kappa ranges from −1.0 (perfect disagreement) to 1.0 (perfect agreement). Values of 0.41 to 0.60 indicate fair agreement, 0.61 to 0.8 indicate moderate agreement, while levels above 0.8 indicate good agreement (Frank-Stromborg & Olsen 2004).

Equivalence also refers to the degree to which two different forms of a particular scale are able to produce similar results when completed by the same participant/s on different occasions (Burns & Grove 2009). In practice there are few scales that have alternative forms, so this type of reliability is seldom able to be assessed.

Homogeneity or internal consistency is the extent to which all items in the scale measure the same variable (Burns & Grove 2009). The most commonly used test of consistency is the Cronbach's alpha coefficient. The value for the coefficient should range between 0.00 and 1.00. The higher the coefficient the more the measure is internally consistent (Polit & Beck 2008). A reliability coefficient of 0.70 is considered acceptable for a newly developed instrument with values of 0.8 and above desirable (Frank-Stromborg & Olsen 2004). The Kuder-Richardson (KR20) coefficient is the same as Cronbach's alpha and is used when the items on the scale are dichotomous (yes/no).

Stability or test-retest reliability refers to the ability of a scale to produce the same or similar results with the same group of participants on two (or more) occasions. The two sets of scores are compared using a correlation coefficient. Reliability coefficients (r) range from 0.0 to 1.0 and a high correlation between the scores supports the stability of the measure. Test-retest reliability assumes that the concept or variable being measured has not changed during the measurement period (Burns & Grove 2009).

Validity of existing tools

The validity of a scale refers to the extent to which it measures what it is supposed to measure. If a researcher wishes to measure self-esteem in a group of adolescents, a scale that truly measures self-esteem and not some other construct such as resilience is needed. Three types of validity are considered: content, criterion and construct.

Content validity refers to the extent to which the items or questions reflect the concept being measured. It is subjective and usually based on prior research and expert opinion (Burns & Grove 2009).

Criterion validity is used to evaluate whether or not a scale measures what it is supposed to measure by comparing it with another measure known to be valid. Criterion validity can be subdivided into two types: concurrent and predictive. If a researcher wished to test whether or not a newly developed 10-item scale measured fatigue, they could ask participants to complete the scale and at the same time (concurrently) ask them to rate their fatigue on a Visual Analogue Scale measuring 0–10. If the scores from the scale closely match the scores from the visual analogue, the researcher could conclude that there is some evidence for the concurrent validity of the scale. Predictive validity refers to the ability of a scale to predict a future occurrence (Burns & Grove 2009).

Construct validity is the extent to which the instrument measures what it is supposed to measure (Macnee & McCabe 2008). Construct validity is established over time with an accumulation of evidence. Methods to establish construct validity include convergent, divergent and multitrait-multimethod.

The convergent approach involves the use of two instruments that are supposed to measure the same variable or construct (two measures of depression). Participants are asked to complete both measures and then a correlation analysis is used to assess whether the scores change in the same direction. If one goes up, the other should go up. The divergent approach uses measures that are theoretically opposite (fatigue and vitality) and examines the correlation between them, which should be negative. The multitrait-multimethod approach is based on the premise that different measures of the same construct should produce similar results while measures of different constructs should produce dissimilar results (Elliot 2007). Statistical methods such as factor analysis can also be used to measure construct validity. Factor analysis identifies and groups together items in a scale that measure the same underyling attribute. For further reading on the use of factor analysis to demonstrate construct validity, see Polit and Beck (2008).

Using a hand-held device

Innovative ways to engage potential participants should be considered by all researchers, to ensure maximal participation. A hand-held device can be used for most types of data collection (Bobula et al. 2004; Fahey & Ranse 2010) and observation of practice. The most common hand-held devices are personal digital assistants and tablet personal computers.

Personal digital assistant (PDA)

A PDA is a small hand-held device commonly used in today's society to store the owner's personal information. In research, PDAs are primarily used for data collection and capture. PDAs are convenient because the researcher can enter real-time information into an electronic form (Figure 10.1). Once data is entered into the PDA, it is synchronised with a personal computer and imported into a database, removing the need for paper forms and later transcription (Guadagno et al. 2004).

Fahey and Ranse (2010) used PDAs at a large agricultural show in Australia to collect information about the types of advice, clinical interventions and activities that health care professionals undertook.

Figure 10.1   Examples of PDA screens used to collect data

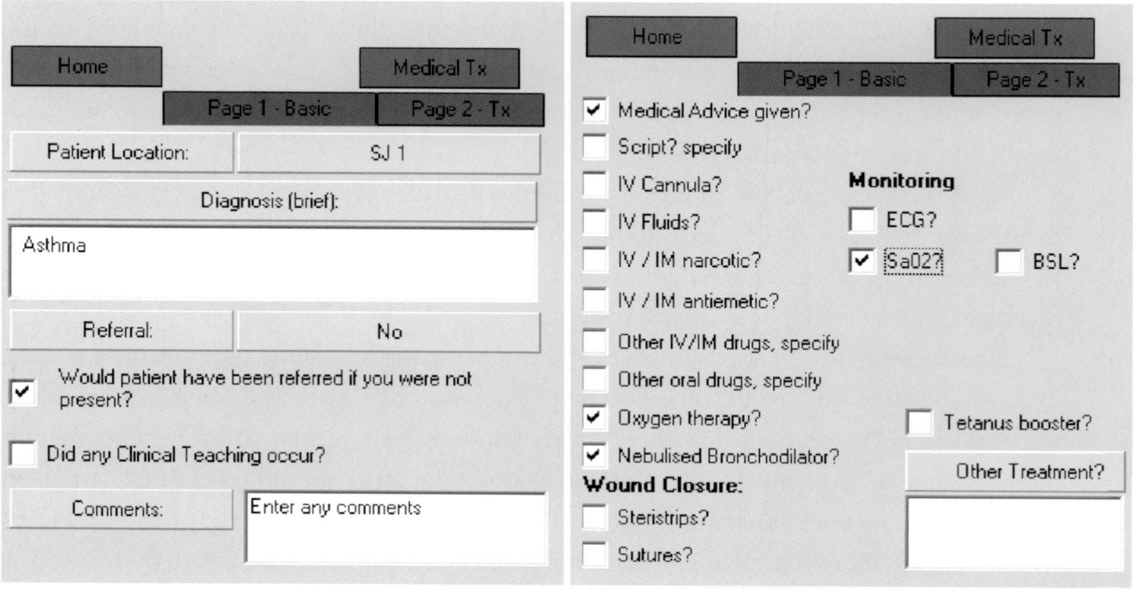

Source: Fahey & Ranse 2010

PDAs do not restrict researchers to single-centre studies; in fact they allow for the use of multiple PDAs, which have the ability to link their data.

Guadagno and associates (2004) used hand-held devices in four emergency departments to undertake a multicentre study on elder neglect. Information collected from participants included an individual interview and a physical examination. Once data had been entered by the data collectors at the various sites, the data were transferred to a central location via a telephone line.

The use of technology relies on the acceptance of the users, adequate testing of the technology before usage and a back-up strategy in the event of equipment failure (Guadagno et al. 2004). If designing a survey for use with a PDA, a computer software program is needed to create the data entry form in a compatible format. Such software programs are available online, and include Pendragon Software (www.pendragon-software.com) and HanDBase (www.handbase.com). In some instances, forms can be generated using Microsoft Access or similar programs and then transferred from the researchers' personal computer to the PDA.

Tablet personal computer and laptops

A tablet personal computer (tablet PC) is similar to a laptop computer. It differs from the PDA in that it is a fully functioning personal computer, whereas the PDA is a small compact computer with limited capacity and functionality. The tablet PC has a larger touch screen, which allows participants to engage in interactive functions. Unlike the PDA, the tablet PC does not require specialised programs to create data collection forms or to collect data. Microsoft programs such as Excel and Access will function to their normal capacity, reducing the need for specialised information technology knowledge. Like a PDA, multiple devices can be used simultaneously that collectively synchronise to create a single database.

Summary

The methods used to collect quantitative data are a crucial element in determining the quality of the research. There are a number of quantitative methods that may be used and the task for the beginning researcher is to choose a method or methods that are consistent with the purpose of the research and the chosen design. If the data collection methods are not appropriate then the research findings can be challenged.

IMPLICATIONS FOR EVIDENCE-BASED NURSING AND MIDWIFERY

Evidence-based practice has become an expected standard in health care. The evidence from any research will only be as good as the data from which it was drawn. The method chosen to generate the data is therefore a crucial component. There are a variety of data collection methods commonly used in quantitative research and choosing the right one for the research question, the problem, the design, and the accuracy and consistency of results is at the centre of successful data collection.

Practice exercise 10.1

The SF-36 Health and Well-Being is a standard questionnaire which can be used to assess an individual's general well-being. There are 36 questions which evaluate physical and mental health. One of the questions is shown below.

In general, would you say your health is:

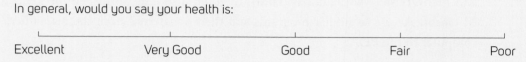

Excellent   Very Good   Good   Fair   Poor

Two team members will collect data by the personal face-to-face interviewing method. They have tested the questionnaire by asking 10 patients admitted to the hospital with chest pain as their chief complaint. They have found that interrater reliability of the questions ranges between 0.80 and 0.95. Does this confirm that the questionnaire has reliability? Explain.

Source: J. E. Ware 2010. SF-36® health survey update. Retrieved 2 September 2010, from <www.sf-6.org/tools/sf36.shtml>

Practice exercise 10.2

Create a survey using SurveyMonkey. To do this exercise, readers will need to be at a computer with active internet access.

1   In your desired internet browser, go to <www.surveymonkey.com>
2   Click on 'Join now for free!'
3   Enter your details to obtain a username and password.
4   Plan what you would like to ask your respondents and list the variables.
5   Once you have logged on using your username and password click on 'create survey'.
6   Design a survey with 10 questions:
    a   the first 5 should relate to participant demographics, such as age, gender, sex, postcode, income, highest level of education, religion
    b   the next 5 questions should explore a topic of interest to you.
7   Once your survey is complete, send it to five colleagues.

Practice exercise 10.3

a   You are a member of a team of researchers investigating the factors influencing increased turnover rates among nurses and midwives working in a large community health centre. The team is aware of research that links emotional exhaustion, a component of burnout, with decreased job satisfaction and seeking employment elsewhere (voluntary turnover). You have been asked to locate a scale to measure emotional exhaustion, and a search of the databases of available instruments identifies an existing scale that could be used. Outline the steps you would take in deciding whether or not this instrument is suitable for your study.

b   Below are two fictitious studies that use a structured telephone interview to collect data. What factors do you need to consider when using the telephone for collecting data? The research has ethics approval and potential participants have consented to take part in the study.

Study a:

The maternity unit where you work has recently revised the discharge information given to women following the birth. The topics include breastfeeding, infant care and behaviour, physical changes and self-care, emotional changes, resuming sexual activity, and community supports and services. Information is provided in hard copy and online. You have been asked to evaluate women's satisfaction with the information using a rating scale ranging from very satisfied to very dissatisfied for each topic. You decide to collect the data using a structured telephone interview four weeks after the birth.

Study b:

The medical ward in the country hospital where you work has recently developed a structured discharge information program for patients in rural areas living with a chronic illness. The program includes information about managing chronic illness as well as links to sources and websites that deal with particular illnesses. The information is provided in hard copy and online. You have been asked to evaluate client satisfaction with the information using a rating scale ranging from very satisfied to very dissatisfied for each topic. You decide to collect the data using a structured telephone interview four weeks after discharge from hospital.

Answers to practice exercises

10.1

Yes. Interrater reliability more than 0.80 indicates that all three researchers have a similar way of collecting information from participants. No or little bias will occur from having more than one person collect the data.

10.3 a

The following factors should be considered when evaluating an existing scale.

Does the scale measure what we want to measure?

Is the scale designed to measure emotional exhaustion? Does the content contain items that we would expect in a measure of emotional exhaustion based on our understanding of the literature? Is it reliable and valid?

Examine the reliability and validity statistics reported for the scale. Are the appropriate measures reported? Homogeneity or internal consistency is an important measure of reliability. This will be reported as a Cronbach's alpha coefficient. A coefficient of 0.8 or above is desirable. Hint: Refer back to Quality of Measures for other forms of reliability and validity.

Has it been used with this population (nurses and midwives) previously?

Look at the samples used in previous studies. If the scale was designed to use with health professionals it should be suitable.

Will our participants understand the language used in the scale?

Are there some words that may need to be changed for the Australian context? For example, perhaps the scale uses the word 'recipient' where we might use the word 'patient'.

Will we need permission to use the scale?

If the scale is not in the public domain we will need permission from the developer.

Is it available for free or will there be a cost involved?

If there is a cost, factor that cost into the budget for the research.

Is it easy to score or do we need specialised knowledge or expertise?

Some scales (especially scales used in psychological research) require a person with particular knowledge/expertise to administer them. Is there someone on the team who can provide that expertise?

The decision to use a scale requires judgment on a number of factors. If the answer to most of your questions is yes, and you think that the scale will meet the needs of the study, then use it. Otherwise, find another scale or trial the scale in a pilot study (Frank-Stromborg & Olsen 2004). For more information read *Instruments for Clinical Health-Care Research* by Frank-Stromborg and Olsen (2004).

10.3b

Participant factors

Contact the participants to confirm a mutually suitable date and time for interview. Tell them approximately how long the interview will last. Provide them with a toll free number to call if they subsequently wish to change the time/date of the call, ask questions or raise concerns.

Researcher factors

Develop the interview schedule. Ensure questions are easy to understand, deal with only one issue at a time and have an easy response format. For example, using the same response format for the majority of questions (very satisfied to very dissatisfied) means that participants do not have to remember different potential responses (now I want you to rate your satisfaction on a scale from 1 to 10 with 1 being the least satisfied and 10 being the most satisfied).

Develop a data entry sheet based on the interview schedule. Have the research team review the questions and data entry sheet and revise where necessary.

Pilot-test the schedule and the data entry sheets using participants who will not be part of your sample. Ask them for feedback on clarity of questions, how you communicate during the interview, as well as timing the interview so you can inform the study participants how long it will be. Ask a researcher who is experienced in telephone interviewing to sit in on two or three pilot interviews to give feedback on the process. Based on the feedback, revise your questions, data entry sheet and/or how you conduct the interview.

Finally, when calling participants you may be asked questions about current health concerns. You should not give advice to participants that is outside your scope of practice. Follow the processes for this situation, which were approved by the ethics committee. Musselwhite et al. (2007) suggest the following:

- When participants seek general reassurance that their symptom is not unique make a general statement such as 'women often experience fatigue following birth' or 'experiencing fatigue after surgery is not uncommon'.
- Be aware of signs of serious or urgent conditions requiring medical care and either refer to the usual health provider or encourage the participant to contact a support person for immediate help, and/or call emergency services.
- If necessary undertake to make this call with the participant's permission.

Further reading

Frank-Stromborg, M., & Olsen, S. (2004). *Instruments for Clinical Health-Care Research*. Boston: Jones & Bartlett Publishers.

Polit, D., & Beck, C. (2008). Developing and testing self-report scales. In D. Polit & C. Beck (eds), *Nursing Research: Generating and Assessing Evidence for Nursing Practice* (pp. 474–505). Philadelphia: Lippincott Williams & Wilkins.

Walonick, D. (2004). Survival Statistics StatPac Inc. Retrieved 2 August 2009, from <www.statpac.com/surveys>

Weblinks

<http://freeonlinesurveys.com>

Free online surveys; provides a service to develop, distribute and collate free online surveys.

<http://handbase.com>

HanDBase, a software platform that allows for the development of form and the collection of data on a hand-held device, such as a personal digital assistant.

Jan Taylor and Jamie Ranse

<www.ovid.com/site/catalog/DataBase/866.jsp>

Health and Psychosocial Instruments (HAPI) contains a variety of measurement instruments suitable for use in nursing and midwifery research including questionnaires, interview schedules, scales and checklists.

<www.kwiksurveys.com>

Kwik surveys provides a service to develop, distribute and collate free online surveys.

<www.ovid.com/site/catalog/DataBase/120.jsp>

Mental Measurement Yearbook covers more than 4000 commercially available tests in categories such as personality, developmental, behavioural and sensory motor assessment.

<www.pendragon-software.com>

Pendragon Software, a software platform that assists the researcher in development of forms and the collection of data on a hand-held device, such as a PDA.

<www.gravic.com/remark>

Remark has a number of products that will assist with data collection and analysis.

<www.surveymonkey.com>

SurveyMonkey is a service to develop, distribute and collate free online surveys. The most popular web-based survey.

References

Ahern, N. (2005). Using the internet to conduct research. *Nurse Researcher* 13(2), 55–70.

Australian Bureau of Statistics. (2007). *Patterns of Internet Access in Australia, 2006.* (publication no. 8146.0.55.001). Canberra: Australian Government.

Bobula, J., Anderson, L., Riesch, S., Canty-Mitchell, J., Duncan, A., Kaiser-Krueger, H., Brown, R., & Angresano, N. (2004). Enhancing survey data collection among youth and adults: Use of handheld and laptop computers. *Computers, Informatics, Nursing* 22(5), 255–65.

Burns, N. & Grove, S. (2009). *The Practice of Nursing Research: Appraisal, Synthesis, and Generation of Evidence.* St Louis, MI: Elsevier.

Burns, R. (2000). *Introduction to Research Methods.* Sydney: Longman.

Courtney, K. L., & Craven, C. K. (2005). Factors to weigh when considering electronic data collection. *The Canadian Journal of Nursing Research* 37(3), 150–9.

Creedy, D., Cantrill, R., & Cooke, M. (2008). Assessing midwives' breastfeeding knowledge: Properties of the Newborn Feeding Ability questionnaire and Breastfeeding Initiation Practices scale. *International Breastfeeding Journal* 3, 7.

Dillman, D. A., Tortora, R. D., & Bowker, D. (1998). Principles for constructing web-surveys. SESRC Technical Report 98-50, Pullman, Washington. Retrieved 18 November 2010, from <www.sesrc.wsu.edu/dillman/papers/websurveyppr.pdf>.

Duffy, M. E. (2002). Methodological issues in web-based research. *Journal of Nursing Scholarship* 34(1), 83–8.

Elliot, D. (2007). Assessing measuring instruments. In Z. Schneider, D. Whitehead & D. Elliot (eds), *Nursing and Midwifery Research: Methods and Appraisal for Evidence-Based Practice.* (pp. 206–24). Sydney: Elsevier.

Elliot, D., & Schneider, Z. (2007). Quantitative data collection and study validity. In Z. Schneider, D. Whitehead & D. Elliot, *Nursing and Midwifery Research, Methods and Appraisal for Evidence-Based Practice* (pp. 192–205) Sydney: Elsevier.

Fahey, D., & Ranse, J. (2010). The role of medical officers at mass gathering events. Unpublished research.

Frank-Stromborg, M., & Olsen, S. (2004). *Instruments for Clinical Health-Care Research.* Boston: Jones & Bartlett Publishers.

Gerdtz, M. F., & Bucknall, T. K. (2001). Triage nurses' clinical decision making. An observational study of urgency assessment. *Journal of Advanced Nursing* 35(4), 550–61.

Guadagno, L., Vandeweerd, C., Stevens, D., Abraham, I., Paveza, G. J., & Fulmer, T. (2004). Using PDAs for data collection. *Applied Nursing Research* 17(4), 283–91.

Houser, J. (2008). *Nursing Research: Reading, Using and Creating Evidence.* Boston: Jones & Bartlett Publishers.

Im, E. O., & Chee, W. (2002). Issues in protection of human subjects in internet research. *Nursing Research* 51(4), 266–9.

Jirojwong, S., & MacLennan, R. (2004). Do people in rural and remote Queensland delay using health services to manage the episodes of incapacity? *Health and Social Care in the Community* 12(3), 233–42.

Kermode, S., & Roberts, K. (2007a). Quantitative methods. In B. Taylor, S. Kermode & K. Roberts (eds), *Research in Nursing and Health Care: Evidence for Practice* (pp. 200–43). Australia: Thomson.

Kermode, S., & Roberts, K. (2007b). Quantitative data collection and management. In B. Taylor, S. Kermode & K. Roberts (eds), *Research in Nursing and Health Care: Evidence for Practice* (pp. 244–67). Australia: Thomson.

Kitchenham, B., & Pfleeger, S. (2002). Principles of survey research: part 3: Constructing a survey instrument. ACM SIGSOFT Software *Engineering Notes* 27, 20–4.

MacLennan, R. (2009). Project Planning: Projects and protocols. In S. Jirojwong & P. Liamputtong (eds), *Population Health, Communities and Health Promotion* (pp. 123–33) Melbourne: Oxford University Press.

Macnee, C., & McCabe, S. (2008). *Understanding Nursing Research: Reading and Using Research in Evidence-Based Practice.* Philadelphia: Lippincott Williams & Wilkins.

Morris, D. L., Fenton, M. V., & Mercer, Z. B. (2004). Identification of national trends in nursing education through the use of an online survey. *Nursing Outlook* 52(5), 248–54.

Musselwhite, K., Cuff, L., McGregor, L., & King, K. M. (2007). The telephone interview is an effective method of data collection in clinical nursing research: A discussion paper. *International Journal of Nursing Studies* 44, 1064–70.

Nielsen Media Research. (2001). *Size of Internet Universe by Country.* Retrieved 14 August 2009, from <http://en-us.nielsen.com/content/nielsen/en_us/industries/media.html>

Nieswiadomy, R. M. (2008). *Foundations of Nursing Research.* New Jersey: Prentice Hall.

Norman, R. (2001). Have you got an attitude problem? Caring for illicit drug-using patients. *Contemporary Nursing* 10, 83–90.

Polit, D., & Beck, C. (2008). *Nursing Research: Generating and Assessing Evidence for Nursing Practice,* 8th edn. Philadelphia: Lippincott Williams & Wilkins.

Smith, E. (2005). Telephone interviewing in healthcare research: A summary of the evidence. *Nurse Researcher* 12(3), 32–41.

Stewart, S. (2003). Casting the net: Using the internet for survey research. *British Journal of Midwifery* 11(9), 543–5.

Thom, B. (2007). Role of the simple self-designed questionnaire in nursing research. *Journal of Pediatric Oncology Nursing* 24(6), 350–5.

White, G. (2003). Intensive care nurses' perceptions of brain death. *Australian Critical Care* 16(1), 7–14.

PART 3

Pathways to Evidence-based Practice

THE HOSPITAL has called for research grant applications. Ann has now decided to use a qualitative research design to explore the experiences of patients with chest pain. Bob on the other hand wants to investigate personal demographic factors impacting on patients' decision to re-present to the emergency department.

Both Ann and Bob have been successful with their respective grant applications. Ann had reviewed each of the different qualitative designs and decided on a phenomenological approach to enquiry which she believes is the most appropriate for her research question concerning a lived experience. Bob decided on a cross-sectional study. Both Ann and Bob have received good support from their colleagues and research team, who have provided constructive feedback throughout the processes of developing a research proposal and collecting data.

As part of her study Ann and her team conducted in-depth interviews with 10 participants. At the completion of the tenth interview, no new information was forthcoming, so Ann decided that no further interviews were required. Bob and his team collected data from 80 patients as planned. Together, Ann and Bob have now gathered a large amount of data that needs to be analysed. In keeping with a phenomenological research design Ann has selected a thematic approach for the analysis of her interviews. Chapter 11 provides a useful guide in selecting an appropriate method of data analysis that is consistent with the research design of the study. Bob has chosen a quantitative analysis approach, which is consistent with his chosen research design. Chapter 12 provides a comprehensive discussion of the various methods of data analysis used in quantitative research.

After the data are analysed, and the results interpreted, it is important that Ann and Bob compare their results to other similar studies through a critical review of the research literature on the topic. Part of a critical review is an evaluation of the researcher's own study, including a self-evaluation by the researcher, and a critique of the rigour of the study—all processes and procedures used as part of the study. Chapter 13 provides important information on how to conduct a critical review of research literature. ▶

A study is not complete until the findings are presented to your peers. The presentation of findings is an obligation that is part of conducting research. There are several ways by which the findings of a study can be communicated to the broader community of scholars and health care professionals. Chapter 15 explores some ideas about how the research results can be shared with others. The important reason for disseminating results of research studies is to share with colleagues the development of new knowledge and its usefulness in applying the results to current clinical practice. Through the application of research results to clinical practice, current practices can be evaluated and new and improved approaches to practice can be developed supported by the best available evidence. The results of research can play an important role in the development of clinical guidelines and protocols for establishing best practice. As part of choosing the best research evidence to support quality change, a systematic review of available research is needed. Chapter 14 provides a comprehensive description of the steps in synthesising available research on a particular research topic as well as providing a critique of the quality of the research.

The results of Ann and Bob's studies can now be included in the synthesis of research results. Their results have the potential to contribute to a review of current pain management practices in emergency departments. The findings of these studies also have the potential to generate new research questions leading to new research on pain management. The journey Ann and Bob have embarked on is one important step along the pathway of research, a pathway that will lead to new horizons of understanding and the advancement of nursing and midwifery practice.

CHAPTER 11

Qualitative Data Analysis

WITHDRAWN

Lisa Whitehead

Chapter learning objectives

By the end of this chapter you will be able to:

▸ understand the differences between various approaches to qualitative data analysis, including grounded theory, ethnography and phenomenology

▸ apply information on data analysis by working through the early stages of analysis

▸ generate awareness of processes that can be used to improve and demonstrate trustworthiness in qualitative analysis

▸ understand the practicalities and resource demands involved in qualitative data analysis

▸ become familiar with the functions of qualitative data analysis software.

KEY TERMS
Code
Constant comparison
Familiarisation
Methodology
Theme
Theoretical saturation
Theory

Introduction

All data that are collected in the course of a research study require some form of analysis. In qualitative research, data collection can take many forms: face-to-face interviews, focus groups, photographs and explanation (photo voice), objects, video, diaries, field notes and internet-based interviews. There are a number of approaches to qualitative data analysis and the approach taken for any given study will be determined by the methodology guiding the study (see Chapter 5). The researcher is likely to take one of three broad approaches to qualitative analysis:

- The number of times a particular word or concept, for example, fatigue, occurs in narrative would be counted. The qualitative data can then be categorised and if required statistical analysis undertaken. This kind of analysis is referred to as content analysis.
- A thematic analysis would explore data further than the first example. All data referring to a concept, for example, 'stigma', would be given a code, extracted and examined in more detail.
- In a theoretical analysis such as grounded theory, the researcher would analyse the data further to generate an emerging theory. The theory may be tested against existing theories or against further analysis of the data, a process referred to as analytic induction (Strauss & Corbin 1990).

Regardless of the approach to qualitative data analysis, there are a number of general considerations.

The stages of qualitative analysis

Analysis of qualitative data usually goes through some or all of the following stages:

- familiarisation with the data through reading, watching and/or listening
- transcription of recorded material
- organising and indexing of data for easy retrieval and identification
- anonymisation of sensitive data
- coding
- identification of themes
- re-coding
- development of provisional categories
- exploration of relationships between categories
- refinement of themes and categories
- development of theory and incorporation of pre-existing knowledge.

Theories and methods

Where a researcher has adopted a design, such as grounded theory, to inform a study, the process of data analysis will be driven by the framework of that design. The researcher may choose to follow general inductive principles of qualitative research and in this case may choose to draw on a generic approach such as thematic analysis. The particular approach chosen will be guided by a number of considerations including the research question and the sampling method. This section explores the process of data analysis as it relates to a general approach through thematic analysis and then on to three key designs in qualitative research: grounded theory, phenomenology and ethnography.

Thematic analysis

Many qualitative researchers draw on thematic analysis to analyse qualitative data. This may be as part of a wider methodological design such as ethnography, or as a stand-alone design. There are several approaches to thematic analysis in circulation and this section will outline the general features of an inductive thematic analysis.

An interview is generally prepared for analysis by a verbatim transcription. A numbering system such as line numbers is often applied to help locate text throughout the analysis and reporting process. The transcript may be printed out for analysis or imported into a software package such as NVivo and viewed electronically. Once the text has been read a number of times and the researcher is familiar with this, the next step is to identify specific sections of the text. This is termed 'coding' and refers to highlighting sections of the text. These sections may be a word, a phrase or a whole passage; it depends on the researcher's approach and the data as to how much data is highlighted in order to maintain the context of the situation or experience described. Once the transcript has been read a number of times and coding done, often on a number of transcripts, codes are reviewed and, if appropriate, themes generated. Themes may be developed in one of three ways: theory-driven, where the researcher seeks to explore the application of a theory to the data collected; from previous research, where the researcher seeks to explore and compare themes generated through previous research; or inductively (from the raw data), to explore the data without any consciously expressed predetermined interest. The three approaches can be considered on a continuum from theory-driven at one end to data-driven at the other. The former approach is the most common and is discussed further below.

Inductive themes may be derived from the research aims of the study and more specific themes derived from multiple readings of the raw data. One section of text may be coded into more than one theme and sections of text may not be coded at all if they do not relate to the aims of the study (see Practice exercise 11.4). Generally, the creation and assignment of themes to the text continues through a number of readings and undergoes revision as the analysis evolves. A number of sub-themes may emerge as the meaning of an initial theme becomes more complex through the analysis of further texts. Quotations are usually selected to illustrate the essence of the theme. While there are no rules about the number of themes that may be developed in a given study, when a large number of themes are generated the researcher should carefully evaluate that true differences between the themes exist and where there is overlap that this is clear to the reader. The researcher may be able to combine themes with significant overlap to enhance clarity. Depending on the aims of the study, the researcher may choose to present the themes descriptively or interpret them in the context of a theory or conceptual framework as befits the method employed in the study.

While presented as a linear, step-by-step process (Figure 11.1), thematic analysis is an iterative and reflexive process.

Table 11.1   Stages of thematic analysis

Stage 1	Stage 2	Stage 3	Stage 4	Stage 5
Multiple readings of the data to generate familiarisation	Recognising and noting important, interesting and relevant data	Generating themes to capture the qualitative richness of the phenomenon noted in stage 2	Refining of themes and development of relationships between themes through reading and comparison with further data	Interpretation of themes in the context of theory or conceptual framework

Example of inductive coding

In a study analysing qualitative data on the role that families play in supporting a member living with heart failure (Whitehead 2009), analysis of the response to the question 'What impact has living with heart failure in your family had on your life?', one participant gave the response: 'I ring mum and dad every morning to check that they are OK…If I ring and no one answers the phone, I worry because I think something has happened.' This response could be considered to contain two different meaning units and could be assigned two different codes relating to two different themes. The first text segment of meaning, 'I ring mum and dad every morning to check that they are OK', could relate to a theme labelled 'Feelings of responsibility'. The second, 'If I ring and no one answers the phone, I worry because I think something has happened', could be labelled 'anxiety related to deterioration in health'. A large number of themes can be assigned to a single transcript, but often these 'open' themes are combined as analysis continues. Practice exercise 11.4 works through the process of coding using excerpts of transcripts from the heart failure study.

Grounded theory

Grounded theory is a research design where data analysis is viewed as part of a wider approach beginning with the research question, sampling and data collection (see Chapter 5 for a review of grounded theory). Grounded theory analysis is inductive in that the resulting theory emerges from the data through a process of structured analysis. The aim of generating theory as the final output distinguishes grounded theory from other designs that may aim to generate a description of the data or a level of interpretation. The aim of grounded theory is theoretical development (Strauss & Corbin 1998).

Figure 11.1 Description, interpretation and theoretical development

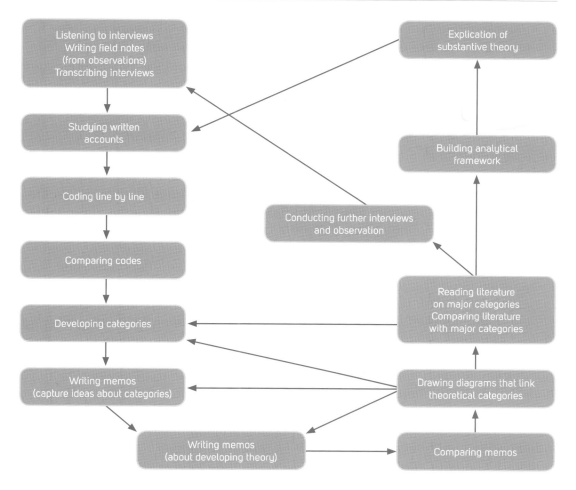

Source: Adapted from Coyne & Cowley 2006

A 'grounded theory' consists of 'plausible relationships' (Strauss & Corbin 1998) between sets of concepts directly developed from the data analysis. Theory provides a set of testable propositions to advance understanding of the social world more clearly, rather than 'absolute truths'.

Grounded theory analysis follows a structured process and normally starts with a broad research question. It then proceeds in stages, with analysis carried out after each stage of data collection to inform understanding of the concept of interest and possibly to reframe the question and so the sampling. A paper by Coyne and Cowley (2006) illustrates this process (see Box 11.1).

Lisa Whitehead

BOX 11.1

STAGES OF DATA COLLECTION

Stage 1

The study started with a broad subject area, 'parent participation in hospitalised child's care'.

Stage 2

The data indicated that 'time' could be a significant condition linked to categories labelled 'relationships' and 'knowing'. The links were tentative, which indicated the need for further sampling. Therefore it was decided to collect data from another research site where the children would experience lengthy admissions (longer than four days) in order to develop and extend the category of time.

Stage 3

The data analysis indicated that additional data needed to be collected in a theoretical manner to clarify the properties of the main categories. The criterion for when to stop sampling the different groups pertinent to a category is the category's theoretical saturation. At this stage of the analysis, the major categories appeared to be 'being there', 'uncertainty', 'disruption', 'environment', 'involvement', 'knowing', 'trusting', 'relationships', 'balancing' and 'controlling'. The links between the major categories needed to be checked with more nurse participants. Three more interviews were conducted.

Stage 4

This phase did not involve more data collection from participants. The researcher reread all the interview transcripts and theoretically sampled for the properties of time (a major category). This helped to identify the links between time and the major categories as time emerged as a sub-category of the categories 'being there', 'disruption' and 'balancing'. This stage helped to clarify that knowing and trusting were both properties and sub-categories of balancing. Concurrent with the theoretical sampling of the data, the sampling of the literature helped to clarify the core processes in the study.

At the core of grounded theory data analysis is the concept of constant comparison. This involves comparing the concepts or categories emerging from one stage of data collection with those emerging from the next. The researcher looks for relationships between the concepts and categories by constantly comparing them to form the basis of the emerging theory (Figure 11.1). The researcher continues with the process of constant comparison until they reach 'theoretical saturation', that is, no further concepts or categories emerge from the data. The process of grounded theory analysis is cumulative and can mean revisiting the data as new ideas emerge and as data collection and analysis progress. 'Theoretical sensitivity', the ability 'to see the research situation and its associated data in new ways, and to explore the data's potential for developing theory' (Strauss & Corbin 1990, p. 44), is important and although creative, remains grounded in the process.

Table 11.2   Grounded theory analysis process

Open coding (initial familiarisation with the data)
Delineation of emergent concepts
Conceptual coding (using emergent concepts)
Refinement of conceptual coding schemes
Clustering of concepts to form analytical categories
Searching for core categories
Core categories lead to identification of core theory
Testing of emerging theory by reference to wider literature and factors (such as cultural or social factors) related to the area of study

An example of how grounded theory analysis was carried out in a research study is given in the example below (Wilson & Crowe 2008).

RESEARCH IN PRACTICE 11.1

Data analysis followed Glaser's (1978) guidelines. Early data were coded with words or a conceptual label for the action in the setting. The smallest text analysed was a paragraph, and sentences relating to a topic were examined collectively rather than separately. This broad grouping ensured that data were not forced into predetermined patterns but rather allowed to speak for themselves (Glaser & Strauss 1967). Categories emerged from the clustering of codes that seemed to fit together and these were constantly compared with each other to ensure that they covered variations. The coding began after the first interview and it soon became apparent that what was of particular importance to the community mental health nurses (CMHN) was the nature and extent of their relationships with service users, with colleagues, with their managers, and hence with the wider organisation.

The core category that emerged described the process by which these nurses actively balance satisfying aspects of their job with unsatisfying aspects. The term that best described this dynamic process of balance and counterbalance was maintaining equilibrium. Maintaining equilibrium meant bridging any disparities that occurred in the category role performance. This category had three properties: working for the organisation, maintaining a personal life and belonging to a team; all had the potential to be dissatisfying or satisfying and subsequently impacting on the category therapeutic relationships. The category of therapeutic relationships had three properties: being therapeutic, knowing oneself and knowing how, which could be positively or negatively affected by the properties in role performance. Therapeutic relationships could be the primary source of satisfaction for CMHNs if the properties of role performance remained predominantly positive. The process of ensuring job satisfaction rather than dissatisfaction required the nurse to maintain an equilibrium between the properties of both categories.

Phenomenology

Researchers undertaking a phenomenological study draw on a variety of philosophical sources (Gadamer 1989; Heidegger 1996; Husserl 1970; Merleau-Ponty 1964). They can use an open approach to data analysis or choose one of the methods developed to guide phenomenological data analysis such as Colaizzi's (1978) seven-stage method or Giorgi's (1985) four-step method.

Researchers such as Gadamer (1989) and van Manen (1994) take an unstructured approach to data analysis with emphasis on the generation of insight that is rooted in life-world experiences and a belief that a structured process of analysis may constrain insight. Others have set out a process for data analysis and one of the most commonly used approaches is that of Giorgi (1985), which includes:

- reading to get a narrative sense of the text as a whole dividing the text into 'meaning units' that differentiate changes in meaning
- expressing the meanings in more general and transferable ways
- formulating a narrative structure that highlights the common themes across experiences and cases
- illustrating the common themes with quotations and drawing out the variety of experiences within a theme.

Box 11.2 illustrates the process of analysis following Giorgi's approach (Giorgi 1986) in a study on concepts of learning (Morgan 1993). The first part contains data from the interview. Following this a basic description of the interview that aims to remain faithful to the specifics of each individual's experience was written. Three key learning concepts were identified in this description.

BOX 11.2

I.   Can I ask you what do you mean by learning? When you think of learning something, what does it mean to you?

S.   To gain some knowledge, I think is learning. We're learning all the time, not necessarily by sitting down and studying. I think there are all kinds of ways. But to me learning is gaining knowledge.

I.   Can you explain what you mean by gaining knowledge?

S.   I suppose just picking up bits of information really. I think if you do it quite basically that's what it is. We do that every day in our way of life, perhaps do it to a greater degree by doing a course. We obviously want to learn more. I obviously want more knowledge about things and I've got an interest in things and I want to know as much as possible about them.

I.   So it is gaining bits and pieces of knowledge.

S.   Yes, yes.

BOX 11.2

For S, learning means to gain knowledge (1), and S affirms that we are learning all the time and that learning (2) can mean more than 'schoolwork'; indeed, S states that there are many ways to learn, but picks 'gaining knowledge' as its meaning. When pressed by the researcher concerning the meaning of 'gaining knowledge', S gives a synonymous answer: 'picking up bits of information', and he repeats it: S again expresses that learning is pervasive in life (3), but allows that it may be more apparent in a course. While S believes everyone wants to learn more, he refers to himself to answer and says that he wants to know as much as possible about things that interest him.

Ethnography

Ethnography focuses on the study of cultures and subcultures. Large-scale ethnographic studies explore large-scale institutions, communities and value-systems. Small-scale ethnographic studies explore single social settings such as a community health centre or staff working in a single ward (Seneviratne et al. 2009). Data collection involves immersion in the setting through observation, interviews with key informants, and often field notes. The aim is to generate the 'emic' or insider view of the members of the culture under study. The presentation of results involves 'thick' description to deliver a detailed account of the patterns of cultural and social relationships.

There are two main approaches to ethnography: descriptive and critical ethnography (Thomas 1993). The approach chosen has implications for the process of analysis where the outcome of a descriptive ethnographic study is to describe cultures and groups and the outcome of critical ethnographic studies is to explore the macro-social issues such as power, control and hidden agendas, drawing in a political element (Thomas 1993). Further detail on ethnography is set out in Chapter 5.

The outcome of an ethnographic analysis has been described as presenting a piece of writing that is artistic, complex and like a story so that the reader can access the complexity of data and see the social action in context (Geertz 1973). Data analysis is described as being time- and energy-intensive (Robertson & Boyle 1984) and requires that the researcher is first familiar with the data collected through field notes, interviews and/or observation. Analysis begins early, as soon as some data have been collected. Researchers then work through the stages of thematic analysis described in detail in the next section. Through the process of thematic analysis, themes are developed and related to one another, a process requiring critical thinking and skills as themes are synthesised (Fetterman 1989). Analysis of ethnographic data involves re-analysing data, moving backwards and forwards through the data and writing, and rewriting the findings. Researchers are active participants in the process of data collection and analysis, and it is necessary to acknowledge the role and influence of the researcher (see the section on trustworthiness for further details).

In presenting the analysis, quotations and examples of field notes are presented for the reader as a window on the findings and to demonstrate the process through which the researcher has gone in arriving at the finding. Ethnographic studies sometimes result in the development of theory but more commonly generate typologies or a classification system. For example, a study on communication in the operating room (Gardezi et al. 2009) identified three forms of recurring 'silences': absence of communication; not responding to queries or requests; and speaking quietly. The silences were classified as defensive or strategic and may have been influenced by larger institutional and structural power dynamics as well as by the immediate situational context. The ethnographic report, the result of the analysis, should present the main features of the group and the setting and uncover the relationships discovered through analysis. Fetterman (1998) describes this process as one 'of compression as the ethnographer moves from field notes to written text' (p. 123). It is important that the participants recognise their own social reality generated by the analysis; this would involve revisiting participants to discuss this or sending out the report for review and discussion.

Analysing visual data

Visual data may take the form of photographs, objects, hand-drawn pictures or video. Visual data may be collected to support other forms of data collection methods or to stand alone. Ethnographic research has a tradition of using visual data, usually photographs, often to illustrate major differences in the culture under study, for example dress (Ball & Smith 1992). Photographs and video allow the researcher to collect data that goes beyond words only, but there are limitations to be aware of. Both represent a snapshot in time, only what the lens can capture and often staged, particularly in the case of historical photographs; permission should be sought to photograph or video such material. Analysis of photographs and video must consider these issues in the generalisation of any analysis to a wider field. Photographs and video can be used for a number of applications in research including documentation, for instance in wound management (Swann 2000), to evaluate teaching and learning for patients and health care professionals (e.g. Krouse 2001), to promote empowerment (e.g. Baker & Wang 2006), and to promote understanding, mainly of patient experience (e.g. Gaskins & Forte 1995). The process of analysis itself can take a structured or unstructured approach depending on the researcher's stance, the research question and the research method adopted for the study. Photographs and videos can be analysed using a structured list of questions or a coding list (e.g. Anderson & Adamsen 2001). Alternatively, the researcher may choose to take an unstructured approach and note down everything that relates to the research question (e.g. Olsson et al. 1998). In a study with older adults on the pain experience, Baker and Wang (2006) asked people to take the photographs themselves and then write narratives to describe how the photograph depicted their experience of pain.

The use of drawings in the study of health and illness is limited and to date largely undertaken with children (Guillemin 2004). There has been a strong focus on the use of drawings for diagnostic or therapeutic purposes (Diem-Wille 2001). Guillemin has conducted studies with women to explore their understanding of heart disease and of menopause using drawing as a method of data collection (Guillemin 2004). Participants were first interviewed, then asked to create a drawing. They were then asked to describe their drawing, which led to reflection on links between the drawing and statements made in the interview.

Building trustworthiness in qualitative data analysis

In building trustworthiness in data analysis, a number of approaches can be taken (see also Chapter 9). The first is setting out a decision trail that documents each step of the data analysis process, effectively creating an audit trail (Whitehead 2004). This transparency allows others to follow and evaluate your process. The transcription of data is held by many, though not all, qualitative researchers as important. Transcription of recorded data reduces reliance on the selective memory and recording of notes by the researcher during data collection. It also allows the sharing of raw data with others to enhance consistency in data analysis. The researcher may instigate independent coding where an independent coder is given the research objectives and some of the raw text from which the themes were developed and asked to create themes from this raw text. Another approach would be to make coding consistency checks where an independent coder is given the research objectives, the themes and descriptions of each theme without the raw text attached. They are then given a sample of the raw text, previously coded by the initial coder, and asked to assign sections of the text to the themes that have emerged. The raw text selected has sections of text from which the initial themes were derived.

Using a qualitative data analysis program such as NVivo, the researcher may open up the data analysis process to others outside the research team to develop external credibility of the analysis process. This could include stakeholder checks, providing the opportunity for people with a specific interest in the research, such as participants and service providers, to comment on themes or the interpretations made (Erlandson et al. 1993, p. 142). Stakeholder checks may be carried out throughout the research process, for example, providing a summary of the data at the completion of interviews and allowing respondents to immediately correct errors of fact or challenge interpretations. Checks may occur during subsequent interviews by asking respondents to verify interpretations and data gathered in earlier interviews. Before submission of the final report, researchers may provide copies of a preliminary analysis version, or specific sections of the research report, to stakeholder groups, asking for a written or oral commentary. A stakeholder check may be conducted by providing a complete draft copy for review by respondents or other persons in the setting being studied.

In qualitative data analysis most approaches recognise the role of the researcher in shaping data collection and in data analysis. The researcher can reflect on their role in data generation and subsequent analysis and make this explicit to the reader of the research report or paper rather than attempt to remove themselves (known as 'bracketing') out of the process or to ignore this. For example Whitehead states in her study of the experience of living with chronic fatigue syndrome:

> [M]y experience as a nurse taught me to recognise patients' symptoms as 'real' to them. One quote that stayed with me after my training seemed particularly relevant: 'pain is what a patient says it is and exists when he says it does' (McCaffery 1983, p. 95). Inherent in this is the acceptance, without prejudice, of what the patient says. I found the treatment that some of the participants had experienced unacceptable and detrimental to their welfare. A review of the notes at a later stage helped to show how my horizon was operating during and shortly after the interview, and prompted reflection on the horizon of the text and the prejudices that I brought, and continued to bring, to the analysis. (2004, p. 517)

Computer software packages for qualitative analysis

The use of computer software packages to aid qualitative data analysis has been growing since the mid-1990s. Current packages include NVivo and AtlasTi, and while they have different interfaces, all facilitate the same processes, namely data storage and management, coding, data searching and retrieval, and developing and testing theory.

Data storage and management

Software packages allow the researcher to import raw data and file these. Data can comprise text files such as transcriptions but also visual material, such as photographs, videos and scanned documents. Files can be labelled and indexed accordingly and text files can be annotated once imported into the software.

Coding

During analysis of the data, themes can be created easily and assigned to small or large sections of the data as the researcher chooses. Figure 11.2 shows a section of a transcribed interview with themes assigned to parts of the text within NVivo.

As analysis evolves, themes can be renamed, deleted or moved into a hierarchical framework without losing any of the data or any analysis. An example of a coding scheme for a study on the experience of fatigue in chronic illness is set out in Figure 11.3.

Following inductive analysis the tree nodes (higher-order nodes) were developed. The theme of impact of fatigue has been 'exploded' to show the sub-themes within the main theme of the impact of fatigue.

Figure 11.2 NVivo screenshot of a transcribed interview

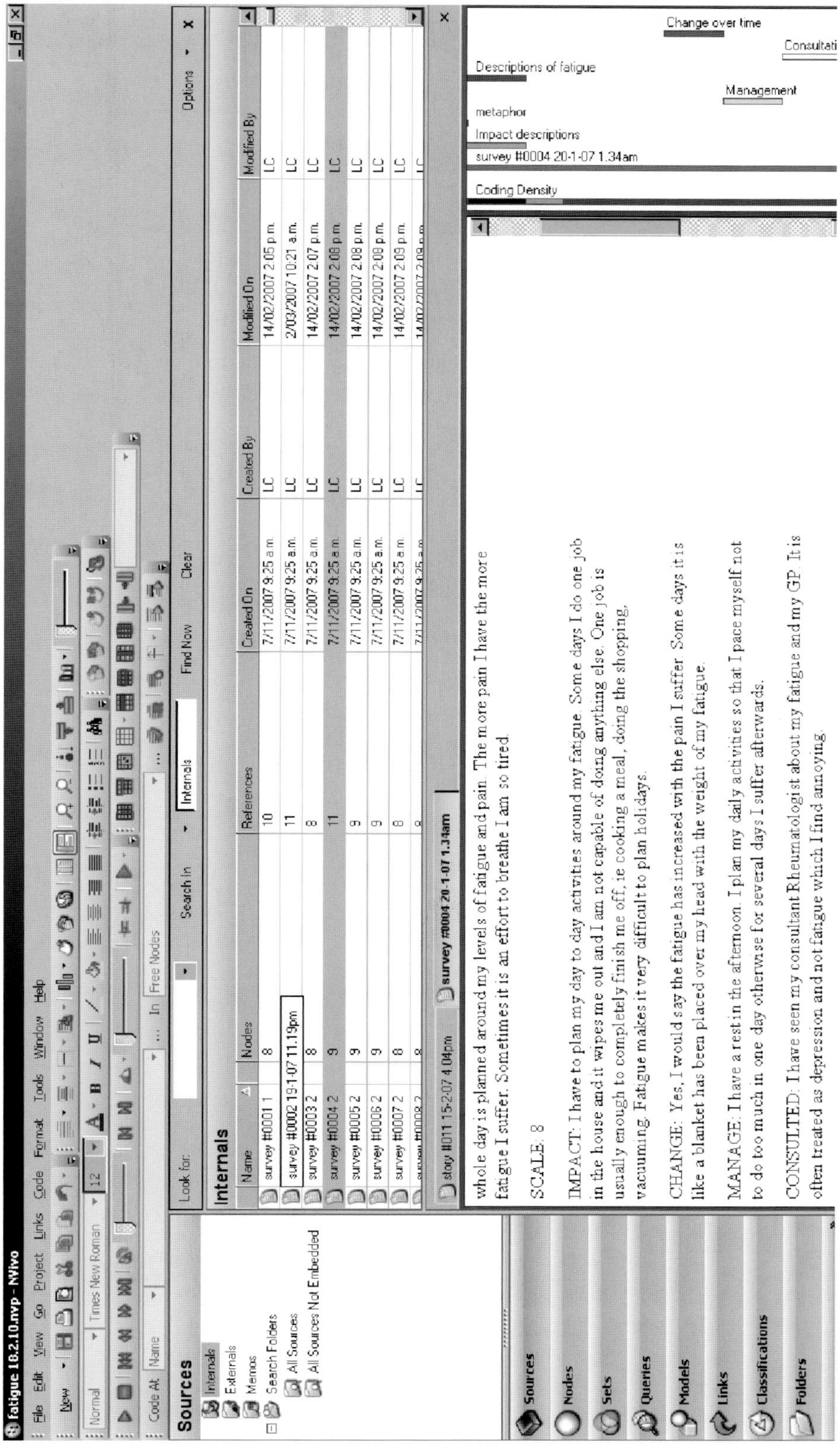

Figure 11.3   NVivo screenshot of an example coding scheme

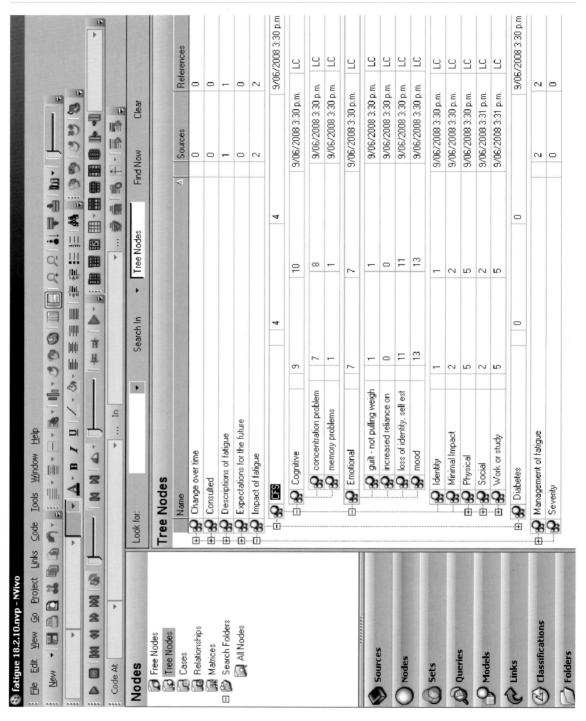

Data searching and retrieval

Computer programs allow the researcher to search the text for particular words or phrases. Data coded under each theme can be displayed easily and if attributes have been assigned to each participant such as gender, occupation and age, the researcher can display data coded under a theme by a given attribute, for example, all data coded under the theme 'stigma' for men under the age of 35 years.

Developing and testing theory

Software packages can facilitate theoretical modelling by allowing relationships between themes to be explored and displayed. This can take the form of building a hierarchical system or producing a diagrammatic representation. Hutchison and colleagues (2009) created a model in NVivo (Figure 11.4) to summarise conceptual development as analysis progressed in a study on how people successfully change their physical activity habits in order to improve their own personal health and/or well-being.

Figure 11.4   Model showing conceptual development

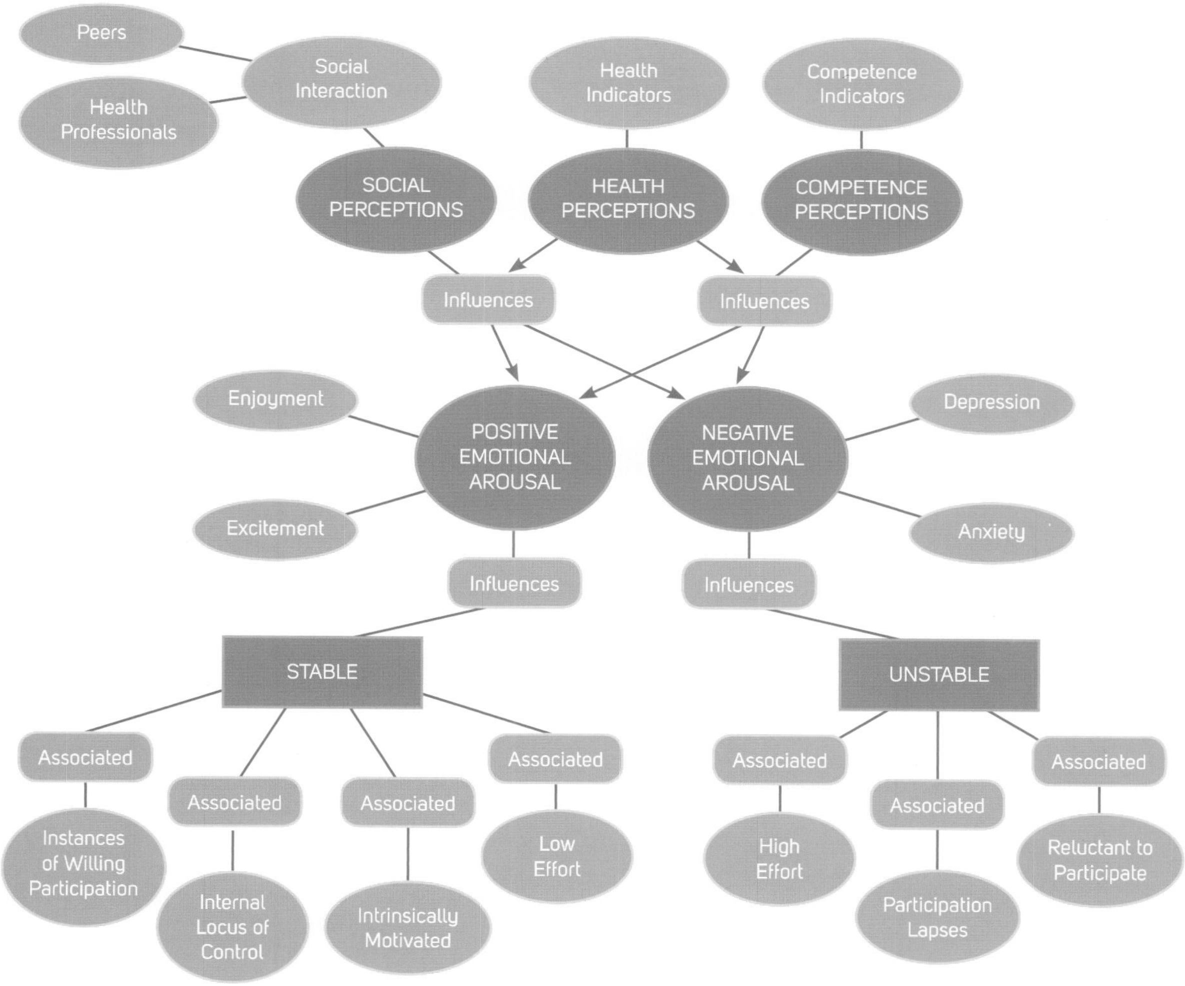

In deciding whether or not to invest in a software package consider:

- the cost of the software and licence
- the hardware required to run the system
- your level of computer self-efficacy and those of others who may be working with you on the data analysis
- the amount of data for analysis.

Links for further information on qualitative data analysis software packages are given at the end of the chapter.

Summary

Qualitative data analysis in nursing research is a creative and complex process, but one wholly grounded in the data collected. All data collected require some form of analysis. In qualitative research, data can take many forms. There are a number of approaches to qualitative data analysis and the approach taken for any given study will be determined by the methodology guiding the study. Analysis begins early in the study and continues until the final report is written. The chosen research method will drive the process of analysis and the choice of approach will be guided by a number of considerations including the research question and the sampling method. The researcher may choose to follow general inductive principles of qualitative research and choose a generic approach such as 'thematic analysis', or else analysis may be embedded in a grounded theory, phenomenological or ethnographical design. Software such as NVivo is increasingly used to support analysis in larger qualitative research studies. An important consideration is the development of trustworthiness of the analytic process in order to achieve and demonstrate a thorough, systematic and transparent process to the reader.

IMPLICATIONS FOR EVIDENCE-BASED NURSING AND MIDWIFERY

Researchers need to ensure that qualitative data analysis is appropriate for their philosophy, research question and design. Different stages are used by researchers to analyse the data so that their research results have rigour and trustworthiness. A number of computer programs can be used to facilitate the data analysing process. These programs also make it easier to conduct complex data analysis with a large data set from different sources. However, the researchers still play important roles in every stage. Detailed activities they used, such as an audit trail, need to be clearly explained so that users have confidence in their use of research evidence.

▸▸▸ **PROBLEM SOLVING 11.1**

Ann and her team conduct a phenomenology study among patients who re-present themselves to the emergency department with chest pain within six months. They interview 10 patients at their homes using open-ended questions. They ask participants to tell how they felt when they experienced pain and what they did before coming to the hospital. Following are transcripts of participant A and participant B.

Participant A: 'I had this sharp pain on my right shoulder when I was working in the garden. I usually start at about 4 or 5-ish in the afternoon. I did not think much about it (pain) so I just stopped what I was doing for a while. The pain's just gone. Ten minutes later, the pain came back. This time it was quite painful and then it went to my heart. (A pointed her finger underneath the left side of her chest, slightly underneath her breast.) I was frightened and I did not have anyone to talk to. Because this pain was worse than the pain I had last time when I went to the hospital. I lay down but the pain persisted. I was scared and decided to go to the hospital.'

Participant B: 'My work (running a restaurant) is so stressful and busy. I have to make sure that all bills are paid, my workers turn up on time and they look after the clients well. I also have to make sure that my family have what they should have similar or more than our friends. I had this pain, not that too painful or anything but it did not go away. I put up with it for about an hour or so and then I sweated and the pain moved from my right arm to left arm. I told my wife and she kept on telling me to go to the hospital. Once I get there, they (health care personnel) checked and I had to be in hospital for about a week. My business almost stopped while I was in hospital. Last time, I had the same pain and I thought I'd better have it checked rather than leaving it too late. This time I did not talk to anyone, even my wife. I did not want to be (admitted) in the hospital again. I was scared.'

Based on the interview transcripts of A and B, what are possible common themes? List two. From the transcripts, the interviewer makes their own note or self-reflection. Discuss whether this is useful or not. Why?

Practice exercise 11.1

Many adults living with type 2 diabetes find it hard to maintain optimum glycaemic control. A group of researchers are interested in exploring this important area and pose the question, 'what factors influence glycaemic control from the perspective of those living with type 2 diabetes?'

From the scenario above on glycaemic control, what qualitative data collection methods could be used to explore this question? List five different sources of data that could be collected.

Practice exercise 11.2

For the two studies outlined below, how would you go about collecting data for each and how would you analyse the data collected?

A study of nursing culture in the intensive care setting

The experience of living with multiple sclerosis.

Practice exercise 11.3

Try conducting an interview, transcribing this and coding.

Find a friend, colleague or family member and ask them to take part in an informal interview with you. Choose a topic they feel comfortable with, such as health, illness or service provision. You may wish to use the following suggestion, 'How do you define a healthy lifestyle?' Conduct the interview for 10 minutes, using a broad, open question to start the interview and using more focused questions to explore responses as the interview progresses. Record the interview and transcribe this yourself into a word processing package. Immediately after the interview write a memo to record your initial response to the interview and your perception of it. The memo can include a summary of the interview, unexpected events such as reaction to questions, or an interruption. The memo will help to prompt your recall when analysing the interview, and facilitates exploration of your position (e.g. beliefs, emotions, viewpoints) during the analysis.

How long did it take to transcribe the interview? Typing skills vary but it is likely to take you considerably longer to transcribe the interview than it took to conduct it.

Review the questions you asked. Did you lead the interviewee in a particular direction in any way? In hindsight, would you have asked follow-up questions to explore a concept further?

Read through the data several times until you become familiar with it. Then highlight or mark in some way those parts of the text that relate to the question driving the interview (e.g. the definition of a healthy lifestyle) and name these. You have started to identify codes. These are likely to be revised as analysis continues and are the first steps in qualitative data analysis.

Practice exercise 11.4

The following extracts are from interviews with people living with a family member with heart failure (Whitehead 2009). The following responses are in relation to the question 'what impact has living with a family member with heart failure had on your life?'

> Leah: We've had a few scary times when he cannot get his breath you know you wonder now is this going to be anything but we have the phone number of the hospital, the doctor the heart staff and that there and had a few bad days but on the whole he's improved a

wee bit, he wasn't sleeping before, he couldn't lie down in bed or anything. When I got him laying down even trying to get pillows up high can't help him, he can't stand up, he can't stand being too warm. He's sleeping a bit better now so it's really keep my fingers crossed you know.

Mary: Well I just worry what's going to happen to him yeah, but now he's got the phone on yeah I'm a bit more peaceful yeah I think like if his breathing is not good at night-time I'm awake you know, if he goes to the toilet I'm instantly awake.

Highlight those areas of the interviews that relate to concern for the family member living with heart failure. You now have your first provisional code called 'concern'. It is likely to be adapted later in the analysis but begins the process of categorising and analysing the data. Concern for the family member takes a number of forms in both interviews. Further analysis may lead to the creation of a number of areas of concern, for example, concern around an exacerbation requiring hospitalisation and concern around the ability to get quality sleep.

Answers to problem solving 11.1

a
Emotion or fear, self-assessment or comparison of pain, consultation with others or help-seeking behaviours, experience of pain and normal daily activities.
b
It is useful as it establishes the rigour of the study including credibility, auditability, fittingness (transferability), dependability and confirmability.

Answer to practice exercise 11.1

Potential data sources include:
Transcripts from interviews with people living with type 2 diabetes
Focus group transcripts
Field notes of observations
Copies of diary entries people living with diabetes have been asked to complete.
Video recordings
Research memos
Recordings of critical incidents around 'difficult moments' in managing glycaemic control.

Lisa Whitehead

Weblinks

The Computer Assisted Qualitative Data Analysis Networking Project (CAQDAS) provides information on available software packages:
<http://caqdas.soc.surrey.ac.uk>

ATLAS.ti:
<www.atlasti.com/index.html>

HyperRESEARCH:
<www.researchware.com>

NVivo:
<www.qsrinternational.com>

References

Anderson, C., & Adamsen, L. (2001). Continuous video recording: A new clinical research tool for studying the nursing care of cancer patients. *Journal of Advanced Nursing* 35, 257–67.

Baker, T., & Wang, C. (2006). Photovoice: Use of a participatory action research method to explore the chronic pain experience in older adults. *Qualitative Health Research* 16, 1405–13.

Ball, M., & Smith, G. (1992). *Analyzing Visual Data*. London: Sage.

Banks, M. (2007). *Visual Methods in Social Research*. London: Sage.

Colaizzi, P. F. (1978). Psychological research as the phenomenologist views it. In R. S. Valle & M. King (eds), *Existential Phenomenological Alternatives for Psychology*. New York: Oxford University Press.

Coyne, I., & Cowley, S. (2006). Using grounded theory to research parent participation. *Journal of Research in Nursing* 11(60), 501–15.

Diem-Wille, G. (2001). A therapeutic perspective: The use of drawings in child psychoanalysis and social science. In T. V. Leeuwen & C. Jewitt (eds), *Handbook of Visual Analysis* (pp. 119–33). Thousand Oaks, CA: Sage.

Erlandson, D., Harris, E., Skipper, B., & Allen, S. (1993). *Doing Naturalistic Inquiry: A Guide to Methods*. Newbury Park, CA: Sage.

Fetterman, D. M. (1984). *Ethnography in Educational Evaluation*. Beverly Hills, CA: Sage.

Fetterman, D. M. (1989) *Ethnography: Step by Step*. Newbury Park, CA: Sage.

Fetterman, D. M. (1998). *Ethnography: Step-by-Step*, 2nd edn [Applied Social Research Methods Series, vol. 17]. Thousand Oak, CA: Sage.

Gadamer, H. (1989). *Truth and Method*, 2nd edn. London: Sheed & Ward.

Gardezi, F., Lingard, L., Espins, L., Whyte, S., Orser, B., & Baker, G. R. (2009). Silence, power and communication in the operating room. *Journal of Advanced Nursing* 65(7), 1390–9.

Gaskins S., & Forte L. (1995). The meaning of hope: Implications for nursing practice and research. *Journal of Gerontological Nursing* 21(3), 17–25.

Geertz, C. (1973). Thick description: Toward an interpretive theory of culture. In *The Interpretation of Cultures: Selected Essays*. New York: Basic Books.

Giorgi, A. (1985). Sketch of a psychological phenomenological method. In A. Giorgi (ed.), *Phenomenology and Psychological Research* (pp. 8–22*)*. Pittsburgh: Duquesne University Press.

Giorgi, A. (1986). A phenomenological analysis of descriptions of conceptions of learning obtained from a phenomenographic perspective. *Publications from the Department of Education*, Göteborg University, Retrieved 9 October 2010, from <http://www.ped.gu.se/biorn/phgraph/misc/constr/giorgi.html>.

Glaser, B. (1978). *Theoretical Sensitivity: Advances in the Methodology of Grounded Theory*. Mill Valley, CA: Sociology Press.

Glaser, B., & Strauss, A. (1967). *The Discovery of Grounded Theory: Strategies for Qualitative Research*. Chicago: Aldine.

Guillemin, M. (2004). Understanding illness: Using drawings as a research method. *Qualitative Health Research* 14, 272–89.

Heidegger, M. (1996). *Being and Time*, transl. Joan Stambaugh. Albany, NY: State University of New York Press.

Husserl, E. (1970). *The Idea of Phenomenology*. The Hague: Nijhoff.

Hutchison, A., Halley Johnston, L., & Breckon, J. (2009). Using QSR-NVivo to facilitate the development of a grounded theory project: An account of a worked example. *International Journal of Social Research Methodology* 13(4), 283–302.

Krouse, H. (2001). Video modelling to educate patients. *Journal of Advanced Nursing* 33, 748–57.

McCaffery, M. (1983). *Nursing the Patient in Pain*. London: Harper & Row.

Merleau-Ponty, M. (1964). *The Primacy of Perception, and Other Essays on Phenomenological Psychology, the Philosophy of Art, History, and Politics*. Evanston, IL: Northwestern University Press.

Morgan, A. (1993). *Improving Your Students' Learning: Reflections on the Experience of Study*. London: Kogan Page Ltd.

Olsson, P., Jansson, L., & Norberg, A. (1998). Parenthood as talked about in Swedish ante and postnatal midwifery consultations. *Scandinavian Journal of Caring Sciences* 12, 205–14.

Robertson, M., & Boyle J. (1984). Ethnography: Contributions to nursing research. *Journal of Advanced Nursing* 9(1), 43–9.

Seneviratne, C. C., Mather, C. M., & Then, K. L. (2009). Understanding nursing on an acute stroke unit: Perceptions of space, time and interprofessional practice. *Journal of Advanced Nursing* 65(9), 1872–81.

Strauss, A., & Corbin, J. (1990). *Basics of Qualitative Research: Grounded Theory Procedures and Techniques*. London: Sage.

Strauss, A., & Corbin, J. (1998). *Basics of Qualitative Research: Techniques and Procedures for Developing Grounded Theory*, 2nd edn. Thousand Oaks, CA: Sage.

Lisa Whitehead

Swann, G. (2000). Photography in wound care. *Nursing Times* 96, 9–12.

Thomas, J. (1993). *Doing Critical Ethnography.* London: Sage.

Van Manen, M. (1994). Pedagogy, virtue, and narrative identity in teaching. *Curriculum Inquiry* 4(2), 135–70.

Whitehead, L. (2004). Enhancing the quality of hermeneutic research: Decision trail. *Journal of Advanced Nursing* 45(5), 512–18.

Whitehead, L. (2009). *Living with Chronic Illness: Exploring the Role of the Family in Supporting Members Living with Heart Failure.* Families Commission, New Zealand.

Wilson, B., & Crowe, M. (2008). Maintaining equilibrium: A theory of job satisfaction for community mental health nurses. *Journal of Psychiatric and Mental Health Nursing* 15(10), 816–22.

CHAPTER 12

Quantitative Data Analysis

Petra Buettner, Reinhold Muller and Monika Buhrer-Skinner

Chapter learning objectives

By the end of this chapter you will be able to:

▶ understand how to describe quantitative data

▶ describe the main functions of inferential statistics

▶ explain how to interpret a confidence interval

▶ explain statistical hypothesis testing and the uncertainties involved

▶ outline some fundamentals of and key steps towards multivariable statistical analysis.

KEY TERMS

Alpha error
Beta error
Confidence interval
Confounding
Measures of central tendency
Multivariable procedures
p-value
Research hypothesis
Statistical hypothesis
Statistical inference

Introduction

Nurses and midwives working in the clinical, education or research field are called upon to provide information or data about how effective nursing is in improving patient outcomes. Quantitative data analysis using statistics has the potential to provide the necessary information to demonstrate the effectiveness of nursing and midwifery interventions.

Like sampling and research design, there are many new terms and formulae associated with statistics. This chapter introduces the nurse or midwife to areas of importance in quantitative data analysis that are relevant to practice, education and research. Many other aspects of complex statistics are beyond the scope of this chapter and further reading is provided where appropriate.

Why statistics?

In our modern world we are inundated with statistics to an unprecedented degree. Statistics are used in the media to provide information, for example, on economics, employment, road accidents, opinion polls and surveys. Health professionals are even more likely to be confronted with statistics than the general public—the books and publications we are all required to read to remain on top of our profession are jam-packed with statistics.

For example, a study reported on the evaluation of strategies to improve postnatal care for women in Australian hospitals. The study found that time was a major issue, with 57% of women saying they had received 10 minutes or less of uninterrupted time with a midwife, and only 11% reported having spent 20 minutes or more time with a midwife (Schmied et al. 2009). In December 2008 Norman Swan reported on Radio National about a trial that investigated the effect of breathing exercises aiming to reduce the severity of asthma symptoms. The study compared physiotherapist-supervised breathing training with nurse-delivered education on asthma. The study concluded that statistically, breathing training significantly improved asthma-specific health status ($p=0.002$), though this training does not negate the need for inhalers (Thomas et al. 2009).

These examples show that, broadly speaking, statistics provide us with (1) numbers, and numbers are an unambiguous language understood by everybody in the same way, and (2) tools to measure the uncertainty or random error involved when inferring from a sample to the wider target population. This uncertainty is expressed in the p-value, which we will introduce later. The ability to assess the uncertainties involved when deducing from a sample to the target population is the main reason for the ongoing triumph of statistics in the health sciences. Statistics is a core tool of the scientific method that helps the acquisition of knowledge in a standard and universally accepted manner and thus forms the basis of today's gold standard: evidence-based practice.

First, let us begin by introducing a study conducted by nurses in Queensland. Edwards and others (2009) described a randomised controlled trial of quality of life in a community nursing intervention for patients with chronic leg ulcers. Overall, 67 patients with venous leg ulcers were randomly allocated to either the Lindsay Leg Club® model of care or the traditional community nursing model. The study showed that patients who received care under the Leg Club® model demonstrated significantly improved outcomes in quality of life, morale, self-esteem, healing, pain and functional ability. The authors concluded that this model of care should be evaluated further and should eventually be implemented by community health organisations involved in the care of this group of patients.

Descriptive versus comparative statistics

Statistics allow us to address descriptive as well as comparative quantitative research questions. In the first instance descriptive statistics will stay with the sample data and describe these data in a comprehensive way without drawing any statistical inferences. In the second instance comparative or inferential statistics will be used with the aim of drawing inferences from the sample to the wider target population.

All quantitative research should start by formulating a research hypothesis—the scientific question the study will be designed to answer with statistical confidence. A research hypothesis includes a precise quantitative statement about the hypothesised result (see Chapters 1, 2 and 6 for further information).

BOX 12.1

RESEARCH HYPOTHESIS

A quantitative research hypothesis is a precise statement about the question the study will be designed to answer. It must be plausible and falsifiable. The research hypothesis should clearly state study factor and outcome variables and should give a quantitative statement about the expected result of the study.

Example: In the Lindsay Leg Club® model study introduced above, the authors investigated whether participants receiving care under the Leg Club® model would show improved quality of life in comparison with participants receiving individual home care. In this study, quality of life was measured with Spitzer's quality of life index (Spitzer et al. 1981) for chronically ill patients, described by mean value and standard deviation. This scale has a range from 0=poor quality of life to 10=excellent quality of life.

A possible quantitative research hypothesis for this study is:

The mean value of the quality of life score in the group receiving the Lindsay Leg Club® intervention will be improved by 1 unit (mean value change from 8 to 9) while the quality of life score for the control group remains unchanged.

Comment: In this research hypothesis the study factors are intervention and control, while the outcome is quality of life. The hypothesis is precise as it provides a quantitative statement of expected results (it gives the mean values) and it is therefore falsifiable. If the study shows the expected improvement in the quality of life of 1 unit or even more in the intervention group compared to the control, then the hypothesis will be supported; if not it is falsified!

Source: Adapted from Edwards et al. 2009

Descriptive statistics

Types of quantitative data

We frequently read or hear information based on descriptive statistics. They are presented in various forms such as percentages or averages. Visually, they are presented in graphs. All quantitative research collects quantitative data, that is, information on characteristics that can be measured, classified and subsequently coded into numbers. These characteristics are usually called variables (e.g. age, gender, concurrent adenoidectomy, number of siblings, quality of life) and the information collected is called the data. Data are analysed using appropriate statistical methods. The correct choice of a statistical method, however, depends on the type(s) of the variable(s) collected.

We need to differentiate two major types of variables: categorical and numerical variables (Table 12.1), and this constitutes the first step in finding 'the' correct statistical procedure for a given data set and a given research question (Altman 1991).

Categorical variables have defined categories (variable gender: categories female/male; variable type of nurse: categories registered/enrolled) and the codes given to these categories in statistical analysis are arbitrary, for example, gender codes could be 1 = male and 2 = female, or vice versa, or any other dichotomous code combination. Categorical data can be further classified as being either nominal or ordinal. In an ordinal categorical variable the categories follow a natural order (such as level of education: primary school, high school, tertiary education), while this is not the case in nominal variables (e.g. gender: either male or female; blood group: O, A, B or AB).

In contrast, the observed numbers in numerical variables have an intrinsic meaning (e.g. age: 16 years). Numerical variables therefore retain quantitative information on measurements. They can be further classified into discrete or continuous. Discrete numerical variables are usually natural counts and can only take on whole numbers (e.g. number of children: 0, 1, 2, 3…) while continuous data are measurements that can take on any value within a meaningful range. The values are limited only by our ability to measure precisely (e.g. weight: 45 kg; height: 145 cm).

Table 12.1   Types of quantitative variables

Categorical		Numerical	
Nominal	Ordinal	Discrete	Continuous
No order of categories	Ordered categories	Integer measurements	Real number measurements
Examples:			
Gender	Level of education	Number of children	Reaction time
Blood group	Developmental stages of a child	Number of partners	Age
Category of nurse	TNM staging of tumours	Number of hospital beds	Height

Please note: Continuous variables are often modified to become discrete or even categorical, but the reverse process is not possible. For example, age of a person might be 18 years, 9 months, 16 days … but we say this person is 18 years old ('age at last birthday'), hence creating a discrete variable from a continuous one. We might even say this person is below or above 20 years, thus creating a categorical variable. As a rule, always collect quantitative information as precisely as possible. Categorisation can easily be achieved later during analysis using statistical software.

Description of quantitative data

All researchers are required to describe their data by applying descriptive statistics. Basic description of the data allows us to assess their sample and whether the conclusions reached by the research apply to our situation. For example, results of a study based on children aged between 10 and 17 years with the average age of 13 years may have different implications for practice, compared to a study focusing on the same health issue but using children aged 6 to 13 years with an average age of 9 years.

Descriptive statistics are needed for all quantitative research questions. They constitute the core component of descriptive research and the base for further comparative statistical analyses in comparative research. Correct descriptive statistics summarise the collected data in a meaningful way and are—as all statistics—dependent on the type of variables (Table 12.2). Descriptive statistics for categorical variables usually only describe the percentages of each category. Numerical variables are summarised using a measure of central tendency together with a measure of dispersion.

The most frequently used measures of central tendency are the arithmetic mean and the median. These measures point to the centre of the distribution of the numerical data. The arithmetic mean by definition is the sum of the values measured divided by the number of values, while the median is the value in the middle of the ordered observations (50%-quantile).

Table 12.2   Decision table for descriptive statistics and univariate graphical display

TYPE of VARIABLE		
CATEGORICAL Nominal or ordinal	NUMERICAL Discrete or continuous	
	Data convex and symmetrical	Data skewed or too few observations to judge
DESCRIPTIVE STATISTICS		
	Measures of central tendency and dispersion	
Percentages of categories	Mean and standard deviation (SD)	Median and inter-quartile range (IQR) or Median and range (few observations)
Examples 42% male	Mean weight 22.5 kg (SD 6.5)	Median number of cigarettes smoked per day 10 (IQR = [5, 20])
GRAPHICAL DISPLAY		
Bar chart	Histogram Stem-and-leaf plot Plot of mean and standard deviation	Histogram Stem-and-leaf plot Box-and-Whiskers plot

BOX 12.2

MEASURES OF CENTRAL TENDENCY

The arithmetic mean of a sample with n observations x1, x2, x3,..., xn is:

$$\overline{X} = \frac{x_1 + x_2 + x_3 + ... + x_n}{n}$$

The age of 7 participants (n=7) in a study was recorded as: 62, 71, 59, 67, 88, 77, 59.

Calculation of the arithmetic mean ($\overline{x}$) for this small example:

$$\overline{X} = \frac{62 + 71 + 59 + 67 + 88 + 77 + 59}{7} = 69$$

The median ($x_{0.5}$) of a sample with n observations x1, x2, x3,..., xn in ascending order is dependent on whether the sample size (n) is odd or even.

If sample size (n) is odd:

$$x_{0.5} = \frac{(n + 1)}{2} \text{ th largest observation}$$

Calculation of the median ($x_{0.5}$) for the small example with sample size n =7.

First sort values in ascending order: 59, 59, 62, 67, 71, 77, 88.

Calculate position of median value:

$$x_{0.5} = \frac{(7 + 1)}{2} = \frac{8}{2} = 4^{th} \text{ largest observation}$$

hence the median is 67, which is the fourth largest value.

If the sample size (n) is even:

$$x_{0.5} = \text{average of } \frac{(n)}{2} \text{ th} + (\frac{(n)}{2} + 1) = \text{th largest observation}$$

Calculation of the median ($x_{0.5}$) for a small example with sample size $n = 6$:

Sorted values in ascending order: 59, 62, 67, 71, 77, 88.

Calculate the position of median value:

$$x_{0.5} = \text{average of } \frac{(6)}{2} \text{ th} + (\frac{(6)}{2} + 1) = \text{th largest observation}$$

$$= \text{average of } 3^{rd} + (3+1)^{th} \text{ largest observation}$$

$$= \text{average of } 3^{rd} + 4^{th} \text{ largest observation}$$

$$\text{hence the median is } \frac{67+71}{2} = 69$$

A measure of central tendency is usually accompanied by a measure of dispersion indicating the spread (variability) of the data. If the arithmetic mean is used as the measure of central tendency, the standard deviation (SD) is the dispersion measure of choice. If the median is used, the inter-quartile range (IQR) is an adequate dispersion measure. Providing minimum and maximum values (i.e. the range) is sometimes informative, in particular when observed values show little variation. Please read the chapter on summary statistics in Burt Gerstman's book (2008) for further detailed information.

The standard deviation is an important measure of variability. The basic idea of the standard deviation is measuring the combined distance between the mean value and each individual observation. In Box 12.2 we showed an example for how the mean is calculated from seven individual age values. The mean was 69 years. The standard deviation for this mean value would take into account the distance, that is, the difference between each value and the mean: 62–69, 71–69, 59–69, 67–69, 88–69, 77–69 and 59–69. If we added up just these seven differences we would end up with 0, because positive and negative differences would cancel each other out—this is the definition of the mean value! Hence the formula for the standard deviation is a little more complicated, but the basic idea is looking at these differences to the mean value as a measure of the variability of the data.

Mean or median—when to use which?

This question can only be answered by checking the distribution of the numerical variable. If the distribution is convex and symmetrical (Figure 12.1a), the mean will be similar to the median and the arithmetic mean and standard deviation are used for descriptive purposes. If the distribution is convex but asymmetrical (Figure 12.1b), or there are too few observations to judge the distribution, then median and inter-quartile range are the descriptive measures of choice. Figure 12.1b below shows negatively and positively skewed data. Non-convex distributions (including bimodal and concave distributions) (Figure 12.1c) are rare and require expert advice.

Figure 12.1a   Convex and symmetrical distribution

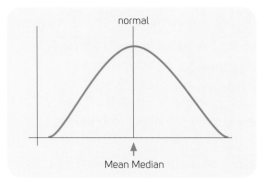

Figure 12.1b   Convex and asymmetrical distributions

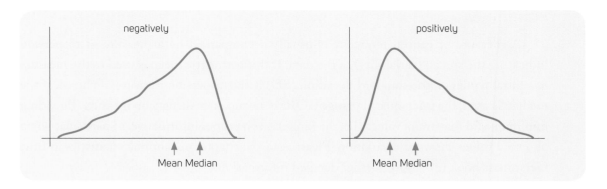

Figure 12.1c   Non-convex distribution

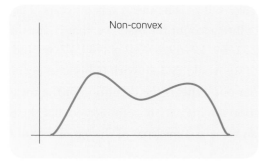

Please note

The mean is notoriously sensitive to outliers; the median, in contrast, is a very robust measure. There are formal statistical processes, such as the Kolmogorov-Smirnov test for normality, to decide whether to use mean or median and subsequently parametric or non-parametric statistics (Zar 2010). However, checking the shape of the distribution under question is a reasonable start and generally provides a good decision base for the choice of descriptive measures.

Graphical display

Graphical displays are often used in the description of variables since they may show complex data and relationships more clearly than tables alone. As before, the correct graphical display depends on the type of variable(s) involved.

Graphical displays for one variable ('univariate')

The standard graphical display for a categorical variable is a bar chart (Figure 12.2a). In bar charts the height of the bar represents the absolute or relative frequency of the category.

The histogram (Figures 12.2b [symmetrical distribution] and 12.2c [skewed distribution]) is the graph of choice for numerical data. In a histogram the bars are not spaced as in a bar chart but joined, indicating that the different categories displayed follow each other directly. In a histogram, the area of the bar indicates the absolute or relative frequency. Please note that in histograms the width of the bars can change and that the impression given by a histogram might vary considerably with the chosen width of the bars.

Figure 12.2a–c   Graphic displays for one variable

a
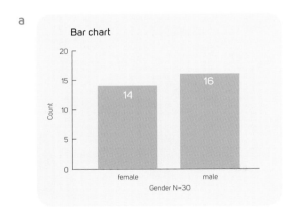

b
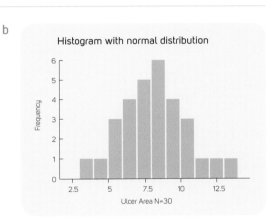

c
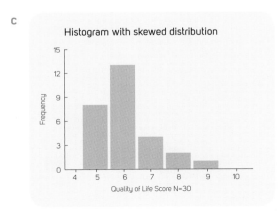

Graphical display involving two variables ('bivariate')

If both variables concerned are categorical the depiction of choice is a cross-tabulation, which is a table where the categories of one variable define the columns and the categories of the second variable define the rows. If both variables are numerical a scatter plot (Figure 12.2d) is used to show their relationship graphically. A scatter plot is a two-dimensional coordinate system with two axes (X-axis and Y-axis) and each participant is marked by a dot where the readings from the X-axis and from the Y-axis intersect.

If one variable is categorical and the second one is numerical there are two options, depending on the appropriate measure of central tendency for the numerical variable. If mean and standard deviation are used, a mean and standard deviation plot (Figure 12.2e) can be created depicting the numerical variable in each category of the categorical variable using mean and standard deviation. In case the numerical variable is described by median and inter-quartile range, a box-and-whiskers plot (Figure 12.2f) can be used where, for each category, the box is defined by the 25%- and the 75%-quantile; the bar in the box is the median, and the whiskers show minimum and maximum value of the distribution.

Figure 12.2d–f   Graphic displays involving two variables

d
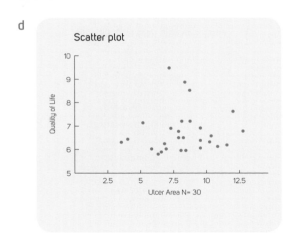

e
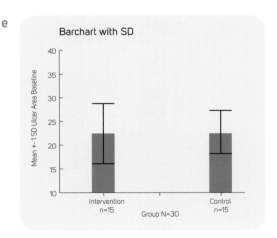

f
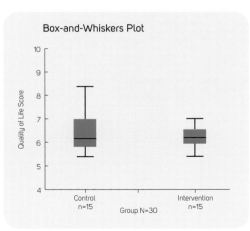

Whenever you use either tables or figures to describe data, never forget to mention the sample size and the extent of missing values. Hardly any data set is entirely without missing values; these might be missing for a reason and the missing values might actually form their own interesting group.

BOX 12.3
DESCRIPTIVE STATISTICS

Percentage of categorical data and measures of central tendency and dispersion for numerical data are used to describe a data set. Descriptive statistics are used in all quantitative studies, because describing the data is always the first step of statistical analysis.

Example: A study investigated the perceived quality of life of patients who underwent coronary artery bypass graft surgery (Ballan & Lee 2007). Quality of life was measured pre- and post-operatively using the validated SF-36 questionnaire separated into physical and mental health. These two scores range from 0 (=worst) to 100 (=best).

An abridged description of the 62 participants is given in the following table, an example of descriptive statistics display.

Variable	Descriptive statistics
Mean age (SD)* [years]	66.4 (10.2)
% Male	87.1%
% Hypertensive	93.5%
Smoking status % Ex-smokers % Current smokers	 42.0% 24.2%
Median number of cigarettes of current smokers smoked per day (IQR)**	10 (5, 20)
Pre-operative SF-36 results Mean physical functioning score (SD) Mean mental health score (SD)	 26.1 (8.0) 53.4 (12.7)

*SD = standard deviation; **IQR = inter-quartile range

Comment: The majority (87.1%) of the 62 participants were male and mean age of participants was 66 years (SD10.2). This implies that the age was approximately normally distributed. The median number of cigarettes smoked was 10. This implies that the distribution of numbers of cigarettes was skewed. It also implies that 50% of current smokers smoked less or equal to 10 cigarettes per day. The inter-quartile range is from 5 to 20 cigarettes, implying that 25% of current smokers smoked less or equal to 5 cigarettes per day while 75% smoked less or equal to 20 cigarettes per day.

Source: Adapted from Ballan & Lee 2007

Inferential statistics

In general, researchers want to use the findings from the data of their participants or sample to apply to the wider population. The ability of statistics to use information from a sample and transfer the results to this wider target population is called statistical inference (see also Chapter 8). It is one of the main reasons for using statistics in the health sciences. Inferential statistics offers two main tools: (1) hypothesis testing and (2) the confidence interval, which are both grounded in the same theory.

Confidence interval

The $(1-\alpha)$-confidence interval is notably a statement about the target population, taking information exclusively from a sample into account. The $(1-\alpha)$-confidence interval is given with some measure of certainty (usually 95%). In general, we have to start from the uncertainty, which is denoted by alpha (α). Alpha can take on any value between 0 and 1. However, it is most often chosen to be 0.05 (or 5%)—a completely arbitrary but internationally accepted choice.

Hence, for example, if a 95%-confidence interval is given, we are 95% sure that the confidence interval includes the true target population parameter. The interpretation of a $(1-\alpha)$-confidence interval is that the true but unknown population parameter of interest (e.g. the mean value) lies within the interval with a probability of $1-\alpha$.

BOX 12.4
CONFIDENCE INTERVAL

A $(1-\alpha)$-confidence interval tells us that the true but unknown population parameter of interest (e.g. the mean value) lies within the interval with a probability of $1-\alpha$.

Example: A study investigated the perceived quality of life of patients who underwent coronary artery bypass graft surgery (Ballan & Lee 2007). Quality of life was measured pre- and post-operatively using the validated SF-36 questionnaire separated into physical and mental health. These two scores range from 0 (=worst) to 100 (=best) and were summarised using mean values and standard deviations.

SF-36	Pre-operation	Post-operation	Difference
Mean physical functioning score (SD)	26.1 (8.0)	33.5 (10.2)	7.4
Mean mental health score (SD)	53.4 (12.7)	53.7 (10.1)	0.3

One can calculate 95%-confidence intervals for the post- to pre- differences in the physical and mental health scores.

Physical functioning score: 95%-confidence interval = (2.8, 12.0)

Mental functioning score: 95%-confidence interval = (-0.35, 0.95)

BOX 12.4

The 95%-confidence interval for the post- to pre- difference in the physical functioning score implies that we can be 95% confident that the true difference in the target population is between 2.8 and 12.0. This interval does not include 0, hence the difference of 7.4 between pre and post is statistically significant.

The 95%-confidence interval for the post- to pre- difference in the mental health score implies that we can be 95% confident that the true difference in the target population is between −0.35 and 0.95. This interval does include 0, hence the difference of 0.3 between pre and post is not statistically significant, as 'no difference' cannot be excluded!

Source: Adapted from Ballan & Lee 2007

Please note

1   Confidence intervals can be calculated for many different parameters, that is, for mean values, proportions, medians, odds-ratios and so on. The respective formulae vary, but they all have in common that an estimation of the variability of the data and the sample size are taken into account.

2   Confidence intervals for the population mean are symmetrically constructed around the sample mean. Generally, all confidence intervals do include the sample estimate (e.g. the sample mean, sample proportion). However, confidence intervals do not refer to the sample but to the population.

3   The larger the sample size the narrower the confidence interval (all else the same). Hence an increase in sample size will make a confidence interval more precise.

4   The smaller the uncertainty (α) the wider the resulting confidence interval (all else the same).

5   All statistical procedures assume true random sampling (see Chapter 8). If random sampling cannot be assumed, standard estimates of variances might not apply. In particular, cluster sampling in survey designs should be acknowledged and sample size as well as statistical analysis requires adjustment.

Statistical hypothesis testing for difference

Many health science researchers conduct research to find out whether one type of care is better than another type of care. The comparison can also be made among three or more groups. A comparative research hypothesis, such as: 'Is there a difference in the quality of life in patients participating in the Lindsay Leg Club® compared to normal community nursing care?' can be answered by judging how likely it is that an observed difference between groups is due to chance alone.

This judgment can be based on either of two statistical tools:

1   Conducting a statistical test which directly gives the probability that the difference arose by chance alone.

2   Calculating the 95%-confidence interval for the difference of the proportions between the groups. If the 95%-confidence interval does not include zero, the groups are called 'statistically significantly different'.

A large number of different statistical tests are available and depending on the types of variables involved, the parameters under study and the research hypothesis, one particular test is usually most appropriate (Figure 12.3).

The result of a statistical test is called the p-value. The p-value gives the probability that the observed difference between groups (or an even larger difference) is due to chance alone. By convention, a p-value below 0.05 is considered statistically significant. Again, allowing 5% uncertainty is completely arbitrary, though internationally accepted. For example, $p = 0.026$ implies that there is a 26 in 1000 probability (or 2.6%) that the observed difference (or an even greater difference) is due to chance alone, assuming that in reality there is no difference.

Please note

1   In the scientific literature the word 'significant' should be used in a statistical context only, that is, if a statistical test was conducted that resulted in a p-value less than 0.05.

2   Statistical significance does not automatically imply medical relevance. Small differences can be statistically significant if only the sample size is large enough, but may not be medically relevant. The medical relevance of an observed difference has to be established before conducting a statistical test! If deemed irrelevant, no statistical test should be carried out. For example, in the Lindsay Leg Club® intervention trial quality of life was measured using Spitzer's quality of life index (1981) for chronically ill patients. This scale has a range from 0=poor quality of life to 10=excellent quality of life. If we consider a difference of 1 unit or larger for this index as clinically relevant but the study reveals only a difference of 0.75, then no statistical test should be performed. Even if this test was significant, it would not relate to a result that was clinically relevant.

Errors in statistical testing and the problem of multiple comparisons

When a statistical test is conducted two types of error can occur (Table 12.3): alpha error (α; type I error) and beta error (β; type II error). Alpha error implies that a statistical test finds a significant difference between groups, when in reality there is none. Beta error implies that a statistical test does not detect an existing difference between groups when in reality there is one.

Table 12.3   Errors in statistical hypothesis testing

		Reality	
		No difference	Difference
Statistical test	No difference	1-Alpha	Beta error (false negative)
	Difference	Alpha error (false positive)	1-Beta Power of test

At first glance, the alpha error seems to be under control as only p-values below 0.05 will be called statistically significant. Hence alpha can maximally be 0.05. However, this is only true if one statistical test per data set is performed. Usually, this is far from being the case! During statistical analysis numerous statistical tests are usually performed and the alpha error increases with each test. This problem is called multiple comparisons.

Naturally one does not know which of the statistical tests conducted are significant by chance alone. One can adjust either (at the design stage) the sample size or (at the analysis stage) the alpha level (e.g. Bonferroni adjustment) to take care of the issue of multiple comparisons. For a broader introduction to the issue and technical details on how to adjust for multiple comparisons please refer to Jerrold Zar's book (2010).

Beta error is only controlled if a sample size calculation was conducted which, for a given research hypothesis, will ensure that there is adequate power to detect a difference of an expected size. The power of a study is the probability that the study will detect an expected difference if it truly exists in the target population (see Chapter 8 for further information). In general, studies should be designed large enough to have a power in excess of 80%.

Please note

1   Confident statistical hypothesis testing can only be performed if an appropriate research hypothesis is specified and a sample size calculation is conducted during the design phase of the study.

2   A study will only be able to confirm or reject the specified research hypotheses with statistical confidence. All other statistical tests performed will be subject to uncontrolled alpha and beta error and require confirmation by an adequately planned independent study.

3   The sample size calculation can be adjusted a priori to take care of multiple comparisons if more than one research hypothesis is considered.

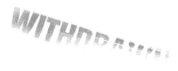

BOX 12.5
THE RESULT OF A STATISTICAL TEST

A p-value is the result of a statistical test. The p-value gives the probability that an observed difference or an even more extreme difference happened by chance alone (given that in reality there is no difference).

Example 1: The Lindsay Leg Club® intervention study investigated whether participants receiving care under the Leg Club model would show improved quality of life in comparison with participants receiving individual home care. In this study, quality of life was measured with Spitzer's quality of life index (1981) for the chronically ill. This scale has a range from 0=poor quality of life to 10=excellent quality of life.

Study results for quality of life (mean and SD)

	Before	After	Difference
Lindsay Leg Club® intervention	7.61 (1.65)	8.96 (1.43)	1.35
Control group	7.86 (2.27)	8.11 (2.10)	0.25

The p-value for comparing the differences between the two groups was 0.014. This p-value implies that the observed difference (or a more extreme difference; 1.35-0.25=1.15) between intervention and control group happened by chance alone with a likelihood of 0.014 (or 1.4%) if in reality there is no difference between the two groups. Hence it is unlikely that the result happened by chance alone. This result is statistically significant.

Source: Adapted from Edwards et al. 2009

Example 2: A study investigated the perceived quality of life of patients who underwent coronary artery bypass graft surgery. Quality of life was measured pre- and post-operatively using the validated SF-36 questionnaire separated into physical and mental health. These two scores range from 0 (=worst) to 100 (=best) and were summarised using mean values and standard deviations.

SF-36 pre- and post-operatively

SF-36	Pre-operation	Post-operation	Difference
Mean physical functioning score (SD)	26.1 (8.0)	33.5 (10.2)	7.4
Mean mental health score (SD)	53.4 (12.7)	53.7 (10.1)	0.3

The p-value for the physical functioning score was less than 0.001; the p-value for the mental health score was 0.902.

The p-value for the physical functioning score implies that the probability that the observed difference between pre- and post-surgery (7.4) occurred by chance alone was less than 0.001 (or less than 0.1%), assuming that in reality there was no difference. Hence it is very unlikely that the observed difference in physical functioning occurred by chance alone. This result is statistically significant.

BOX 12.5

On the other hand, the p-value for mental health implies that the probability that the observed difference between pre- and post-surgery (0.3) occurred by chance alone was 0.902 (or 90.2%) assuming that in reality there was no difference. Hence it is very likely that the observed difference in mental health occurred by chance alone. This result is not statistically significant.

Source: Adapted from Ballan & Lee 2007

Selecting an appropriate bivariate test procedure

The choice of the correct statistical test procedure for a specific bivariate (two variables) test situation is dependent on the types of the two variables involved. Once identified, this information leads to the right group of statistical tests as detailed in Figure 12.3.

1   If both variables are numerical (e.g. age and quality of life score) then the correct statistical test procedures can be found in the correlation/regression group.

2   If both variables are categorical (e.g. type of medication and post-operative vomiting) then the correct statistical test belongs to the chi-square group.

3   If one variable is numerical and the other variable is categorical (e.g. gender and quality of life) then the correct statistical test procedure is either a parametric t-test/Analysis of Variance or a non-parametric Wilcoxon type test.

Figure 12.3 Classification of bivariate statistical tests

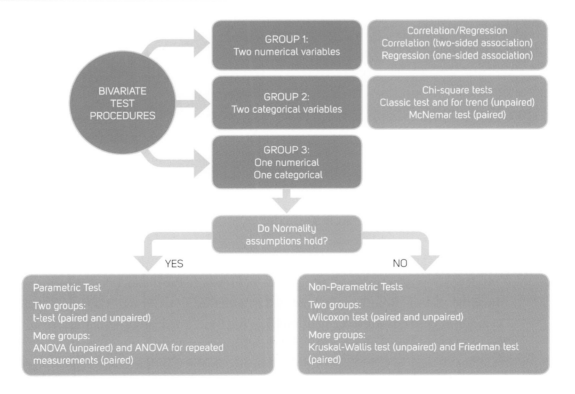

Petra Buettner, Reinhold Muller and Monika Buhrer-Skinner

Based on the types of the two variables involved, Figure 12.3 points to the right group of tests for a given study situation. To reach at one particular test, however, additional decisions have to be made as detailed in Figure 12.3 and outlined below.

Table 12.4   Examples of research hypothesis, types of data and bivariate statistical tests

	Variable 1	Variable 2	Test used
Hypothesis: The mean quality of life improvement is higher in the Lindsay Leg Club® intervention group compared to the control group.			
Variable	Intervention or control	Quality of life score (mean value)	
Type of variable	Nominal	Numerical	t-test comparing mean values
Hypothesis: In the Lindsay Leg Club® intervention trial the improvements in quality of life are associated with the changes in activities of daily living.			
Variable	Quality of life score	Activity of daily living score	
Type of variable	Numerical	Numerical	Correlation (two-sided association)
Hypothesis: In the Lindsay Leg Club® intervention trial the gender distribution is similar between intervention and control group.			
Variable	Intervention or control	Gender	
Type of variable	Nominal	Nominal	Chi-square test
Hypothesis: The median pain severity at baseline is higher in the Lindsay Leg Club® intervention group compared to the control group.			
Variable	Intervention or control	Pain severity at baseline (median value)	
Type of variable	Nominal	Numerical	Wilcoxon test comparing median values

Source: Adapted from Edwards et al. 2009

In the following, further terminology is introduced which is additionally required for deciding which statistical test is adequate.

One-sided versus two-sided scientific question

This decision is relevant for all test groups and refers to the distinction between a situation where the research hypothesis is interested in both directions (group A differs from group B; i.e. group A better or worse than group B) or not (one-sided: group A better than group B). The following example further clarifies this distinction.

The change in quality of life for patients in the Lindsay Leg Club® intervention group is different from the change for patients in the traditional community nursing group (two-sided; result could go either way). The quality of life for patients in the Lindsay Leg Club® intervention group improves more than for patients in the traditional community nursing group (one-sided; result is expected to go one way only).

One-sided statistical tests are more likely to return statistically significant results than two-sided tests. Therefore one-sided testing has to be thoroughly justified. Most research hypotheses are formulated as two-sided questions.

Paired versus unpaired test

If the research hypothesis under consideration involves the comparison of two (or more) groups who are independent from each other (i.e. different people; e.g. comparing patients in the Lindsay Leg Club® group with patients in the control group), then the unpaired version of the statistical test procedure is used. If the research hypothesis involves comparing the same people who were measured twice or more often (e.g. quality of life is assessed in patients in the Lindsay Leg Club® group at baseline and after six months), then the paired version of the statistical test is correct. This distinction is relevant in statistical test groups 2 and 3 only.

Parametric versus non-parametric test

In test groups 1 and 3 a decision is made as to whether a parametric or non-parametric statistical test is required. The answer to this question is linked to the distribution of the numerical variable(s) involved. If the numerical variable is approximately normally distributed (see below) in all categories of the categorical variable (group 3), or both numerical variables are approximately normally distributed (group 1), then a parametric test is used. Otherwise a non-parametric test will be conducted.

As a rule of thumb, a numerical variable is approximately normally distributed if (1) the distribution is convex and symmetrical; (2) mean and median differ by less than 10%; and (3) the standard deviation is less than a third of the mean value (this last criterion is only appropriate for distributions that are not centrally located around zero). One can also test for normality formally by using the Kolmogorov-Smirnov test (Zar 2010).

Regression and correlation: One-sided versus two-sided association

Statistical test group 1 differs from the two other groups as regression and correlation procedures are not deciding on a difference, but rather investigate whether an association exists between the two numerical variables involved. This association can be either one-sided or two-sided. When the association between the two variables is one-sided, that is, one variable may influence the other but the reverse is not possible, then we use a regression approach where the independent variable is depicted on the x-axis. A classical regression example is the association between age and blood pressure. Age influences blood pressure (as we get older, blood pressure usually increases), but blood pressure cannot influence age. Age is the independent variable and is depicted on the x-axis. When the association is two-sided, that is, both variables can influence each other, then a correlation approach is used and the allocation of the variables to the axes of the scatter plot is arbitrary. An example of a two-sided association could be investigating the association between level of physical activity and alcohol consumption. Either characteristic could influence the other; there is no clear independent variable. Hence, this is an example of a correlation problem.

Following the graphical display conventions introduced above, two numerical variables are usually depicted in a scatter plot. Before embarking on regression or correlation analysis we should always look at the scatter plot, as this graph is informative about the nature of the association under study. Standard procedures of regression and correlation statistics assume a linear relationship—that is, as one variable increases, the other increases as well (positive linear relationship: Figure 12.4a); or as one variable increases, the other variable decreases

Figure 12.4   Scatter plots of association

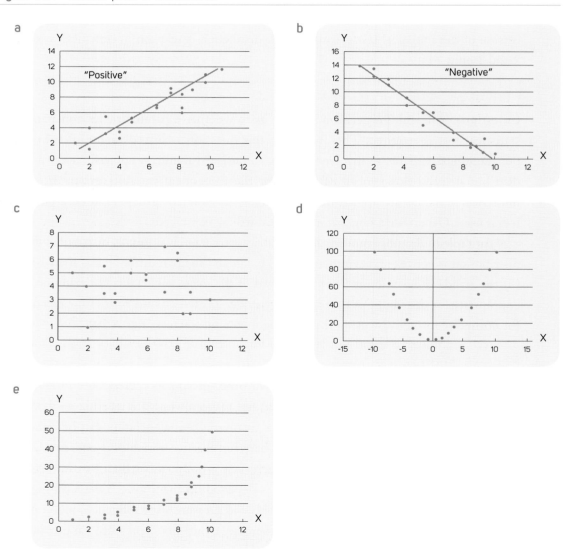

(negative linear relationship: Figure 12.4b). A linear relationship implies that a straight line will be sufficient to summarise the relationship well (see lines in Figures 12.4a and 12.4b).

If the dots of the scatter plot form an indistinct cloud (Figure 12.4c), a negligable association between the two variables exists. This figure shows that whatever value one variable has, the other variable can take any value of its range. Relationships do not need to be all linear, but can be quadratic (Figure 12.4.d), exponential (Figure 12.4.e) or even more complex. In these cases a linear regression or correlation analysis is inappropriate and more complex approaches are necessary.

The strength of linear regression or correlation is assessed by the so-called Pearson's correlation coefficient (parametric) or Spearman's rank correlation coefficient (non-parametric). Please always remember when using these statistics to refer back to the scatter plot, as these statistics can be strongly influenced by outliers.

Survival analysis

One additional bivariate test, the logrank test, is worth mentioning when introducing the most common bivariate test procedures. When a specified event (e.g. death) is observed in a cohort of people who are followed up for a period of time, special statistical procedures (survival analysis) become necessary. The individual survival time (i.e. follow-up time to event) is often unknown for some people in the cohort, because not everybody will have the event during the study period. The cases who do not have the event during the follow-up period or who withdraw from the study are called censored cases. These cases cannot be deleted from the data set because this would lead to an underestimation of the survival probability—as these people did survive for some time. In this situation the logrank test is used to compare survival probabilities between groups. For further details on survival analysis please refer to Douglas Altman (1991).

Please note

1   Refer to the chapter 'Choosing the statistical method' in Martin Bland's (2000) book for further details. A description of how to calculate a bivariate statistical test by hand is provided in all standard statistical textbooks (see e.g. Zar 2010 or Bland 2000).

2   The introduced statistical test procedures above refer to statistical tests for difference or association. However, some comparative research questions might not ask for difference, but rather for equivalence of effects or agreement between observers or instruments. Both situations require special test procedures. Unfortunately, tests or measures for equivalence or agreement are often not part of standard statistical software and require calculation 'by hand'.

Multivariable statistical analysis

Studying health phenomena in human populations is usually more complicated than just relating two characteristics, such as age and blood pressure. Blood pressure might be influenced by other characteristics, for example, gender. That is, bivariate statistical analysis is often insufficient to adequately address the research question under study. The main advantage of multivariable techniques in the health sciences is that they enable the researcher to assess more than one single study factor at a time and therefore allow adjusting for the influence of factors other than the study factor. These 'other factors' are called confounders and they are a common problem in quantitative designs. Confounding occurs when extraneous variables (confounders) that are correlated with both the study factor and the outcome distort the bivariate association under study.

Researchers try to avoid or minimise confounding through randomisation. Randomisation allocates participants of a study into intervention and control groups by chance alone. We randomise participants in order to compare groups that are similar with respect to other influencing characteristics (confounders). A randomised controlled trial such as the Lindsay Leg Club® intervention study has no issue with confounding, since, for example, age and gender distributions are similar for the two groups that are being compared. Therefore, bivariate analysis is completely sufficient for this trial. Multivariate analyses usually become necessary in studies in which one cannot randomise or in which randomisation failed.

For example, if one were to investigate the relationship between the number of sexual partners somebody has had during the last year (= study factor) and the likelihood of having a positive test for *Chlamydia trachomatis* (= outcome), age would need to be considered as a potential confounder. The reasons are that (1) age is related to the number of sexual partners a person has had during the previous year—a younger person is more likely to have changed sexual partners while an older person is more likely to be in a stable relationship. (2) Age is also related to the likelihood of *Chlamydia*—younger people are more likely to be *Chlamydia*-positive than older people. Therefore, one could argue that part of the association found between number of sexual partners and *Chlamydia* is due to age.

Before the actual multivariable statistical analysis can be conducted, several preparatory steps are usually necessary. The first step for any multivariable approach is always a thorough descriptive analysis. At least two additional steps are necessary: a detailed examination of the bivariate associations of all variables involved and the coding of all variables. More detailed advice on preparation for multivariable analysis can be found in Alvan Feinstein's (1996) book.

Selecting an appropriate multivariable method

The selection of a suitable multivariable method is dependent on a number of considerations which include the research hypothesis, the type of the target variable (outcome) and to a lesser degree the types of independent variables, and the statistical assumptions that need to be fulfilled. Table 12.5 provides a commented overview of the multivariable models used most frequently in the health sciences.

Table 12.5   Overview of multivariable methods most frequently used in the health sciences

Target variable	Multivariate model and use	Main assumptions	Comments
Numerical —continuous	Multiple linear regression analysis Assesses strength and direction of relationship	Normality, linearity, homoscedasticity, no outliers	(1) Discrete or ordinal target variables with many categories can also be analysed; (2) Classically all independent variables are continuous, in reality all types can be used; (3) If linearity is violated transform data or use non-linear regression analysis.
Numerical —continuous	Analysis of Variance Assesses whether relationship exists	Normality, homoscedasticity, equal sample sizes, random sampling	(1) Classically all independent variables are nominal (ANOVA), generalisations including continuous variables available (ANCOVA, MANCOVA); (2) Equal sample size requirement per cell might be fulfilled in experimental designs.
Categorical —binary	Logistic regression Assesses strength and direction of relationship	Linearity, homogeneity of variances, homoscedasticity of residuals, no outliers	(1) Preferred over discriminant function analysis because normality of independent variables is not required; (2) Transform data if linearity is violated.
Survival ('moving binary')	Cox proportional hazard analysis Assesses strength and direction of relationship with mortality	Proportional hazards and linearity	(1) Robust method to analyse binary outcome moving in time; (2) Transform data if linearity is violated; (3) Sample size requirements are dependent on expected differences and the event rate.

Two additional analytical techniques should also be mentioned briefly. Factor analysis is used in an exploratory way to extract a few conceptually meaningful independent factors from a larger collection of correlated variables, such as in the development of new psychometric scales (e.g. in the development of a new survey tool to measure quality of life). Cluster analysis is an exploratory method to organise observed data into clusters to give it a meaningful structure (taxonomy).

BOX 12.6

MULTIVARIABLE METHODS

A multivariable model is used to investigate the relationship between study factor(s) and outcome by simultaneously allowing adjustment for confounding. Multivariable methods can assess the effects of several study factors together. Multivariable methods become necessary for randomised trials when randomisation failed.

Example 1: A study investigates the association between number of sexual partners and prevalence of *Chlamydia trachomatis*. This research question implies an observational study design because ethically humans cannot be randomised into groups with different numbers of sexual partners. Therefore, a number of confounders might exist which potentially have an effect on the association under investigation and a multivariable analysis is necessary. The confounders might be age, gender, sexual preference, etc.

The outcome is *Chlamydia trachomatis* (yes/no) and is categorical, binary. Therefore, the multivariable method of choice would be a logistic regression. The logistic regression analysis will assess the effect of the number of sexual partners adjusted for confounding variables.

Example 2: A study on pain management in patients with advanced cancer comparing morning versus evening once only sustained-released morphine sulfate. A Visual Analogue Scale was used to measure pain levels in values ranging from 0=no pain to 100=maximal pain. The study randomised patients into the two groups (morning versus evening), but let's assume that this randomisation did not work out for gender. The morning group has many more female participants than the evening group. We also know from other studies that men perceive pain levels differently from women. Hence gender is a potential confounder.

The outcome level of pain is measured as a numerical variable. Therefore, the multivariable method of choice would be a multiple linear regression analysis. Assumptions for linear regression analysis need to be checked. The multiple linear regression analysis will assess the effect of the intervention on level of pain adjusted for gender.

Source: Example 2 adapted from Currow et al. 2007

For technical details on the above introduced multivariable methods, please refer to Feinstein (1996), Kleinbaum et al. (1988), or Kleinbaum and Klein (2002).

A step-by-step guide to multivariable analysis

In the following a short guide is presented that lists and comments on important steps involved in the preparation, conduct and presentation of a multivariable analysis:

1   Identify the type of the variables (outcome and independent variables) involved (Table 12.1).

2   Conduct a thorough descriptive and bivariate analysis including a correlation matrix; exclude collinear variables.

3   Identify the multivariable model best suited to your study situation (Table 12.5).

4   Check whether the assumptions of the model are fulfilled—and seek remedy if not. Multivariable procedures have diverse assumptions to be met (Table 12.5) and their general discussion is beyond the scope of this chapter (for more details see Feinstein 1996). However, one frequently overlooked assumption for numerical data is linearity; that is, the relationship between two numerical variables is supposed to be linear. Linearity has to be checked and if not given, numerical data should be either categorised (e.g. by taking the quartiles as the cut-offs) and dummy-coded, or mathematically transformed (e.g. by a logarithmic transformation).

5   Prepare all variables for multivariable analysis; dummy-code and transform as appropriate.

6   *The modelling process: Find the 'best' model.*

It is recommended to start with a hierarchically structured full model that includes all independent variables under consideration and their two-way (and possibly higher-order) interactions. An interaction of two variables is the product of these variables (e.g. for two dummy-coded characteristics the product will again be a 0/1 variable, with one identifying the category where both of the initial variables are true).

A stepwise backward elimination process (deleting the interactions and independent variables that are statistically insignificantly related with the outcome) that observes the hierarchy of the model should be used. This elimination process will start considering the highest-order interactions and removing those that are not relevant before looking at single independent characteristics. If an interaction is statistically significant all lower-order terms will have to remain in the model too—irrespective of significance—since interactions can only be meaningfully interpreted if the underlying basic variables are also in the model.

A stepwise forward procedure can then be applied where at each step the most significant variable (out of those not in the model) is added to the model until no further significant variables can be added. Generally, the stepwise forward and backward procedures should result in the same model. If discrepancies occur, variables have to be closely investigated for confounding and collinearity.

For more details please refer to Kleinbaum and Klein's book on logistic regression (2002). The approach described there can be transferred to other multivariable models.

Petra Buettner, Reinhold Muller and Monika Buhrer-Skinner

7   *Assessment of confounding*

Confounding is a systematic error, while statistical significance deals exclusively with random error. Assessment of confounding consequently cannot be based on statistical significance but is assessed by comparing the magnitude of the changes in the estimates of the previously established model when adding or dropping a potential confounder. If the estimate of an independent variable in the model changes by 10% or more (this is again an arbitrary cut-off), this potential confounder is a true confounder and should be kept in the model—irrespective of its own significance.

It is not advisable to simply add all potential confounders into the model since this results in less precise effects (i.e. confidence intervals would be wider) for the independent variables. Only confounders with a proven relevant impact should be added and consequently the check described above has to be conducted for each single potential confounder separately. Please be aware of changes in the estimate caused by changes in sample size (missing values).

The final model will then include all variables and interactions detected by means of the model-building processes plus all relevant confounders. Such a model will provide the most valid estimates for the effects of the independent variables on the outcomes that are achievable by the data set.

Most statistical software packages have automated backward and forward elimination processes. However, these automated approaches cannot take confounding into account (since the identification of confounding does not involve statistical testing). Hence in reality the final model will always be identified 'manually'.

Most statistical software will also include the constant into the model. If not please make sure it is added manually since the meaningful interpretation of every estimate depends on the presence of the constant.

8   *Regression diagnostics*

Steps 1 to 7 will deliver a 'final' model that gives the most valid estimates of the impact of independent variables and their interactions on the target variable. However, there remains the question of whether the model is a good predictive model, that is, whether it fits the observed data well. This fit of the model is checked by regression diagnostics, which can take on a variety of forms mainly depending on the type of model. Regression diagnostics gives an impression of the overall fit but is also used to finally check model assumptions—notably linearity.

In multiple regression analysis, for instance, the observed values can be compared directly with the model estimates. The observed differences, the residuals, should be approximately normally distributed around zero. In logistic regression analysis, numerous statistics have been developed to measure the goodness-of-fit of the model, while the accuracy of the estimated classification can be checked in classification tables and classification plots (for more details see e.g. Feinstein 1996).

9   *Presentation of the results of a multivariable analysis*

A good presentation of the results should not only present the variables that build the final model in tabulated form, but should also give a description of the methods and processes used to build this model. The table should specify all characteristics and interactions identified, together with their appropriate effect measures (e.g. odds-ratio, relative risk, regression coefficient), 95%-confidence intervals and respective p-values. It is important for any valid interpretation to also explicitly state the reference category (baseline) for each effect.

Table 12.6   Example of table of results

A cross-sectional study was conducted to identify risk factors for *Chlamydia trachomatis* infection in young Australian adults. A logistic regression analysis was conducted and the following results were found.

Chlamydia trachomatis				
Risk factor	No (n=698)	Yes (n=78)	Adjusted odds-ratio (95%-CI)	p-value
Gender				
Female	476	58	1	
Male	222	20	0.78 (0.43, 1.3)	P=0.431
Age				
21-25	442	46	1	
18-20	256	32	1.2 (0.75, 2.0)	P=0.585
Number of sexual partners in previous year				
None	168	12	1	
One	328	28	1.1 (0.59, 2.3)	P=0.724
More than one	202	38	2.6 (1.3, 5.3)	P=0.045

Source: Buhrer-Skinner, unpublished data

The results provided in Table 12.6 show that men were 0.78 times as likely to test positive for *Chlamydia* compared to women (= reference category; baseline). One can be 95% confident that the true odds-ratio is somewhere between 0.43 and 1.3. Because the confidence interval includes the null value of the odds-ratio (i.e. 1), this result is statistically non-significant. The p-value is 0.431, implying that this result or an even 'greater' odds-ratio could happen by chance alone with a probability of 43.1%. This result is not statistically significant.

In contrast, the number of sexual partners showed a statistically significant effect. People who had one sexual partner during the previous year were 1.1 times more likely to test positive for *Chlamydia* compared to the people with no sexual partner during the previous year (= reference category; baseline). People who had more than one sexual partner during the previous year were 2.6 times more likely to test positive for *Chlamydia* compared to those with no sexual partner during the previous year (p=0.045). These results show a dose–response relationship: the more partners, the higher the likelihood of *Chlamydia*.

Please note

An odds-ratio is the odds of exposure in the group of interest (e.g. *Chlamydia*-positive group) divided by the odds of exposure in the control group (e.g. *Chlamydia*-negative group in the above example). An odds-ratio of 1 implies that no difference exists between the groups compared.

Use of computer programs for data analysis

Nowadays nobody will conduct serious statistical analysis by hand. The rise of faster and faster personal computers and specialised statistical software allows easy access to complicated statistical methodology for everybody. A cautious note should be introduced here—the ready access to statistical software is no substitute for a comprehensive understanding of the implemented statistical tools. Statistical software is a fantastic tool, but only if users have adequate knowledge of statistical reasoning and its underlying assumptions.

There are a multitude of statistical software packages available, such as STATA, PASW, SAS, BMDP, S-PLUS and EPI-info. Most of these packages are licensed and rather expensive; hence choice might be limited to the software to which your employer or your university subscribed. EPI-info was developed by the World Health Organization and is a free-source software available on the internet. Some programs, for example, SPSS (now PASW), offer student and graduate versions that are much more affordable but that are also limited in their statistical capabilities. Most software programs can be checked out for free on the internet for a limited time.

At the beginner's level differences between the professional statistical software packages are rather more formal than content-based. Programs such as STATA, SPSS, S-PLUS or SAS all cover the basic bivariate and multivariable statistical procedures, and differences come only with the perceived user-friendliness of the program. But this is a personal matter, so you need to find the program that suits you best yourself. All statistical software packages come with handbooks and exquisite help functions. Please read up or ask a specialist, when in doubt.

Summary

Statistics is the tool that allows us to analyse data collected during quantitative research projects. It enables us to confirm or reject quantitative research hypotheses. In our chapter we aimed to provide an introduction to the world of numbers; a world that many perceive as daunting. The chapter gives you guidance on how to describe your data correctly, and it also points you in the right direction for choosing a statistical test relating two characteristics. However, most data analyses require more complex approaches than bivariate statistics and so we also introduced multivariable methods. Don't be scared! Follow our simple rules and try statistics with your own data.

IMPLICATIONS FOR EVIDENCE-BASED NURSING AND MIDWIFERY

The use of appropriate statistical procedures to analyse quantitative data is essential to confirming or refuting research hypotheses posed by nursing or midwifery researchers. The quality of a study and its results is partly judged by the use of adequate statistical methods, that is, the researchers have used an appropriate measure of central tendency for describing sample characteristics and have applied the correct parametric or non-parametric statistical tests or multivariable methods to explore differences in nominal or continuous outcome. Multivariable techniques are complex, but provide researchers with the ability to consider the effect of several study factors on the outcome while simultaneously adjusting for confounding factors.

Nurses and midwives require sufficient knowledge of statistical procedures to be able to design a study appropriately (sample size), understand and use appropriate statistical procedures, and finally report comprehensively on the findings of the analysis. Similarly, nurses reading published research need first to be able to judge whether statistical methods used were appropriate and second to understand the results of a study in order to interpret nursing or midwifery research.

Practice exercise 12.1

You are part of a research team which is investigating whether a difference exists in perceived pain during burns dressing for patients receiving intramuscular injection of Pethidine versus inhaling Entonox.

What characteristics do you need to develop a falsifiable research hypothesis?

Try to formulate a research hypothesis for this scenario.

Source: Adapted from Ruegg et al. 2009

Practice exercise 12.2

You are part of a research team which is investigating whether a difference exists in perceived pain during burns dressing for patients receiving intramuscular injection of Pethidine versus inhaling Entonox.

Data is collected on the following characteristics: age, gender, ethnicity, body mass index, surface area of burns, pain score (measured using a Visual Analogue Scale ranging from 0=no pain to 100=worst pain), and perceived pain tolerance (scale: low tolerance, moderate tolerance, high tolerance).

a   Classify these variables into categorical (nominal/ordinal) and numerical (discrete/continuous).

- A total of 48 patients participated in the study: 32 participants were male (Graphic 1) and 41 were Caucasian (Graphic 2). Low pain tolerance was recorded for 2 patients, 11 patients showed moderate and 35 showed high pain tolerance (Graphic 3).
- Descriptive statistics for body mass index are: mean 29.1, SD 2.6, median 29.4, IQR [27, 31]; range 23.9. to 34.9 (Graphic 4).
- Descriptive statistics for age in years are: mean 57.0, SD 15.8, median 58.8, IQR [47.7, 65.4]; range 18 to 96 (Graphic 5).
- Descriptive statistics for surface area of burns in cm^2 are: mean 8.0, SD 15.3, median 3, IQR [2, 5]; range 2 to 96 (Graphic 6).
- Descriptive statistics for pain score for patients using Entonox are: mean 36.5, SD 15.1, median 37.0, IQR = [26, 51], range 7 to 57 (Graphic 7).

The data are graphically displayed below.

b   Choose the correct descriptive statistics based on the information given for the variables: gender, ethnicity, pain tolerance, BMI, age, wound surface area and pain score.

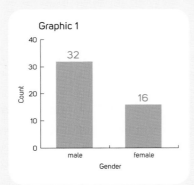

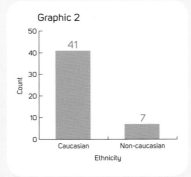

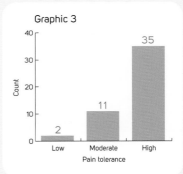

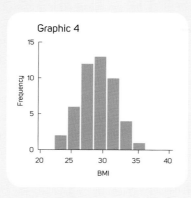

Graphic 4

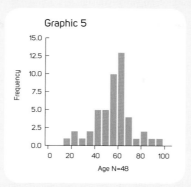

Graphic 5

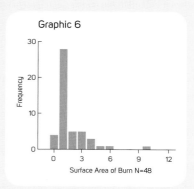

Graphic 6

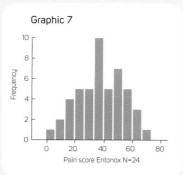

Graphic 7

Source: Adapted from Ruegg et al. 2009

Practice exercise 12.3

Bivariate statistical tests

You are part of a research team that is investigating whether a difference exists in perceived pain during burns dressing for patients receiving intramuscular injection of Pethidine versus inhaling Entonox.

Data is collected on the following characteristics: age, gender, ethnicity, body mass index, surface area of burns, pain score (measured using a Visual Analogue Scale ranging from 0=no pain to 100=worst pain), and perceived pain tolerance (scale: low tolerance, moderate tolerance, high tolerance).

a   Which group of bivariate statistical tests would be appropriate for investigating relationships between the following variables (refer to Figure 12.3)?

- pain score and type of pain relief
- pain score and body mass index
- gender and perceived pain tolerance
- age and gender
- gender and type of pain relief
- ethnicity and pain score
- age and pain score.

Further analysis of the data showed the following: a total of 48 patients participated in the study: 32 participants were male (Graphic 1) and 41 were Caucasian (Graphic 2). Low pain tolerance was recorded for 2 patients, 11 patients showed moderate and 35 showed high pain tolerance (Graphic 3).

Descriptive statistics for body mass index are: mean 29.1, SD 2.6, median 29.4, Interquartile range (IQR) [27, 31]; range 23.9. to 34.9 (Graphic 4).

Descriptive statistics for age are: mean 57.0, SD 15.8, median 58.8, IQR [47.7, 65.4]; range 18 to 96 (Graphic 5). In the category of male gender the descriptive statistics for age are: mean 55.3, SD 15.9, median 57.3, IQR [45.4, 65.4], range 18 to 96 (Graphic 6). In the category of female gender the values are: mean 60.6, SD 15.6, median 59.4, IQR [53.4, 68.8], range 36 to 90 (Graphic 7).

Descriptive statistics for surface area of burns are: mean 8.0, SD 15.3, median 3, IQR [2, 5]; range 2 to 96 (Graphic 8).

Descriptive statistics for pain score (total Graphic 9) using Entonox are: mean 36.5, SD 15.1, median 37.0, IQR = [26, 51], range 7 to 57 (Graphic 10).

Descriptive statistics for pain score using Entonox are: mean 45.5.1, SD 12.8, median 44.8, IQR [39.4, 51.7], and range 17 to 71 (Graphic 11).

Descriptive statistics for pain score in the category of non-Caucasian ethnicity are: mean 45.6, SD 18.1, median 51.1, IQR [30.3, 56.9], range 16 to 71 (Graphic 12), while the descriptive statistics for the total pain score are: mean 41, SD 14.6, median 42.2, IQR [31.3,51.2], and range 7 to 71 (Graphic 9). The data are graphically displayed below.

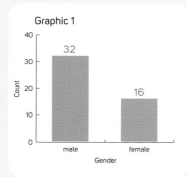

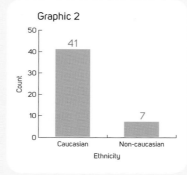

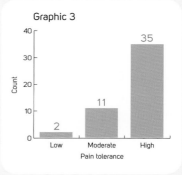

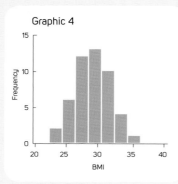

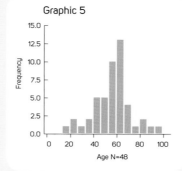

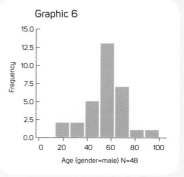

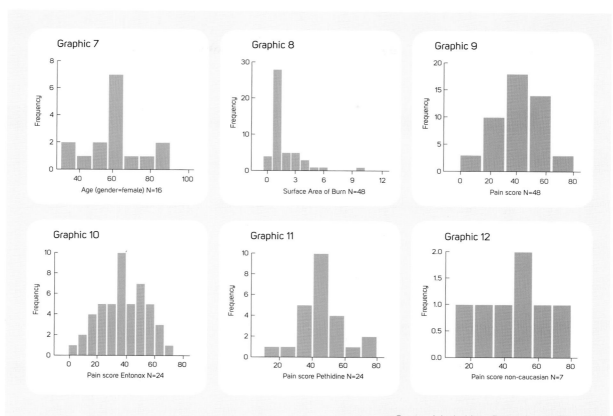

Source: Adapted from Ruegg et al. 2009

b   Based on the information you have, which particular bivariate statistical test would be appropriate for investigating relationships between the above mentioned variables?

Answers to practice exercises

12.1

You would consider defining the following characteristics:

Study factor: Type of pain relief (Pethidine or Entonox);

Outcome: Perceived pain (measure pain using a validated instrument, e.g. Visual Analogue Scale);

Quantitative statement about the expected result: The expected difference can be either expressed as a total difference between average values (either mean or median) of the pain score, e.g. the mean pain scores in the participants who use Pethidine versus those who use Entonox or as a relative difference between the two study groups, e.g. the pain score in the one group will be x% different (possibly higher or lower) from the pain score in the other group. Always remember that the difference that you are trying to detect should be clinically relevant.

In addition a measure of the variability (e.g. standard deviation) of the pain score will be needed. Additionally you would need to clearly define inclusion and exclusion criteria of participants.

Possible research hypothesis: The mean pain score of patients who receive Pethidine during burns dressing is 5 units (standard deviation 3 units) lower than the mean pain score of patients who received Entonox.

12.2a

Characteristic	Type of variable
Age	Numerical Discrete if measured as age at last birthday Continuous if measured as time since birth
Gender	Categorical nominal
Ethnicity	Categorical nominal
Body Mass Index (BMI)	Numerical continuous
Surface area of burns	Numerical continuous
Pain score	Numerical continuous between 0 and 100
Perceived pain tolerance	Categorical ordinal

12. 2b

Characteristic	Values	Rationale
Gender male n=32	66%	Categorical variable with two categories, the second category (female n=16, 33%) is implied
Ethnicity Caucasian n=41	85.4%	Categorical variable with two categories, the other category (non-Caucasian n=7, 14.6%) is implied

Pain tolerance
    Low n=2
    Moderate n=11
    High n=35
	
	4.2%
	22.9%
	72.9%
		Categorical variable with three categories, data is given for all categories

Mean BMI (SD)* [kg/m²]	29.1 (2.6)	Numerical variable, histogram shows a symmetrical distribution (Graphic 4)
Mean age (SD) [years]	57 (15.8)	Numerical variable, histogram shows a symmetrical distribution (Graphic 5)
Median surface area of burns (IQR)**[cm²]	3 (2, 5)	Numerical variable, histogram shows asymmetrical distribution (Graphic 6)
Mean pain score using Entonox (SD)	36.5 (15.1)	Numerical variable, histogram shows a symmetrical distribution (Graphic 7)

*SD = standard deviation; **IQR = inter-quartile range

12.3a

Variable	Type of variable
Age	Numerical
Gender	Categorical/ 2 categories
Ethnicity	Categorical/ 2 categories
Body mass index (BMI)	Numerical
Surface area of burns	Numerical
Pain score	Numerical
Perceived pain tolerance	Categorical ordinal/ 3 categories
Type of pain relief	Categorical/ 2 categories

Variable	Group of bivariate statistical test	
Pain score and type of pain relief	Numerical/ categorical	Group 3
Pain score and BMI	Numerical/numerical	Group 1
Gender and perceived pain tolerance	Categorical/ categorical	Group 2
Age and gender	Numerical/ categorical	Group 3
Gender and type of pain relief	Categorical/ categorical	Group 2
Ethnicity and pain score	Categorical/ numerical	Group 3
Age and pain score	Numerical/ numerical	Group 1

12.3b

Variables	Statistical test	Rationale
Pain score and type of pain relief	Unpaired t-test	Symmetrical distribution of pain score in both categories
Pain score and BMI	Regression	One-sided association: BMI could influence pain score but not the other way around; both variables are symmetrically distributed
Gender and perceived pain tolerance	Unpaired chi-square test or Fisher's exact test (small sample size)	Pain tolerance is an ordinal categorical variable, but the sample size in the example is small
Age and gender	Unpaired t-test	Symmetrical distribution of age in both categories
Gender and type of pain relief	Unpaired chi-square test or Fisher's exact test (small sample size)	Both categorical variables have two categories; small sample size
Ethnicity and pain score	Unpaired Wilcoxon test	Asymmetrical distribution of pain score in one of the categories; small sample size
Age and pain score	Regression	One-sided association: age might influence pain score but not the other way around; both variables are symmetrically distributed

Further reading

Altman, D. G. (1991). *Practical Statistics for Medical Research*. Cornwall: Chapman & Hall, TJ Press.

Feinstein, A. (1996). *Multivariable Analysis. An Introduction*. New Haven, CN: Yale University Press.

Kleinbaum, D. G., & Klein, M. (2002). *Logistic Regression. A Self-Learning Text*, 2nd edn. New York: Springer Verlag.

Kleinbaum, D. G., Kupper, L. L., & Morgenstern, H. (1982). *Epidemiologic Research: Principles and Quantitative Methods*. New York: Van Nostrand Reinhold.

Weblinks

Confidence intervals for binomial distributions:

<http://statpages.org/confint.html>

Statistical calculation pages:

<http://statpages.org>

Equivalence tests (non-inferiority test):

<www.graphpad.com/library/BiostatsSpecial/article_182.htm>

References

Altman, D. G. (1991). *Practical Statistics for Medical Research*. Cornwall: Chapman & Hall, T. J. Press.

Ballan, A., & Lee, G. (2007). A comparative study of patient perceived quality of life pre and post coronary artery bypass graft surgery. *Australian Journal of Advanced Nursing* 24(4), 24.

Bland, M. (2000). *An Introduction to Medical Statistics*, 3rd edn. Melbourne: Oxford University Press.

Currow, D. C., Plummer, J. L., Cooney, N. J., Gorman, D., & Glare, P. A. (2007). A randomized, double-blind, multi-site, crossover, placebo-controlled equivalence study of morning versus evening once-daily sustained-release morphine sulfate in people with pain from advanced cancer. *Journal of Pain and Symptom Management* 34(1), 17–23.

Edwards, H., Courtney, M., Finlayson, K., Shuter, P., & Linday, E. (2009). A randomised controlled trial of a community nursing intervention: Improved quality of life and healing for clients with leg ulcers. *Journal of Clinical Nursing* 18, 1541–9.

Feinstein, A. (1996). *Multivariable Analysis. An Introduction*. New Haven, CN: Yale University Press.

Gerstman, B. B. (2008). *Basic Biostatistics. Statistics for Public Health Practice*. Sudbury, MA: Jones & Bartlett Publishers.

Kleinbaum, D. G., & Klein, M. (2002). *Logistic Regression. A Self-Learning Text*, 2nd edn. New York: Springer Verlag.

Kleinbaum, D. G., Kupper, L. L., & Muller, K. E. (1988). *Applied Regression Analysis and Other Multivariable Methods*, 2nd edn. North Scituate, MA: Duxbury Press, Wadsworth Publishing Company.

Ruegg, T. A., Curran, C. R., & Lamb, T. (2009). Use of buffered lidocaine in bone marrow biopsies: a randomized, controlled trial. *Oncology Nursing Forum* 36(1), 52.

Schmied, V., Cooke, M., Gutwein, R., Steinlein, E., & Homer, C. (2009). An evaluation of strategies to improve the quality and content of hospital-based postnatal care in a metropolitan Australian hospital. *Journal of Clinical Nursing* 18(13), 1850–61.

Spitzer, W., Dobson, A., & Hall, J. (1981). Measuring the quality of life of cancer patients: A concise QL-Index for use by physicians. *Journal of Chronic Diseases* 34, 585–97.

Thomas, M., McKinley, R. K., Mellor, S., Watkin, G., Holloway, E., Scullion, J., et al. (2009). Breathing exercises for asthma: A randomised controlled trial. *Thorax* 64(1), 55–61.

Zar, J. H. (2010). *Biostatistical Analysis*, 5th edn. Upper Saddle River, NJ: Pearson/Prentice Hall.

CHAPTER 13

Critical Review of Research

Jane Warland and Phil Maude

Chapter learning objectives

By the end of this chapter you will be able to:

▶ understand the definition of critical review

▶ describe terms associated with critical appraisal

▶ list strategies for developing critical appraisal skills

▶ describe the use of common appraisal tools and techniques

▶ discuss the basic attributes of high-quality primary studies

▶ analyse how study design and method affect the quality and applicability of clinical-based evidence.

Introduction

It is the responsibility of every registered nurse or midwife (RN/M) to keep up to date with current research (ANMC 2006a,b), but there are a number of widely known barriers to achieving this (Cheek et al. 2005). Many RN/Ms have difficulty understanding the research literature because they are unfamiliar with how to tell the difference between well and poorly conducted research. Learning how to critically appraise literature is therefore a vital skill for all practitioners.

This chapter will guide you through four steps to help you develop your ability to review literature critically:

1   selection and effective reading of the literature
2   critical appraisal and consideration of the level of available evidence
3   collation and description of the literature
4   considering the application of evidence to practice.

A critical review is 'the process of objectively, critically and analytically reading a research report's content for scientific merit and application to practice or theory' (Schneider et al. 2007, p. 53). The objective of a critical review is not to criticise the article but to critique it—to objectively review the research process and verify that the methods the researchers used were sound. A critical appraisal of the literature is essential when considering a rationale for change to practice or when implementing care that is evidence-based.

Selection and effective reading of the literature

A review of the literature is a classification and evaluation of what scholars and researchers have written on a topic, organised according to a guiding concept such as the research objective(s), hypothesis, thesis or the problem/issue. It is an analysis of the current knowledge concerning a topic.

Your objective is not to list as many articles as possible; rather, it is to demonstrate your intellectual ability to recognise relevant information, and to synthesise and evaluate it according to the guiding concept. You want to know what literature exists and you want to make an informed evaluation or critical appraisal of this literature. To meet both of these needs, you must employ two sets of skills:

- *Information-seeking:* the ability to scan the literature efficiently using manual or computerised methods to identify potentially useful articles, books and grey literature.
- *Critical appraisal:* the ability to apply principles of analysis to identify unbiased and valid studies. You need to produce more than just a descriptive list of articles and books. You need to show that you understand the study design, sample size

and key findings and can critique the methods used. It is usually a bad sign when every paragraph of your review begins with the names of researchers. Instead, organise your review into useful, informative sections that present themes or identify trends.

To begin, you explain the search strategy you used so that your approach to finding the literature and deciding what was included and excluded is clear. A list of databases such as MEDLINE, PsycLit, CINAHL or SCOPUS is also needed.

BOX 13.1
EXAMPLE OF SEARCH STRATEGY DESCRIPTION

The literature reviewed was drawn from a search conducted using the Cumulative Index to Nursing and Allied Health Literature (CINAHL), MEDLINE, and PsycINFO electronic databases. The search was limited to primary research articles published between 2005 and 2010, in English and involving different settings in nursing such as psychiatry, emergency nursing and general wards. The search terms used were: 'violence' or 'violent' or 'aggression' or 'aggressive' and 'nurses'. Of the 77 articles that were found 17 were chosen for inclusion in this review as they were research papers that included data from Australia. Articles concerning horizontal violence and nursing were excluded.

When you are planning to review the literature there are a number of questions you could ask yourself, for example:

1. Do I have a specific thesis, problem or research question that my literature review helps to define?

2. What type of literature review am I conducting? Am I looking at issues of theory? methodology? policy? quantitative research (such as studies of a new or controversial procedure)? qualitative research (such as studies determining criteria for allocating health care resources)?

3. What is the scope of my literature review? What types of publications am I using, for example journals, books, government documents, popular media? What discipline am I working in? Is it nursing, psychology, sociology, medicine or a combination of two or more areas?

4. How good are my information-seeking skills? Has my search been wide enough to ensure that I have found all the relevant material? Has it been narrow enough to exclude irrelevant material? Is the number of sources I have used appropriate and reflective of the scope of the available literature?

5. Is there a specific relationship between the literature I have chosen to review and the problem I have formulated?

6. How have I made decisions to include some works and exclude others?

7. Have I critically analysed the literature I use? Do I just list and summarise authors and articles, or do I assess them? Do I discuss the strengths and weaknesses of the cited material?

8   Have I cited and discussed studies contrary to my perspective?

9   Will the reader find my literature review relevant, appropriate and useful?

As you continue with your review, ask these questions about the specific book or article you are reviewing:

1   Has the author formulated a problem/issue? Is this a research paper?

2   Is the problem/issue ambiguous or clearly articulated? Is its significance (scope, severity, relevance) discussed?

3   What are the strengths and limitations of the way the author has formulated the problem or issue?

4   Could the problem have been approached more effectively from another perspective?

5   What is the author's research orientation such as interpretive, critical science or a combination?

6   What is the author's theoretical framework, for example, developmental, feminist or psychoanalytic?

7   What is the relationship between the theoretical and research perspectives?

8   Has the author evaluated the literature relevant to the problem/issue? Does the author include literature taking positions they do not agree with?

9   In a research study, how good are the three basic components of the study design: population, intervention, outcome? How accurate and valid are the measurements? Is the analysis of the data accurate and relevant to the research question? Are the conclusions validly based on the data and analysis?

10   In popular literature, does the author use appeals to emotion, one-sided examples, rhetorically charged language and tone? Is the author objective, or are they merely 'proving' what they already believe?

11   How does the author structure their argument? Can you 'deconstruct' the flow of the argument to analyse if or where it breaks down?

12   Is this a book or article that contributes to our understanding of the problem under study, and in what ways is it useful for practice? What are its strengths and limitations?

13   How does this book or article fit into the thesis or question I am developing?

Making sense of the literature—first pass

When you first come to an area of research, you are filling in the background in a general way, getting a feel for the whole area, an idea of its scope, starting to appreciate the controversies, to see the high points, and to become more familiar with the main authors. This is your starting point.

Is there too much literature to handle?

At this stage there may seem to be masses of literature relevant to your research. Or you may worry that there seems to be hardly anything. As you read, think about and discuss articles and isolate the issues you are more interested in. In this way, you focus your topic more and more. The more you can close in on what your research question or topic of enquiry actually is, the more you will be able to have a basis for selecting the relevant areas of the literature. This is the only way to bring it down to a manageable size and to ensure you have looked at all the literature across disciplines.

Is very little literature available?

If initially you cannot seem to find much at all on your research area, and you are sure that you have used all avenues for searching that the library can present you with, there are a few possibilities:

- You could be right at the cutting edge of something new and it is not surprising there is little around.
- You could be limiting yourself to too narrow an area and not appreciating that relevant material could be just around the corner in a closely related field.
- Maybe your key search terms are not well chosen, are loosely defined or not focused enough. For example, if you type in the search term 'preceptorship and nursing' you will find a great deal of information. However, the term 'preceptorship' is used in the USA to describe the first year a nurse works in the health service after graduating, but in the UK and Australia this is used to describe clinical support of student and novice staff.
- Unfortunately there is another possibility: that there's nothing in the literature because it's not a worthwhile area of research.

Quality of the literature

You learn to judge, evaluate and look critically at the literature by judging, evaluating and looking critically at it. That is, you learn to do something by practising. There are some questions you could find useful and, with practice, you will develop many others:

- Is the problem clearly spelled out?
- Are the results presented new?
- Was the research influential in that others picked up the threads and pursued them?
- How large a sample was used? Was the sample size justified?
- How convincing is the argument made?
- How were the results analysed?
- What perspective are they coming from?

- Are the generalisations justified by the evidence on which they are made?
- What is the significance of this research?
- What are the assumptions behind the research?
- Is the methodology justified as the most appropriate to study the problem?
- Is the theoretical basis transparent?

Critical appraisal and consideration of level of available evidence

Becoming familiar with the process of critical review

Critically appraising literature commonly involves utilising some kind of appraisal tool (see Weblinks). Such tools are designed to help you read and think about the study in a systematic manner. After working your way through the questions in the tool, you should have some idea about the worth of the article you have appraised. But this will only be achieved if you actually can 'tell' the answers to the questions posed in the tool. Frequently, novice reviewers come unstuck using these tools because they actually cannot 'tell' whether the researchers have met the stated criteria or not. Thus they may have little more idea about the quality of the research at the end of the appraisal than at the beginning.

How then do you get the knowledge you need in order to be able to use these appraisal tools adequately? Here we outline some of the strategies you can use to become familiar with the critical review process:

1 Regularly read high-quality research papers. Commonly an article published in a peer-reviewed journal has been critically appraised by someone who is an expert in either content, study design used or both. High-quality peer-reviewed journals often use three or four reviewers. In the case of quantitative studies, most high-impact journals will also use a statistician to check whether the statistical analysis was correctly conducted. What this means is that if you read journal articles published in peer-reviewed journals with high-impact factors, you start to get a sense of how a well-written, well-reported, valid study will read.

2 Practise critical appraisal. In a critical appraisal process, it really is a matter of practice makes perfect. Some ideas for getting you started are to:
   - Practise on your own.
     - Start small and simple.
     - Perform a literature search in the area of your interest.
     - Of these articles, find one that is a few pages long.
     - Find one that has attracted some correspondence to the editor. This will help you see what others have said (for more on this see the next section).

- Skim-read (Schneider et al. 2007) your article through, then go and do something else for a while.
- Read it through more thoroughly again, this time making some notes about any questions that spring to your mind.
- Look up the answers to your questions in a research text or dictionary, or seek out someone with expertise to answer your questions.
- Complete a critical appraisal tool such as CASP for your article.
- Follow this process by telling a colleague or your classmate about the article, the key points, what it found that was new and the significance of these findings for clinical practice.

- Practise with others.
  - A very good way of becoming familiar with critical appraisal is to join a journal club. A journal club typically meets regularly to discuss and critically appraise journal articles. Participating in such a group allows you not only to keep abreast of current literature but also to give you experience in reading and understanding research literature. If you do not have a journal club at your workplace, then seriously consider starting one.

3   Read reviews done by others. There are two ways you can easily access reviews conducted by others. The first is reading reviewer's comments on a manuscript and the second is reading critical reviews posted on the internet.

Read reviewers' comments from open-access published journals

Open-access journals offer free availability to readers and quick online publication of research articles. The review process for these journals is open and provides novice researchers and students with excellent real-world examples of critical appraisal in action.

The 'pre-publication history' of articles allows you to read the manuscript originally submitted, the reviewers' comments, the authors' response, alterations made, follow-up reviewers' comments and the final article.

This gives good insight into the review process and the kinds of comments reviewers typically make. It may be interesting for you to realise that almost invariably the reviewers require the authors to justify some aspect of their study and further refine their article before it can be published, which process improves the articles.

Open-access published journals are listed in Weblinks.

Read critical reviews posted on the internet

Another way of becoming familiar with the critical review process is to read a critical review conducted by another person. One example is the Joanna Briggs Institute site, which has a range of critical reviews in its Rapid Appraisal Protocol internet database (RAPid). Many of the reviews on this site have been conducted by students. Another example is an internet site called Best Bets, developed by the Emergency Department of Manchester Royal Infirmary, UK, to provide quick and easy access to a range of critical reviews of research literature typically conducted by clinicians at this hospital. Visitors can browse 'critical appraisals' in the databases section (see Best Bets at <www.bestbets.org>).

Critique methods

In this section, methods for critiquing quantitative and qualitative articles will be considered. We use a case study of a cohort study to give a practical example of the application of a critical appraisal tool (CAT). We will provide links to web-based resources for the particular method you are interested in later in the chapter.

Use of critical appraisal tools to critique literature

There are a number of critical appraisal tools available (see Further reading and Weblinks). While these look a little different, they all provide you with a step-by-step systematic, logical process for appraising research literature.

Interactive critical appraisal tools

Web-based critical appraisal tools (CAT) have been specifically developed for health care students such as nurses and midwives to help them to organise, conduct and archive summaries of evidence. These include the Critical Appraisal Tool maker (CATmaker) (Badenoch et al. 2004), and RAPid. CATmaker is a free interactive tool that enables you to store research questions, search strategies and/or complete appraisals. However, the RAPid CAT is available to JBI subscribers. In addition to CATmaker features, RAPid is designed to assist users to appraise and summarise evidence from a wide range of sources, including the results of qualitative studies. Once you have completed a RAPid appraisal you are invited to contribute it to the RAPid database. Both of these tools have drop-down boxes that allow users to logically work their way through an appraisal.

Critical appraisal tools

In a systematic review of CATs, Katrak and others (2004) found that there were more than 100 CATs currently in use. Such a wide choice presents the novice reviewer with a problem of which tool to use in which circumstance. They can be broadly classified into design-specific and generic. Both of these have advantages and disadvantages of use. Choosing a design-specific tool can assist you to appraise a specific study design; a generic tool is more flexible but may lack specific items to enable you to determine the quality of a certain design.

BOX 13.2

EXAMPLE CRITICAL APPRAISAL OF A COHORT STUDY

Article appraised: M. Lim, M. Hellard & C. Aitken (2005) The case of the disappearing teaspoons: Longitudinal cohort study of the displacement of teaspoons in an Australian research institute. BMJ 3311498-1500 available online at <www.bmj.com/cgi/content/full/331/7531/1498>. This case study will follow the CASP 12 questions to help you make sense of a cohort study guidelines for critical appraisal of a quantitative research article. Using each of the CASP headings, the article will be critiqued and analysed to answer questions as to whether the research article being studied is credible and worthy of use within evidence-based practice. We have chosen an article that is short and fairly simple. We are not suggesting this appraisal is perfect or even complete, but it should give you an idea of what you need to consider when you conduct a critical appraisal.

Q. Did the study address a clearly focused issue?

Yes   Can't Tell   No

In order to answer this question you need to know what is meant by 'clearly focused'. The kinds of things that need to be considered here are listed in the appraisal tool, but simply put, this aspect of clear focus means that the researchers did not try to do too much. For example, if they were also trying to investigate missing knives and forks then this may have resulted in a much less focused study.

Q. Did the authors use an appropriate method to answer their question?

Yes   Can't Tell   No

A cohort design is used to observe a group that is linked in some way because they share common characteristics—in this case, marked teaspoons. The cohort are studied over a period of time to observe an outcome (in this case, disappearance).

The researchers' principal method was a longitudinal cohort, which was used to study the disappearance rate of a group of teaspoons. But they also used a survey of staff members. While a survey is not normally part of a cohort study, it was an appropriate addition as it adds insight to the study question—why are the teaspoons going missing?

At this point you are asked 'Is it worth continuing?' If your first two answers were anything other than yes then there probably is no point continuing because either the study is not worth reading (if you have circled 'no') or (if you have circled 'can't tell') you may not yet have the necessary skills to complete the appraisal.

The next section of the appraisal tool is all about rigour.

BOX 13.2

Q. Was the cohort recruited in an acceptable way?

Yes	Can't Tell	No

This asks you whether a selection bias might have occurred because if it has then the ability of the researchers to generalise their findings is limited. As we read in Chapter 6 of this book, generalisability means the ability the researcher has to claim that because a certain finding has occurred in one setting the same thing will occur in another similar setting.

The tool then poses the following questions:

- Was the cohort representative of a defined population?
- Was there something special about the cohort?
- Was everybody included who should have been included?

The cohort in this study was artificially constructed and as such all sections of the cohort, such as all teaspoons, were identical and all were present at the commencement of the study.

Q. Was the exposure accurately measured to minimise bias?

Yes	Can't Tell	No

We are looking for measurement or classification bias:

- Did they use subjective or objective measurements?
- Do the measures truly reflect what you want them to (have they been validated)?
- Were the subjects classified into exposure groups based on the same procedure?

Once again you are required to have some knowledge of how a measurement or classification bias may occur. Basically, this section is asking you to determine if the exposure to disappearance was accurately measured. Could something else have happened to the teaspoons? In this case it was difficult for the researchers to determine if the teaspoons had disappeared forever, or only temporarily because they were in use at the time of the count.

Q. Was the outcome accurately measured to minimise bias?

Yes	Can't Tell	No

Q. Did they use objective measurement?

Yes, they counted the presence or absence of the teaspoons from the tearoom every week.

Q. Do the measures truly reflect what you want, i.e. have they been validated?

Yes, the researchers established this as a valid method of data collection by using a pilot study.

Q. Has a reliable system been used to detect all missing teaspoons?

This was reasonably reliable although the researchers don't discuss timing of their weekly teaspoon count. If, for example, the count was conducted at lunchtime this may have resulted in more teaspoons appearing to have disappeared than if they conducted the search in the first or last part of the day.

BOX 13.2

Q. Were the measurement methods similar in the different groups?

Probably: all teaspoons were counted by the same team, although interrater reliability wasn't checked (meaning that some team members may have conducted a more thorough search for teaspoons than others).

Q. Were the subjects and/or assessors blinded to the exposure (does this matter)?

The subjects were inanimate objects. The assessors could not have easily been blinded from the exposure in this instance because they were required to look for the teaspoons. This does matter as they may have had a vested interest in ensuring the teaspoons disappeared to enable them to report their significant findings, and by not conducting as thorough a search as perhaps they might if they had been blinded to the outcome of disappearance being the outcome of interest.

Q.Have the authors identified all important confounding factors? List the ones you think might be important, that the authors missed.

Yes   Can't Tell   No

Much of the correspondence regarding this paper discussed potential confounding factors that the authors missed including:

Teabags and forks (Woodall 2005)

The researchers themselves (Aitken 2005)

Coffee and tea drinkers (Lisse 2005)

Dishwashers (Underwood 2005)

Children (Baker 2005)

Dishes (Grantholm 2006)

Teaspoons used for other purposes (Silver 2006)

Gender of staff (Smith 2005, Cannizzaro 2006)

Attrition rates (Shadbolt 2006)

The weather (Bowler 2006)

The spoon fairy (Scholten 2006)

Q. Was the follow-up of the subjects complete and long enough?

Yes   Can't Tell   No

Probably not. There is no indication that the researchers did anything other than a cursory search; the teaspoons may have been in use when the final count occurred.

Q. What are the results of this study?

The results are reported in an unusual way for a cohort study, i.e. there is no relative risk (RR) reported. However, the researchers report statistically significant findings.

BOX 13.2

Q. How precise are the results?

The 95% confidence interval (CI) is narrow (0.76—1.28), indicating that the results are likely to be precise.

Q. Do you believe the results?

Yes   Can't Tell   No

The results are logical and make sense.

Q. Can the results be applied to the local population?

Yes   Can't Tell   No

Even though teaspoons may differ a little from place to place the results are generalisable across many different workplaces. However, these are not generalisable to other places where teaspoons are used, such as a home.

Q. Do the results of this study fit with other available evidence?

Yes   Can't Tell   No

This is the first reported empirical study to study this phenomenon, but the results fit with anecdotal everyday observation.

Critical appraisal of statistics

Understanding results when statistics have been used is one of the most challenging areas for many novice researchers. Probably a good approach to critique of statistics is to consider the question 'Has the researcher provided justification for the types of statistical tests used?' Most researchers understand that their readers might not necessarily understand the subtleties of the statistical tests they have used and will usually provide an explanation about what their results mean.

A study by Zellner and others (2007) examined quantitative articles published in 13 nursing research journals during 2000. They found that the 10 most common statistics were 'mean, frequency distribution, standard deviation, range, percentiles, percentages, quartiles, t-test, ANOVA, correlation, Cronbach alpha and Chi-Square' (p. 562). These 10 statistics represented 80% of all statistics used in the 462 articles they reviewed. So if you can understand these descriptive statistics you will very likely understand most nursing articles. Thus it would be a good idea to look up and aim to understand the meaning of these statistical tests and terms. When you come across new statistical methods look these up and add them to your knowledge base for the language of statistics.

Jane Warland and Phil Maude

An article by Beitz (2008) offers some very good information about decision-making for statistical tests in nursing research and how to problem-solve and question the statistics being used.

When making an appraisal of a qualitative study the CAT may look a little different from the CASP tool used above. The following questions are typical:

Writing style, author credibility, title and abstract

- Is the journal article well laid out with clear section headings and signposting?
- Are definitions explained and is clear language used?
- Are the researchers' qualifications and affiliations provided?
- Does the title reflect the study design, topic and findings?
- Upon reading the abstract do you have a vivid picture of the research, why it was conducted?

Aim/purpose, literature review and theoretical framework

- Is the aim or purpose of the study clearly articulated?
- Have the author(s) provided the research question(s)?
- Is the literature review extensive, contemporary and does it include key articles?
- Is the literature review critical and unbiased?
- If a literature review is not provided, have the author(s) justified this and do they relate their findings to the literature in the discussion section of the paper?
- Do the author(s) acknowledge their interest in the study and reflect on bias and conflicts of interest?
- Has a conceptual framework been identified and if so is it justified and applicable to the study?
- Has the use of a conceptual framework influenced or biased the reporting of the study findings?

Method, sampling, data analysis, philosophical integration and ethical considerations

- Have the author(s) stayed true to the method they have identified?
- Could you replicate this study from the description provided of sampling and data analysis?
- Is the sampling method adequate and is the sample size justified?
- Could other participants have added breadth of understanding of this phenomenon?
- Does the article advise that a study proposal was considered by an ethics committee and was approved?
- Have the participants been adequately informed of the study risks and has the matter of anonymity and confidentiality of data been addressed?

Rigour, presentation, links to the literature and implications for practice

- Are the findings consistent with other studies?
- Are the findings reported in a clear manner with examples of participant transcripts to support claims for themes?
- Have the aims of the study been addressed, research questions answered or considerations been made for methodological limitations that caused answers to not emerge?
- Were credibility, confirmabilty, transferability, dependability, fittingness and trustworthiness discussed?
- Is the importance of the implications for findings discussed and appropriately considered?
- Is the citation of literature consistent with what is within the text and is it adequate and extensive?

Sources: Adapted from Cutcliffe & Ward 2006; Ryan et al. 2007

Learning to critically appraise: Collating, describing and critiquing

Now that you have 'made sense' of the article you are ready to collate the evidence you have gathered about its worth in order to write a critical appraisal. When students are asked to write a 'critical appraisal' of literature, it is a common mistake to criticise rather than critique. What you are asked to do when you critique literature is to systematically and logically examine the article to look for:

- what was said and how well it was said
- what assumptions underlie the author's argument
- what issues were overlooked
- what implications were drawn
- what consequences for change in practice arise from the study.

The following is an example of a critical appraisal of the 'teaspoon' study and would be the type that would be used in a journal club setting. The sections in block quotes are all that you would actually see in an appraisal. The text provides guidance and insight into what is written.

Introduce article to be reviewed and set in context

This section of your critical appraisal need not be long and can be quite descriptive. For example:

> This study sought to determine the rate of teaspoon disappearance from staff tearooms and whether the rate of loss was influenced by the relative value of the teaspoon. The workplace involved was a research institute.

The next section of your critique is a step-by-step critique of key elements in the article. We commence with the title and work through each of the headings as laid out in the article itself:

The title identifies the phenomenon studied (missing teaspoons), the place the study took place (Australian research institute) and the method used (longitudinal cohort study). The title is therefore both succinct and descriptive, giving the reader a clear idea of what the study is about.

The article should also provide information concerning who the researchers are, their qualifications and if they are appropriate individuals to undertake the research. While the authors' qualifications are not given, their position within the institution is cited as 'director, research assistant and research officer'. This indicates that they probably have the research skills required to have conducted this investigation effectively. Furthermore, all work within the study setting, indicating that all are aware of and interested in the issue of missing teaspoons.

This article was published in the *British Medical Journal*, a respected peer-reviewed journal. The journal was no doubt chosen by the researchers because it is a journal which is used by the target reading population, namely health professionals interested in understanding the phenomenon of missing teaspoons.

Abstract

The abstract should provide a comprehensive and clear summary of the study and should include all its major features. The information in the abstract is a clear and concise summary of the study, making this a well-structured and adequate abstract.

Introduction

The introduction outlines the research problem, in this case that teaspoons are going missing from the researchers' workplace tearooms. With the stated high incidence of teaspoon loss the findings of this study could have significant benefits to workers in understanding the phenomenon of teaspoon loss from workplace tearooms.

Literature review

The literature review should cover all the current theory and research regarding the study and contextualise the paper. The authors state that they did not find any literature concerning the phenomenon of interest. They used three well-known search engines.

While the use of Google as a search engine in a scholarly publication should be questioned, Google Scholar and MEDLINE are suitable search engines to use. The authors' search strategy would seem a little perfunctory, but after replicating their stated strategy and adding the words 'cutlery' and 'misplaced' from the same five-year period (1999–2004) and using the same search engines, verification was achieved. There was no published research concerning the phenomenon of interest at the time the study was conducted.

Research approach (methodology/methods)

The method section is the section of the research article where the author explains in detail exactly how they conducted the study. This section should include how sampling occurred, information about data collection and analysis, validity, reliability and trustworthiness of the data, and ethical issues (Bluff & Cluett 2006). In the case of this study the method was a longitudinal cohort approach. This method is used when the researcher wishes to follow a defined group (marked teaspoons) over a period of time. It is therefore a suitable method to use to answer the research question.

Sampling

The authors used 70 teaspoons. They gave no explanation of why this number was chosen but they did allow for other teaspoons to be added to tearooms by others because they only counted the teaspoons they had marked.

Validity and reliability

The authors addressed reliability and validity issues by conducting a pilot study. It is difficult to determine how rigorous data collection was because the researchers don't discuss the timing of their weekly teaspoon count. If, for example, the count was conducted at lunchtime this may have resulted in more teaspoons appearing to have disappeared than if they had conducted the search during the first or last part of the day. Furthermore, while all teaspoons were counted by members from the same team, they do not discuss if or how interrater reliability was established. This leaves the reader wondering if some team members may have conducted a more thorough search for teaspoons than others.

Ethical issues

The only ethical consideration mentioned in this paper was the statement that approval for the study was given by the 'director of the institute' (p. 4). This is problematic because this authorising person was also one of the stated researchers. In a study of this nature that involves inanimate objects there might be a prima facie case for no ethical considerations. However, after the data collection period ended, workers were made aware of the study and asked to complete an anonymous survey. It is possible that teaspoon thieves may have felt guilty at this point in the study and non-thieves may have thought they were being accused of theft. Therefore, this study should have been reviewed by a properly formed institutional ethics committee in order to ensure that there was careful and sensitive revelation of the study and the fact that there were missing teaspoons. Anonymity of participation should have been examined by an impartial third party to ensure ethical compliance. Counselling should have been offered for traumatised staff members vicariously accused of theft. Furthermore, no details were given of what would happen to the anonymous surveys such as how long they would be retained, where, and who would have access.

Jane Warland and Phil Maude

Findings/results

The results are reported in an unusual way for a cohort study: the researchers use percentages of disappearance and there is no Relative Risk (RR) reported. However, the researchers report statistical significance at $p \leq 0.05$ difference between communal tearooms and those that are not. The 95% CI is narrow (0.76—1.28), indicating that these results are likely to be precise. Overall the results are logical and make sense.

Conclusion/recommendations/implications for nursing

The conclusions should be clear and concise and derived from the findings of the study (Bluff & Cluett 2006). While the researchers do confuse the reader with talk of teaspoons 'slipping away' to another planet and spoonoid lifestyle, generally speaking the conclusions are logically presented and in keeping with the findings of the study.

Some recommendations are not made by the authors but have since been suggested by other *BMJ* readers including:

* chaining teaspoons to the tearoom wall via a 'strongly mounted wall bracket' or
* forcing staff to provide their own teaspoon.

Furthermore, the authors do become a little carried away with recommending that the findings of their study have implications for the national research agenda.

Conclusion

The conclusion to your critique should effectively and succinctly summarise the main findings of the critique process to establish the significance of the study's findings:

> This study addresses a previously unidentified gap in research literature. However, there are some shortcomings related to rigour and attention to detail which leave the reader wondering about some aspects of the study design. Overall, the findings were both logical and likely.

Collation and description of the literature

In practical terms, it is necessary to have an overall picture of how the thread runs through your analysis of the literature before you can get down to actually describing the literature. One strategy that many writers use as a way to begin the literature review is to proceed from the general, wider view of the research they are reviewing to the specific problem. This is not a formula but is a common pattern and may be worth trying. Maybe use a summary sheet for each paper you review or at least write notes and highlight important sections that you need to review. These notes may be attached or even written onto the paper directly so that your opinion on each section is not lost. You may use a grid-like system to make short notes of your articles and the information that is coming out of each to assist you to use and collate all the literature.

Article	Concept 1	Concept 2	Concept 3	Concept 4
	How the literature defines the issue	Extent of the problem in contemporary times	Interventions and their levels of effectiveness	Attitudes of clinicians to change to practice
Abercrombie 2009	Does not define	Provides extensive statistics from 3 key countries	Sample size was large across 3 locations	Not included
Finch 2010	Differs from all other texts	Focus on Australia	Large cohort study	Considerations made
Gozzo 2008	Similar to Myer	Focus on Australia	Large cohort study	Included in limitations section
Myer et al. 2008	Similar to Gozzo	Focus on Australia	Large cohort study	Not included

Whatever the pattern that fits your work best, you need to keep in mind that what you are doing is writing about what was done before. But you are not simply reporting on previous research. You have to write about it in terms of how well it was done and what it achieved. For example, a series of paragraphs of the kind:

> 'Green (1975) discovered…'
>
> 'In 1978, Black conducted experiments and discovered that…'
>
> 'Later Brown (1980) illustrated this in…'

demonstrates neither your understanding of the literature nor your ability to evaluate other people's work.

Maybe at an earlier stage, or in your first version of your literature review, you needed a summary of who did what. But in your final version, you have to show that you have thought about it, can synthesise the work and can succinctly pass judgment on the relative merits of research conducted in your field. So, to take the above example, it would be better to say something like:

> 'There seems to be general agreement on x (White 1987; Brown 1980; Black 1978; Green 1975), but Green (1975) sees x as a consequence of y, while Black (1978) suggests that x and y are interrelated.
>
> While Green's work has some limitations in that it…, its main value lies in…'

Jane Warland and Phil Maude

Approaching your writing in this way forces you to make judgments and, furthermore, to distinguish your thoughts from assessments made by others. It is this whole process of revealing limitations or recognising the possibility of taking research further that allows you to formulate and justify your writing.

A literature review is not just a summary, but a conceptually organised synthesis of the results of your search. It must

- organise information and relate it to the argument you are developing
- synthesise results into a summary of what is and isn't known
- identify controversy when it appears in the literature
- develop questions or recommendations for further research.

Although we value 'unbiased' scientific research, the truth is that no author is free from outside influence, such as a particular theoretical framework or model (e.g. a feminist examination of gender inequity in medical research), the author's rhetorical purpose (e.g. a researcher's reasons for advocating the effectiveness of a certain drug) or an experience-based practical perspective (e.g. the belief that one approach to pain management is more effective than another). The value of your review depends not simply on how many sources you find, but also on your awareness of how these different perspectives affect the way that research on your topic is conducted, published and read.

In critically evaluating, you are looking for the strengths of certain studies and the significance and contributions made by researchers. You are also looking for limitations, flaws and weaknesses of particular studies, or of whole lines of enquiry.

Indeed, if you take this critical approach to looking at previous research in your field, your final literature review will not be a compilation of summaries but an evaluation. Then it will reflect your capacity for critical analysis.

You can then continue the process of making sense of the literature by gaining more expertise, which allows you to become more confident, and by being much more focused on your specific research. You are still reading and perhaps needing to reread some of the literature. You are thinking about it as you are analysing texts or other data. You are able to talk about it easily and discuss it. In other words, it is becoming part of you. At a deeper level than before,

- you are now not only looking at findings but are looking at how others have arrived at their findings
- you are looking at what assumptions are leading to the way something is investigated
- you are looking for genuine differences in theories as opposed to semantic difference
- you are gaining an understanding of why the field developed in the way it did
- you have a sense of where it might be going.

Considering the application of evidence to practice

Using appraisal tools can help you make sense of studies to understand application to practice. Research is a word that often puts us off. Research often occurs by an individual or small group; it costs dollars because it diverts people from their normal roles and it is often of interest but not applied to practice. Evidence-based practice is focused on the recognition and uptake of the best available evidence to support practice. In many ways the findings of research studies can challenge clinicians and managers to consider change. There are many resources readily available, but at a local level clinicians need good critique skills to evaluate what they are reading and managers need confidence in the evidence to embark on the often difficult process of change to practice.

Summary

Like most procedures that health care professionals need to learn, the more you practise reading and writing about research literature the better your familiarity and accuracy will be. The critical appraisal of research is a fundamental skill to help in the uptake of contemporary evidence and facilitates practice development. This chapter has provided background information, defined terminology, and offered examples and links to valuable print-based and web-based resources. We hope this will assist the reader to be critical of the literature and make better decisions about health interventions. Certainly the CATs assist but the final work the clinician must do is make sound decisions about the value of the literature. Recommendations for change or no change to practice are only as good as the reader's knowledge base. We have suggested that a journal club is an excellent way to bring novices and experienced clinicians together and improve decision-making. A final point to make is that evidence may indicate a need to change practice, but it also needs to be implemented after careful consideration of the clinical significance, that is, the impact on service users, clinical staff and the organisation's overall plan and budget. If the procedural change reduces care and active intervention or is not culturally or fiscally sound it may deliver poorer results in the long run.

IMPLICATIONS FOR EVIDENCE-BASED NURSING AND MIDWIFERY

The level of evidence is based on a study research design (see Table 1.1) because it indicates the rigour of the overall research process. However, research users still have to be able to critically review research reports (journal articles, conference proceedings and conference presentations) in order to identify their strengths and weaknesses. As users, clinicians then will have the confidence to apply the research evidence in their own practice.

Jane Warland and Phil Maude

▶▶▶   **PROBLEM SOLVING 13.1**

a

Bob and his team review publications relating to chest pain. Following is a part of an article:

'Fifteen hospitals agreed to participate in the study. Of these, data were provided by ten senior nurse managers who completed questionnaires of 55 patients who presented to the hospitals with chest pain.'

What information do Bob and his team need to further explore the quality of this article? List two.

b

Ann and her team also review the literature. Following is a part of the article:

'Seven patients who presented at the hospital with chest pain were approached and invited to participate in the study. They were individually interviewed at their homes using open-ended questions. Interviews were recorded by audiotape and transcribed verbatim. Four themes were derived from the data...'

What information do Ann and her team need to further explore the quality of this article?

Practice exercise 13.1

Think about the research topics that you are interested in. List these and consider:

1   Why have you chosen these topics?
2   What personal and professional bias do you bring to each topic?
3   Consider ways you may overcome these biases.

Practice exercise 13.2

Use your library home page or favourite database to search the online databases for a topic that is of interest to you.

Identify a research paper by looking at the abstract or the description of the paper within the indexing.

Identify the methodological approach used. If you are not sure ask a colleague to assist you.

Go to one of the internet web pages and choose an appropriate tool to critically appraise this article.

Note how this helps you to read and understand the article as well as be critical about the strengths and limitations presented.

Write a brief summary of this article using your notes from the critical appraisal tool.

What themes have come out of this paper? If you are unsure consider what key points have been presented.

Now consider how you would use this work to critique other articles concerning this topic and compare and contrast the strengths and limitations within a paper.

Answers to problem solving 13.1

a

How many hospitals did the 10 senior nurse managers collect data from? Did they represent all 15 hospitals? If not, what bias could occur? (sampling and representativeness)

What method did the researchers use to ensure that 10 senior nurse managers used the same process when they collected data, e.g. training and having a manual for data collectors? (interrater reliability)

How were the questionnaires designed? Was it necessary to have a standard tool? Were they piloted before the actual use? (validity and reliability of research instrument)

Was the number of the sample (55) sufficient? It could be compared to an expected number from 10 hospitals (assuming 10 senior nurse managers from 10 hospitals). Would there be any bias? For example, only patients presented at a particular time or day were included.

b

What research design did the researchers use? (A particular research design has certain characteristics; do they match with the above information?)

Were there any sources of data to triangulate the results?

Who conducted the interviews? What strategy was used to make sure that participants have trust or tell the truth?

What were the steps used by the researchers to ensure the credibility, auditability, fittingness (transferability), dependability and confirmability of the results?

Further reading

Borbasi, S., Jackson, D., & Langford, R. (2007). *Navigating the Maze of Nursing Research.* Sydney: Mosby.

Burns, N., & Grove, S. (2005). *The Practice of Nursing Research: Conduct, Critique, and Utilization,* 5th edn. Philadelphia: Saunders.

Burns, N., & Grove, S. (2006). *Understanding Nursing Research: Building and Evidence Based Practice.* St Louis, MI: Elsevier Saunders.

Corbin, J., & Strauss, A. (2008). *Basics of Qualitative Research: Techniques and Procedures for Developing Grounded Theory.* Los Angeles: Sage.

Coughlan, M., Cronin, P., & Ryan, F. (2007). Step by step guide to critiquing research. Part 1: Quantitative research. *British Journal of Nursing* 16(11), 658–63.

Creswell, J. (2007). *Qualitative Inquiry and Research Design: Choosing Among Five Approaches.* London: Sage Publications.

Crombie, I. (1996). *The Pocket Guide to Critical Appraisal.* London: British Medical Journal Publishing Group, pp. 23–9.

Liamputtong, P. (2007). *Researching the Vulnerable: A Guide to Sensitive Research Methods*. London, Thousand Oaks, CA: Sage Publications.

LoBiondo-Wood, G., & Haber, J. (2006). *Nursing Research: Methods and Critical Appraisal for Evidence-Based Practice*. St Louis, MO: Mosby Elsevier.

Newell, R., & Burnard, P. (2006). *Vital Notes for Nurses: Research for Evidence-Based Practice*. Oxford: Blackwell.

Ryan, F., Coughlan, M., & Cronin, P. (2007). Step by step guide to critiquing research. Part 2: Qualitative research. *British Journal of Nursing* 16(12), 738–44.

Streubert Speziale, H., & Carpenter, D. (2007). *Qualitative Research in Nursing: Advancing the Humanistic Imperative*. Philadelphia: Lippincott.

Taylor, B., Kermode, S., & Roberts, K. (2006). *Research in Nursing and Health Care: Evidence for Practice*. Melbourne: Thomson Learning.

Weblinks

The following websites have useful information for critically appraising a research article.

CASP—The Critical Appraisal Skills Program:

<www/phru.nhs/casp/casp.htm>,

Part of the United Kingdom's National Health Service Public Health Resources Unit. Once within these web pages, click on 'Learning Resources' and you will find critical appraisal tools for various research designs. CASP offers links to additional resources and evidence-based web pages, making it a one-stop shop for critical appraisal.

Evidence Based Nursing Guides and Tools originates at McGill University in the USA and offers downloadable critique tools and examples of critical appraisals using these tools:

<www.muhc-ebn.mcgill.ca/EBN_tools.htm>

Evidence Based Practice Checklists, available from the University of Glasgow:

<www.gla.ac.uk/departments/generalpractice/crit_ap.htm>

Offers several downloadable critical appraisal checklists and a useful section with key terms called 'jargon buster'.

Some additional internet web pages are worth looking at if you are searching for grey data or systematic reviews. You will have extensive access if you locate these via your library web page and not as an individual:

Australian Digital Thesis Collection:

<http://adt.caul.edu.au>

CDBSR—Cochrane Data Base of Systematic Reviews:

<www.cochrane.org>

DARE—Data Base of Reviews of Effectiveness Centre for Reviews and Dissemination:

<www.crd.york.ac.uk/crdweb>

JBI—The Joanna Briggs Institute:

<www.joannabriggs.edu.au/about/home.php>

The University of Sheffield, School of Health and Related Research (ScHARR):

<www.shef.ac.uk/scharr>

Open-access journals available in the field of nursing and midwifery include:

BMC-nursing:

<www.biomedcentral.com/bmcnurs>

BMC-pregnancy and childbirth:

<www.biomedcentral.com/bmcpregnancychildbirth>

International Breastfeeding Journal:

<www.internationalbreastfeedingjournal.com>

References

ANMC. (2006a). National competency standards for the registered nurse. Available at <http://anmc.org.au/docs/Competency_standards_RN.pdf>

ANMC. (2006b). National competency standards for the midwife. Access through <http://en-us.nielsen.com/content/nielsen/en_us/industries/media.html>

Badenoch, D., Sackett, D., Straus, S., Ball, C., & Dawes, M. (2004). CATmaker version 1.1, Retrieved 9 October 2010, from <www.cebm.net>

Beitz, J. (2008). Statistical test selection and analysis: Demystifying a 'mysterious' process. *Journal of Wound Ostomy and Continence Nursing* 35(6), 561–8.

Bluff, R., & Cluett, E. (2006). Critiquing the literature. In E. Cluett & R. Bluff (eds), *Principles and Practice of Research in Midwifery*, 2nd edn (pp. 243–61). Edinburgh: Churchill Livingstone.

Cheek, J., Gillham, D., & Ballantyne, A. (2005). Using education to promote research dissemination in nursing. *International Journal of Nursing Education Scholarship* 2(1), Article 31. Doi: 10.2202/1548-923X.1191 available at <www.bepress.com/ijnes/vol2/iss1/art31>

Cutcliffe, J., & Ward, M. (2006). *Critiquing Nursing Research*. Salisbury, UK: Quay Books.

Katrak, P., Bialocerkowski, A., Massy-Westropp, N., Kumar, S., & Grimmer, K. (2004). A systematic review of the content of critical appraisal tools. *BMC Medical Research Methodology* 4(22) Doi: 10.1186/1471-2288-4-22.

Lim, M., Hellard, M., & Aitken, C. (2005). The case of the disappearing teaspoons: Longitudinal cohort study of the displacement of teaspoons in an Australian research institute. *British Medical Journal* 331, 1498–500.

Rochon, P. A., Gurwitz, J. H., Sykora, K., Mamdani, M., Streiner, D. L., Garfinkel, S., Normand, S.-L.T., & Anderson, G. M. (2005). Reader's guide to critical appraisal of cohort studies: 1. Role and design. *British Medical Journal* 330, 895–7.

Ryan, F., Coughlan, M., & Cronin, P. (2007). Step by step guide to critiquing research. Part 2: Qualitative research. *British Journal of Nursing* 16(12), 738–44.

Schneider, Z., Whitehead, D., Elliot, D., LoBiondo-Wood, G., & Haber, J. (2007). *Nursing and Midwifery Research: Methods and Appraisal for Evidence-Based Practice*. Sydney: Mosby Elsevier.

St Pierre, J. (2005). Changing nursing practice through a nursing journal club: As hospitals seek to promote evidence-based nursing practice and improve the quality of bedside nursing care, formation of a nursing journal club can be one strategy to accomplish both goals. *MedSurg Nursing* 14(6), 390–2

Zellner, K., Boerst, C., & Tabb, W. (2007). Statistics used in current nursing research. *Journal of Nursing Education* 42(2), 55–9.

CHAPTER 14

Undertaking a Systematic Review

Ritin Fernandez, Maree Johnson and Rhonda Griffiths

Chapter learning objectives

By the end of this chapter you will be able to:

▸ understand how to formulate a focused clinical question

▸ explain the development of a comprehensive literature search strategy on a specific clinical question

▸ explore the various sources of evidence

▸ appreciate the importance of critically appraising the processes of conducting a meta-analysis

▸ understand the processes of conducting a meta-synthesis.

KEY TERMS

Critical appraisal

Data extraction

Meta-analysis

Meta-synthesis

Review protocol

Searching the literature

Systematic review

Introduction

A systematic review is a compilation of all scientific studies on a particular topic according to predetermined criteria (Cullum et al. 2008). Systematic reviews are recognised as the highest form of evidence (NHMRC 2009) because (1) they include all available evidence, (2) the conclusions are based only on research that passes a rigorous critical appraisal and (3) the methods used in the review are explicit and open to the criticism of readers. The outcome of the systematic review is the presentation of the findings in a summary format. Results of a review may validate current practice or provide evidence to change practice or identify that more research is necessary in the area (Fineout-Overholt et al. 2008). Systematic reviews are of specific relevance to clinicians because they incorporate a large body of evidence in a manner that is accessible and available to clinicians. Systematic reviews are the basis of clinical practice guideline or policy development in nursing and midwifery. In addition, they are increasingly required by funding bodies as the first step in any research proposal.

The process of a systematic review

Although systematic reviews are considered to be secondary research, they involve a formal process that is transparent and reproducible. A robust and credible systematic review provides the basis for clinical guideline and policy development.

Planning the review

The first step in undertaking a systematic review is the formation of the review team. There is no ideal number of reviewers that are required in order to complete a systematic review, but the number will be influenced by the scope of the topic and the support and resources available. Nevertheless, it is essential that the review team has extensive clinical experience in the topic under consideration, experience of the systematic review process, and an interest and commitment to developing evidence as a basis for practice (Littell et al. 2008).

Developing the protocol

As in any scientific endeavour, a protocol should be established beforehand. A protocol for a systematic review is equivalent to a proposal for a research study. A developed protocol ensures that the systematic review is as rigorous as possible within practical limits.

Systematic reviews that are published on the Cochrane Library or the Joanna Briggs Institute databases require that the protocols are registered and approved before the review is conducted (see Weblinks). This is a means of informing other researchers and clinicians of the systematic reviews currently in progress, thus avoiding duplication (Higgins & Green 2008). In addition, the peer review process for approval ensures that the systematic review protocol is well defined and provides explicit strategies to reduce the risk of bias and/or misuse. The steps in developing a protocol for a systematic review include:

- formulating a research question
- developing criteria for the inclusion of studies
- defining the search process
- identifying the methods that will be used to assess the quality of the studies
- defining the methods that will be implemented to collect/extract the data
- detailing the process for data analysis and summary of the evidence.

Figure 14.1 Steps in undertaking a systematic review

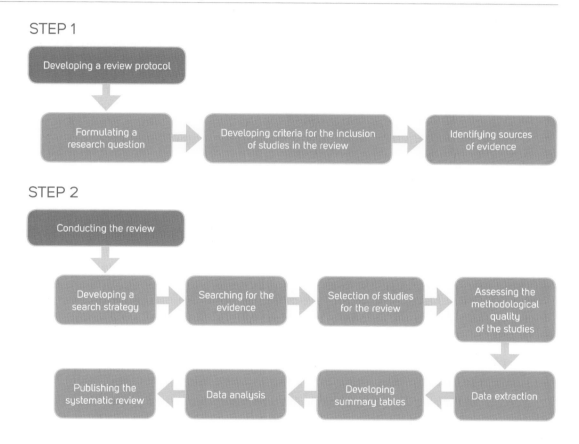

Formulating a research question

To design and execute a systematic review successfully the researcher must be very clear about what is being studied and the nature of the research question (Polit & Beck 2008). Poorly developed questions will result in a large number of citations, many of which will not be relevant to the question under investigation; or they may result in few citations and the ones that are relevant may not be identified. Well-formulated questions that are specific and focused will direct the development of a search strategy for identification of relevant studies (Armstrong 1999). A well-designed research question is a precise statement, based on the characteristics of the Patient/Population, Intervention, Comparison and Outcome (PICO) (Richardson et al. 1995). Studies have shown that the use of the PICO framework improves the specificity and breakdown of clinical problems and leads to more complex search strategies and more precise search results (Davies 2007). The PICO format has also been used to develop questions for qualitative studies. In this case the P stands for participants, the I for phenomena of interest and CO for Context. Examples of poorly designed and well-designed questions are presented below.

Table 14.1   Examples of poorly developed clinical questions

Is tap water effective in cleansing wounds?
Does a baby's birth weight have an impact on their subsequent development?

Table 14.2   Example of a precise clinical question for quantitative studies

Patients or problem	Intervention	Comparison intervention (if any)	Outcome	Well-formulated question
Patients with chronic wounds	Cleansing with tap water	Cleansing with normal saline	Infection rate Healing rates	What is the effect of cleansing with tap water compared to normal saline on the infection and healing rates of chronic wounds?

Developing criteria for the inclusion of studies in the review

The criteria for the inclusion of individual studies must address issues of relevance and validity. Relevance is related to the ability of the selected article to answer the research question posed by the systematic review. Therefore, in order to be relevant, the eligibility criteria are based on the components of the review question. The eligibility criteria therefore consist of the participants/population, interventions, comparisons and outcomes of interest. For systematic reviews, the validity of a trial or an individual study is the extent to which its design and conduct are likely to prevent systematic errors or bias (Crowther et al. 2010). Validity in systematic reviews is therefore largely dependent on the study design. For example, the most reliable research design that will provide the evidence for the effectiveness of an intervention is the randomised controlled trial or RCT.

▶▶▶   TERMS, TIPS AND SKILLS

The prior specification of the eligibility criteria (inclusion and exclusion criteria) is one of the main characteristics that distinguishes a systematic review from a traditional literature review (Nasseri-Moghaddam & Malekzadeh 2006).

Types of participants/populations

The criteria for considering types of participants included in the individual studies should encompass the likely diversity of studies as well as ensure that a meaningful answer can be obtained when studies are considered in aggregate. This can be done by first, identifying a clear definition of the disease or condition and second, by considering the broad population and setting. Both these criteria are present in the following:

> Potable tap water may not be available in all countries or settings, therefore a recent review on water for wound cleansing included studies that used all types of water including boiled and cooled water.

▶▶▶ TERMS, TIPS AND SKILLS

Care should be taken to avoid criteria that will automatically exclude studies.

As systematic reviews are carried out to provide evidence for a global audience, a reason should be given for excluding studies with specific population characteristics or settings. For example, in the systematic review on water for wound cleansing, patients with burns were excluded as the initial management of burns requires a sterile environment (Fernandez & Griffiths 2008).

Types of interventions

The criteria for considering the interventions of interest and the comparators should be made explicit. Particular attention should be given if the interventions are being compared with an inactive control (e.g. placebo, no treatment or usual care), or with an active control (e.g. a variation of the same intervention or a different drug). Complex interventions such as behavioural or educational should have their core components clearly articulated. The mode, frequency, duration and person delivering the intervention should also be clearly stated (Higgins & Green 2008):

> The RCT on wound cleansing stated that tap water was collected from a designated faucet after letting the water run for three minutes.

Types of outcomes

The outcomes investigated in the systematic review should be meaningful to clinicians, patients, the general public, administrators and policy-makers. The primary outcome of interest and the secondary outcomes should be clearly identified. In addition, the methods used to measure these outcomes should also be specified before commencing the review. In some cases, the reviewers might decide to include studies that have used only objective measures (e.g. wound culture results) rather than subjective methods (wound assessment criteria) for outcome measurement. Another important consideration in deciding the criteria for types of outcomes is the timing of the outcome measurement. It is important to give this considerable thought as it can influence the results of the review (Gøtzsche et al. 2007):

> The results of infection rates in all wounds cleansed with either tap water or normal saline cannot be grouped together as there are different types of wounds. Individual studies could have measured outcomes for different types of wounds. Therefore a strategy could be to group the wounds into pre-specified types such as acute or chronic wounds.

It is important to include all outcomes in a review as it will identify the gaps in the primary research and provide researchers with priorities for future studies (Higgins & Green 2008).

Types of studies

It is important to pre-specify the study designs that will be included in the review, taking into account that certain study designs are more appropriate than others for answering particular questions. For example, reviews that ask questions about the effects of health care interventions are best answered by including RCTs (Jadad & Enkin 2007). Other aspects that need to be considered when deciding the types of study are matters relating to language and publication status. A rationale for excluding studies due to language or publication status should be provided.

> In a systematic review on the infection control management of Methicillin-resistant Staphylococcus aureus (MRSA) in acute care (Halcomb, Fernandez, Griffiths, Newton, & Hickman, 2008) studies that were published prior to 1985 were excluded from the review. The rationale reported for the exclusion of these studies was that the use of universal precautions only became mandatory after that year and the inclusion of studies prior to that would have resulted in flawed findings.

RESEARCH IN PRACTICE 14.1

14.1 DECIDING WHAT TO REVIEW

Your manager has asked you as a clinical nurse specialist to review the evidence for the use of tap water compared to normal saline for cleansing wounds. You have formulated the following question:

In patients with acute or chronic wounds, what is the effect of cleansing with tap water compared to normal saline on the infection and healing rates?

What types of studies would be suited for a systematic review on the above question? Give a reason.

Answer: Randomised controlled trial studies, quasi-randomised trial studies, cohort studies, pre-test and post-test studies, case-control studies and qualitative studies.

Identifying sources of evidence

The aim of the search strategy is to undertake a comprehensive search to facilitate retrieval of all published and unpublished clinical trials (Patrick et al. 2004). A comprehensive literature search, which minimises the risk of bias, is another difference between a systematic review and a traditional review (Crowther et al. 2010). A comprehensive and unbiased literature review incorporates both published and unpublished works and should include:

- relevant studies/reports from a variety of databases (e.g. MEDLINE, CINAHL, Cochrane Library, Cochrane Controlled Trials register, Healthstar) and the internet (Montori et al. 2005)
- a review of the reference list of the retrieved articles
- hand-searching journals that are relevant to the research question (Hopewell, Clarke et al. 2007)
- personal communication, which is a valuable source for locating grey literature such as conference papers, theses and government reports (Hopewell, McDonald et al. 2007a)
- consultation with content specialists
- attempts to locate studies/reports in other languages.

▶▶▶ TERMS, TIPS AND SKILLS

A comprehensive search is the foundation for a valid and reliable systematic review and should include both published and unpublished works where possible. Failure to identify a diversity of literature from a wide range of sources could result in a biased review (Hopewell, Clarke et al. 2007; Hopewell, McDonald et al. 2007).

Conducting the systematic review

Developing a search strategy

A clearly defined search strategy is needed to direct an effective literature review and ensure efficient use of resources. The benefits arising from a search strategy include the ability for others to replicate the study, thus reducing the potential for systematic bias.

▶▶▶ TERMS, TIPS AND SKILLS

Optimal search strategies are vital for detecting clinically sound studies.

A precisely described search strategy should include identification and documentation of all steps of each phase of the search for later reference. These are:

- the date, the time period, search terms and combinations of search terms used
- the sources searched and the number of articles located

- the searcher's identity, designation and contact number, and finally
- whether assistance from the librarian for the development and implementation of the search strategy was obtained (Weller 2004).

Retaining the computer search printouts and saving a copy for future reference is recommended (Yoshii et al. 2009).

As each database has its own unique indexing terms, individual search strategies should be developed for each database. During the development of the search strategy, consideration should also be given to the diverse terminology used and the spelling of keywords as this will influence the identification of relevant trials. Search terms can be identified from the keywords used in the individual publications. The PICO model is a good guide to devising a logical list of the search terms. This procedure is likely to result in an extensive volume of literature, which then has to be systematically filtered to identify relevant articles and reports for the study.

Searching for the evidence

Electronic database search

The success of an electronic search is strongly related to the skill of the searcher in using effective strategies. Electronic database searching can be performed using various methods such as searching using textwords, subject headings, truncation and wild cards. Textword searching will retrieve all articles on the database that contain the relevant word in the title or abstract, so the search is likely to include a number of articles that are irrelevant to the question. However, the search can be made more sensitive by using wild cards at any point within the word. This will ensure that the search retrieves articles with all versions of the word (Cullum 2000; Cullum et al. 2008).

Most databases develop their own subject headings to enable searches to be more focused than free text searches. Articles are categorised under subject headings that are deemed to be significant topics in the article. This method provides a consistent way to retrieve information that may use different terminology for the same concepts.

Truncation is another method used to retrieve all possible suffix variations of a root word. For example, the search 'ultraso$' will retrieve the words ultrasound, ultrasonography, ultrasonogram, ultrasound, etc. However, unlimited truncation should be used with care, since documents with unwanted words will be accidentally retrieved (Zhang et al. 2006). For example, the search 'Card$' would retrieve documents with the words 'cardiac', 'cardiology', 'cardiothoracic', etc., but also 'cards' and 'cardigan'.

Searching using wild cards is another strategy that can be used to retrieve all relevant studies. The wild card character '#' (hash sign) can be used within or at the end of a query word to substitute for one required character. It is useful for some plural forms, i.e. 'wom#n', which would retrieve both 'woman' and 'women'. Another wild card character is a

'?' (question mark). It can be used within or at the end of a query word to substitute for one character or no characters. This wild card is useful for retrieving documents that are spelt differently in Australia and America. For example, the search 'randomi\$ed' would retrieve documents with the words 'randomized' and 'randomised'.

Following the search using the key terms, the use of Boolean operators is a way of constructing the research question, indicating the relationships between the search terms as well as limiting the search. The common Boolean operators used are AND, OR, NOT. For example, combining searches for the text words 'diabetes OR IDDM' will yield articles containing either of these words in the title or abstract. Alternatively, by typing in 'diabetes AND insulin' the search can be narrowed to only those articles that have both of these words in the title or abstract, thereby reducing the number of retrieved records.

Manual searching

It is important to be aware that not all journals are indexed by an electronic database, so manual searching may be a very important part of the search strategy. Manual searching involves searching through the reference list of articles that have been found to throw light on the clinical question. It may also involve searching the indexes of journals that are likely to publish articles relevant to the question. It is, however, labour-intensive and time-consuming (Hopewell, Clarke et al. 2007).

Searching the grey literature

Grey literature is information that is either unpublished or has been published in non-commercial form. Publication bias is a common problem identified in systematic reviews, which arises when only published data is included. Researchers have indicated that including grey literature in systematic reviews helps to overcome the problem of publication bias (Hopewell, McDonald et al. 2007). In particular, RCTs that result in no significant difference being found are often difficult to publish in refereed journals, but are nonetheless important to include in systematic reviews. Grey literature is now freely available on many websites and is selectively indexed by numerous commercial database vendors.

Examples of grey literature include:

* government reports
* policy statements and issues papers
* conference proceedings
* pre-prints and post-prints of articles
* theses and dissertations
* market reports
* working papers
* newsletters and bulletins.

Cochrane reviewers receive support with database searching from the Collaborative Review Group. Each review group has a database of all published and unpublished clinical trials that are both electronically identified and hand-searched according to their specialty. The review group librarian searches this database and provides the reviewer with a list of all eligible trials.

Selection of studies for the review

The searching processes locate all citations that reflect the research question, and in many instances the citations may be listed in more than one database. Importing the references and abstracts identified from the search into a bibliographic software such as EndNote and removing duplicate citations will therefore prevent unnecessary waste of time.

Not every study remaining after the removal of duplicates will be eligible for inclusion in the systematic review. Selection for the potential inclusion of the studies is made in a two-stage process. First, the titles and abstracts of the individual studies are verified against the inclusion and exclusion criteria and the full text obtained of relevant citations. Some citations will be rejected at that stage. If the title and abstract are inconclusive, full text should be obtained for further assessment. The second stage is applying the inclusion and exclusion criteria to the full text of the citation. Publications that pass the relevance test are then tested for validity, which means assessing the methodological quality of the study.

Assessing the methodological quality of individual studies

Reliable and systematic methods for the assessment of the methodological quality of the studies are imperative. Numerous assessment tools and checklists have been published to assess the validity of the methodological quality of individual studies (Moher et al. 1995). Systematic reviews published in the Cochrane Library and on the JBI database require the use of their own quality assessment tools for assessing risk of bias in studies (Higgins & Green 2008). An example of the critical appraisal form used by the Joanna Briggs Institute is shown in Appendix 14.1.

▸▸▸ TERMS, TIPS AND SKILLS

Critical appraisal helps to eliminate methodologically poor studies.

The common elements of these quality assessment tools include questions to determine the extent to which the design and conduct of the study are likely to prevent the four causes of systematic errors (Table 14.3).

Table 14.3 Causes of systematic error

Level	Intervention
Selection bias	Systematic differences in comparison groups Knowledge of treatment assignment
Performance bias	Systematic differences in care provided apart from the intervention being evaluated
Attrition bias	Systematic differences in withdrawals from the trial
Detection bias	Systematic differences in outcome assessment Systematic differences in self-reported and objectively measured outcomes

The assessment of the methodological quality of the studies for the review should be conducted independently by two reviewers, with disagreements or indecision being referred to a third person. The name of the author(s) and the journal source should be concealed from the reviewers to reduce bias. The reason for rejecting articles should be documented for future reference. In Cochrane reviews each study is weighted to reflect its design and methodology. An average weight is subsequently calculated as a guide to the quality of the studies in the review.

Data extraction

Data extraction involves the collection of relevant information from the publications using a data collection form to enable a standardised approach. The type of information collected is determined by the review question and so the data collection form will vary between systematic reviews (Leong 2007). Development of the data collection form is an onerous task, so enough time should be set aside for it. Caution should be exercised when developing the data extraction form to ensure that the form is succinct and captures the relevant information (Jones et al. 2005). The form should be pilot-tested and the information obtained should be closely examined for relevance to the question. Spreadsheets are useful tools when designing a data collection form. Appendix 14.2 shows an example of a data extraction form used by the Joanna Briggs Institute.

▶▶▶ TERMS, TIPS AND SKILLS

- Invest sufficient thought and time in designing the data extraction form.
- A data extraction form should include information that will identify the primary study and the reviewers such as study citation, reviewer information/code, participant demographics, participant inclusion/exclusion criteria, description of the interventions, description of the outcome measures, follow-up period, and the number and reasons for withdrawals and dropouts.
- Pilot-test the data extraction.
- Train and assess data extractors.
- Consider blinding the reviewers to the authors of each paper to reduce bias.
- Data collection using the data collection form should be performed by more than one reviewer as it increases the rate of interrater reliability and reduces the risk of bias.
- In the event of a disagreement, an independent arbitrator should intervene prior to data synthesis.
- Attempts should be made to obtain missing data by contacting the authors.
- Documentation of the process and the outcome of the arbitration should be maintained for future reference.

Developing summary tables

The aim of systematic reviews is to present the best available evidence in an easily understood summary form. These summaries are presented in a table built specifically from data detail. The summary table assists in the data analysis. A range of aspects can be presented including study citation, country and year, study design, study sample size, interventions, outcome measures, overall rating of study quality, and study findings. The tabular format is concise but comprehensive, enables comparison of the critical elements, identifies similarities and dissimilarities in the articles, and facilitates interpretation of the results by the target audience (see Table 14.4).

▶▶▶ TERMS, TIPS AND SKILLS

Summary tables provide an overview of vital information from individual studies.

Table 14.4   Example of a summary table

Author, year and country	Study type/ Level of evidence	Participants	Interventions	Results Outcomes	Notes
Griffiths 2001 Australia	RCT/II	35 patients with 49 chronic wounds	Group A: wounds irrigated with tap water Group B: wounds irrigated with normal saline	Infection Group A: No infection was found among 23 wounds Group B: 3 infections were found among 26 wounds Healing Group A: 8 healed among 23 wounds Group B: 16 healed among 26 wounds	Allocation performed using a list of random numbers nominated by person not entering patients into the trial. Both patients and outcome assessors were blinded to the treatment. Criteria for wound infection: Presence of pus, discolouration, friable granulation tissue, pain, tenderness, pocketing or bridging at base of the wound, abnormal smell and wound breakdown. 4 patients in each group withdrew from the study. Wounds were assessed at the end of 6 weeks. Quality of tap water reported to meet Australian National Health and Medical Research Council requirements.

Data analysis

Systematic reviews were initiated to present pooled data from randomised controlled trials reporting the results of medical research. In contrast to medical research, nursing research uses both qualitative and quantitative methods, so the resulting systematic reviews will incorporate a variety of research designs. The methods used for data analysis depend largely on the design of the studies. For quantitative studies the summary is generally presented as a meta-analysis, while evidence from qualitative studies is presented as a meta-synthesis.

Meta-analysis: The synthesis of quantitative data

A meta-analysis is a statistical method that synthesises the findings of multiple small studies as if they were one large, powerful study to draw conclusions about a specific research question (Chamberlain 2007). In the medical literature the terms meta-analysis and systematic review are often used interchangeably, although meta-analysis is only one component of a systematic review (Ioannidis et al. 2008). Meta-analysis can be undertaken using the Review Manager (RevMan), software from the Cochrane Collaboration or any other commercially available software.

Ritin Fernandez, Maree Johnson and Rhonda Griffiths

Carrying out a meta-analysis

Meta-analysis can only be carried out if the studies included in the review are sufficiently homogeneous. Studies are assumed to be clinically homogeneous if they are similar enough in design, population and outcomes to permit the data to be combined (Perera & Heneghan 2008).

Studies that are clinically homogeneous can be combined in a meta-analysis to determine a summary estimate of effect. The effect is summarised in different ways with relative risks (RR) or odds ratios (OR) calculated for dichotomous data and weighted mean difference (WMD) for continuous data (Egger et al. 2001).

Relative risk is used when the outcome of interest has relatively low probability. It is used to compare the risk of developing side effects in people receiving a placebo versus people who are receiving an established (standard of care) treatment (Egger et al. 2001). The odds ratio is the ratio of the odds of an event occurring in one group to the odds of it occurring in another group. The weighted mean difference is used to combine measures for continuous variables when the mean, standard deviation and sample size in each group are known. Each study is given a weight depending on the amount of influence it has on the overall results of the meta-analysis. This method assumes that all the trials have measured the outcome

Figure 14.2   Meta-analysis graph for dichotomous data

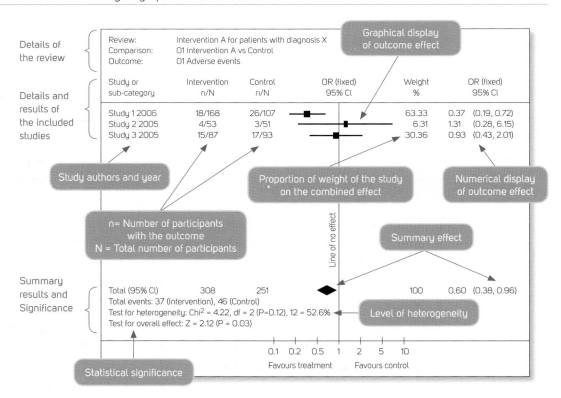

Source: Fernandez & Tran 2008. Reprinted with permission from the publishers

Figure 14.3 Meta-analysis graph for continuous data

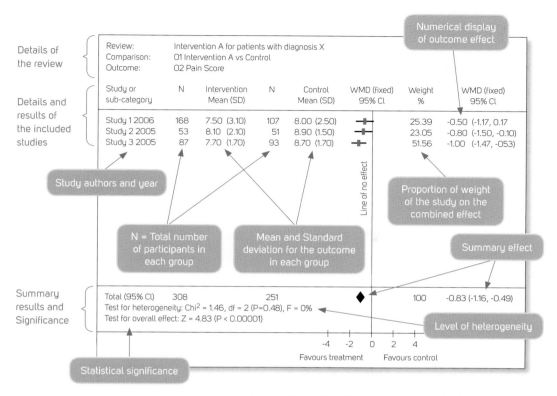

on the same scale. The calculation of these and other subsequent statistics relevant to meta-analysis is undertaken using RevMan, Meta Analysis of Statistics Assessment and Review Instrument (MAStARI) or any other commercially available software.

After deciding on the effect measure, heterogeneity across the studies should be investigated to examine statistically the degree of similarity in the outcomes of the studies. Simply averaging the odds ratios from all the studies would give misleading results, due to equal weight given to all studies, although smaller studies are more subject to chance. To overcome this error, the studies included in the meta-analysis should be combined using either the fixed or random effects model. Choosing the appropriate effects model for the combination is vital. The fixed effects model answers the question whether the studies included in the meta-analysis show that the treatment or exposure produced the effect on average. On the other hand, the random effects model answers the question, On the basis of the studies that are examined, is it possible to comment that the treatment or the exposure will produce a result? For studies that are homogeneous, combining studies using the fixed effects or random effects models will produce similar results.

Statistical homogeneity indicates that the variation in results is larger than what would have been expected by chance (Perera & Heneghan 2008). The commonly used statistical test to measure the statistical heterogeneity is the I2 test, which is independent of the number of studies included in the meta-analysis (Higgins et al. 2003). The I2 is a statistic that measures the proportion of inconsistency in individual studies that cannot be explained by chance (Higgins et al. 2003). An I2 value of less than 25% indicates that the studies are homogeneous and so can be combined using a fixed effects model, while an I2 value of more than 75% indicates that the studies are highly heterogeneous and should be combined using a random effects model (Higgins et al. 2003).

▸▸▸   TERMS, TIPS AND SKILLS

- Ask a statistician for help.
- Use a data analysis program like RevMan or MAStARI.
- Viewing the data is informative.

Meta-synthesis: The synthesis of qualitative data

Qualitative studies should not be disregarded because they provide substantial evidence for clinical decision-making. Meta-synthesis has been developed for the same reasons as meta-analysis, that is, to overcome discrepancies associated with individual qualitative studies (Flemming 2007). Meta-synthesis involves examining research findings from individual qualitative studies and creating summary statements that authentically describe the meaning of these themes (Pearson et al. 2007). The Joanna Briggs Institute has developed software called Qualitative Assessment and Review Instrument (QARI) that enables researchers to carry out systematic reviews and meta-synthesis of qualitative data (see Weblinks).

Carrying out a meta-synthesis

The process of meta-synthesis entails identifying relationships between the findings of existing studies and making interpretations across comparable studies (Barnett-Page & Thomas 2009). This has three distinct phases: identification of the key findings of each study, determining how these findings relate to those of other studies, and combining common findings into themes to generate a description of the phenomenon (Evans 2002).

Identification of the key findings of each study

This phase involves careful reading and rereading of each primary study to search for phrases, metaphors and themes that occur repeatedly across the included studies (Downe 2008). The illustrations from the text that demonstrate their origins are also recorded. This process is a form of confirming the authenticity of the association between each finding in terms of how clearly and/or directly it can be attributed to participants in the primary research (Pearson et al. 2007).

Relate themes across studies

Once the findings have been identified it is important to combine these using methods appropriate to the specific type and nature of data that have been extracted. The key findings from the primary studies are grouped on the basis of similarity in meanings into categories or areas of similarity. The categories are re-examined to interpret the content of each, and to identify consistencies and incongruities.

Description of the phenomenon

These categories are then subjected to a meta-aggregation in order to produce a single comprehensive set of synthesised findings. A synthesised finding is an overarching description of a group of categorised findings that allows for the generation of recommendations for practice (Pearson et al. 2007).

An example of a meta-synthesis is presented in Figure 14.4. This meta-synthesis was undertaken to identify the characteristics of nursing teams. A total of five findings grouped in three categories demonstrated that nursing teams exhibit accountability for their actions, commitment to the nursing team and an enthusiastic, motivating attitude (Pearson et al. 2006).

Figure 14.4   Meta-synthesis characteristics of nursing teams

Synthesis	Category	Finding
Characteristics of nursing teams The function of a nursing team requires nurses to exhibit a variety of characteristics such as accountability for their actions, commitment to the nursing team and an enthusiastic, motivating attitude.	Commitment to the nursing team produces cohesiveness among the groups.	A successful, cohesive team can be produced when individuals are committed to the nursing unit.
	Nurses become accountable for the actions when working within a team functioning approach to care delivery.	Nurses practising with a primary care team describe a feeling of responsibility of the patient's care. There is an increased awareness of accountability for nurses practising in a team of primary care.
	The effectiveness of a team can be improved when members are enthusiastic and motivated towards the team's goals.	Individual enthusiasm and supportive culture encourage teamwork. Motivation improved among team members as a result of awareness of shared problems.

Source: Pearson et al. 2006

Narrative synthesis

Summarising evidence or knowledge in the form of a meta-analysis is not always possible and in these cases the evidence is presented as a narrative synthesis. In addition, a narrative synthesis can be complementary to a meta-analysis or meta-synthesis. In narrative synthesis the findings are explained in a text format. The drawbacks of narrative synthesis are that it lacks transparency and reproducibility and that currently no process is available to guide this form of analysis. The systematic review on the infection control management of MRSA in acute care (Halcomb et al. 2008) is an excellent example of a narrative review in which the complete process of a systematic review was carried out. However, because of the lack of homogeneity in the studies, a narrative synthesis of the results was the best way to present the evidence within the systematic review.

Where to publish the completed systematic review

Once the systematic review has been completed, the findings need to be published so that they can be used in the development of guidelines to be used in clinical practice. If the initial protocol is published in the Cochrane Library or the JBI database, the complete review is also published in the same database. But systematic reviews can also be published on other health databases such as MEDLINE and CINAHL. The Joanna Briggs Institute and the Cochrane Collaboration have developed software that consists of a predeveloped format for the standardised reporting of systematic reviews.

Joanna Briggs and the Cochrane Collaboration

The Joanna Briggs Institute was established in 1996 to provide an evidence base for nursing practice and to devise strategies for the effective dissemination and implementation of that information within the health care setting. The JBI is a growing, dynamic international collaboration involving nursing, medical and allied health researchers, clinicians, academics and quality managers across 40 countries in every continent. The JBI has made evidence available at the point of clinical care by providing nurses with clearly presented summaries of research findings called 'Best Practice Information Sheets' (www.joannabriggs.edu.au/pubs/best_practice.php).

The Cochrane Collaboration is an international not-for-profit organisation that has been established to provide up-to-date, accurate information about the effects of health care on the global health community. The Cochrane Collaboration is named after the British epidemiologist Archie Cochrane and was founded in 1993. The Cochrane Library consists of more than 3500 reviews on various health-related topics. The systematic reviews published in the Cochrane Library are carried out by a global network of dedicated volunteers who are supported by a small number of staff from within the Collaboration.

Summary

Like all research methods, systematic reviews involve a formal process that is transparent and reproducible. Undertaking a systematic review requires both knowledge of the topic under investigation and skills in searching for the literature, critical appraisal and data analysis/synthesis. A robust and credible systematic review provides the basis for clinical guideline and policy development.

This chapter has provided information on the process of undertaking a systematic review, defined terminology, and offered examples and links to valuable web-based resources. We hope this will assist the reader to be able to better understand other published systematic reviews as well as undertake their own reviews.

Finally, even though evidence obtained from systematic reviews is considered to be the highest level of evidence, the systematic review needs to be critically appraised before the evidence is implemented. The evidence should also be carefully considered according to its clinical significance, impact on service users, and costs.

IMPLICATIONS FOR EVIDENCE-BASED NURSING AND MIDWIFERY

Nursing practice is largely based on tradition and rituals (Bachle 2007; Zeitz & McCutcheon 2005). According to various bodies (NHMRC 2009), a systematic review is considered to be the highest level of evidence because of the rigorous methods used and the unbiased results. The findings are therefore used for the development of evidence-based guidelines and policies for clinical practice. For example, findings from the Water for Wound Cleansing Systematic Review are being used by the Cochrane Collaboration as an evidence aid source for wound management in disaster areas. One of the most important aspects of evidence-based nursing is that patients and their families are informed about the various options available to them in relation to their treatment and care. The results of evidence searches should be shared with them so that joint decision-making can result. Information should be shared on a partnership basis, with the practitioner providing explanations so patients are able to decide what will work best for them.

In addition to providing evidence for clinical practice, systematic reviews also provide implications for further research. Students taking higher degree courses often commence with a systematic review, identify the gaps in the literature and then undertake other primary research. Furthermore, funding bodies require evidence from systematic reviews in applications that seek grants for primary research.

The systematic review forms a crucial part of evidence-based nursing and midwifery. Results of the review are made available to health practitioners in a briefly described document. In Australia, this document, the Best Practice Information Sheet, is prepared by the Joanna

Briggs Institute and is widely available through the internet. However, relevant information including the research team and the process used to develop this Best Practice information sheet is included in JBI's Technical Reports. The use of a Best Practice Information Sheet can also vary from one organisation to another organisation (Fineout-Overholt et al. 2004; Melnyk et al. 2004; Melnyk & Fineout-Overholt 2006). Ongoing development to conduct systematic reviews of qualitative research will further assist nurses and midwives to apply the evidence in their care delivery.

▶▶▶   **PROBLEM SOLVING 14.1**

Betty is a registered nurse working at a large volunteer organisation which provides health and social services to homeless people. Betty has been asked by her supervisor to find out about available evidence that the organisation can use to provide health promotion services to homeless women with or without children. Betty can gain access to more than three libraries in her local communities and uses many databases for her search.

a   What are keywords that Betty can use to begin her search? Please also use an asterisk when applicable. It is expected that Betty can discuss this task later with librarians.

b   List three databases that Betty uses for her search. It is suggested that health promotion services can be for physical health, mental health, early disease prevention or early disease detection such as screenings.

Practice exercise 14.1

As a graduate nurse, you have observed an increasing use of restraints by staff in a busy nursing home. You would like to know what types of restraint can be used and their relevant guidelines. You intend to introduce changes within the organisation and would like to know potential barriers so you can discuss the issues with your supervisor.

Start your search by:

•   identifying the Best Practice Information Sheet relating to the use of restraint

•   searching databases to explore whether health organisations have adopted the best practice

•   listing potential barriers

•   analysing whether the identified barriers will be applied in your organisation or not.

Practice exercise 14.2

You are required to develop a search strategy to identify the relevant papers relating to wound cleansing. Which of the following databases would you search?

MEDLINE, CINAHL, EmBaSE, PsycInfo, PEDRO, Cochrane

Compile a search strategy using the search terms listed below

Search history

1)	Wound$	2)	lacerat$	3)	bruis$
4)	Ulcer$	5)	Infect$	6)	Heal$
7)	Solution$	8)	Saline	9)	Sodium Chloride
10)	water	11)	Clean$	12)	Irrigat$
13)	Swabb$	14)	Scrub$	15)	Soak$
16)	bath$	17)	Shower$		

Answers to problem solving 14.1

a

Homeless*, homeless person*

health care worker, nurs*, medical, dental, mental health

health behaviours, compliance, motivation*, outcomes

intervention*, health promotion

women, women NOT men

b

CINAHL, Cochrane, York, JBI, PsycLit, Sociolit, Scopus, MEDLINE, Embase, Google scholar

Appendix 14.1
JBI Critical Appraisal Checklist for Experimental Studies

Reviewer ....   Date ....

Author ....   Year ....   Record Number ....

	Yes (3)	No (2)	Unclear (1)
1. Was the assignment to treatment groups random?			
2. Were participants blinded to treatment allocation?			
3. Was allocation to treatment groups concealed from the allocator?			
4. Were the outcomes of people who withdrew described and included in the analysis?			
5. Were those assessing outcomes blind to the treatment allocation?			
6. Were the control and treatment groups comparable at entry?			
7. Were groups treated identically other than for the named interventions?			
8. Were outcomes measured in the same way for all groups?			
9. Were outcomes measured in a reliable way?			
10. Was there adequate follow-up (>80%)?			
11. Was appropriate statistical analysis used?			

Overall appraisal: ☐ Include   ☐ Exclude   ☐ Seek further info

Comments (Including reasons for exclusion)

....

....

....

....

Joanna Briggs Institute Quantitative Data Critical Appraisal Scale reproduced with Permission of the Joanna Briggs Institute

Appendix 14.2
Data Extraction Form (Quantitative Data)

Author ....   Record Number ....

Journal ....   Year ....

Reviewer ....

Method ....

Setting ....

Participants ....

....

Number of Participants ....

Group A ....   Group B ....

Interventions

Intervention A ....

....

Intervention B ....

....

Outcome Measures

Outcome Description	Scale/Measure

Results ....

Dichotomous Data

Outcome	Treatment Group Number/total number	Control Group Number/total number

Continuous Data

Outcome	Treatment Group Mean & SD (number)	Control Group Mean & SD (number)

Authors Conclusion ....

....

....

Reviewers Conclusion ....

....

....

Joanna Briggs Institute Quantitative Data Extraction Tool reproduced with Permission of the Joanna Briggs Institute

These tools are found within the Joanna Briggs Institute Meta Analysis of Statistics Assessment and Review Instrument (JBI MAStARI) http://mastari.joannabriggs.edu.au/

Further reading

Craig, J. V., & Smyth, R. L. (eds), *The Evidence-Based Practice Manual for Nurses*, 2nd edn. Edinburgh: Elsevier.

Grol, R., & Grimshaw, J. (2003). From best evidence to best practice: Effective implementation of change in patients' care. *Lancet* 362(9391), 1225–30.

Joanna Briggs Institute for Evidence Based Nursing and Midwifery. (2009). The JBI approach to evidence-based practice. Retrieved 10 June 2009, from <www.joannabriggs.edu.au/about/documents/JBI%20Approach%20to%20EBP%20Levels%20of%20Evidence%20Grades%20of%20Recommendation.pdf>

NHMRC. (2009). NHMRC additional levels of evidence and grades for recommendations for developers of guidelines: Stage 2 consultation. Retrieved 10 June 2009, from <www.nhmrc.gov.au/_files_nhmrc/file/publications/synopses/cp30.pdf>

Portney, L. G., & Watkins, M. P. (2009). *Foundations of Clinical Research: Applications to Practice*, 3rd edn. New Jersey: Pearson Education.

Weblinks

Cochrane Collaboration:

<www.cochrane.edu.au>

Evidence-Based Nursing Journal:

<http://ebn.bmj.com>

Searchable database about current ongoing clinical research studies, The U.S. Institutes of Health

<www.clinicaltrials.gov>

Meta-register of worldwide clinical studies

<www.controlled-trials.com>

The New York Academy of Medicine–Library–Grey Literature Report

<www.nyam.org/library/pages/grey_literature_report>

The Grey Literature Network Service widely known as GreyNet

<www.greynet.org/greysourceindex.html>

Information about ongoing health services research and public health projects

<wwwcf.nlm.nih.gov/hsr_project/home_proj.cfm>

References

Armstrong, E. C. (1999). The well-built clinical question: The key to finding the best evidence efficiently. *Wisconsin Medical Journal* 98(2), 25–8.

Bachle, B. (2007). [Rituals in pediatric nursing: Possibilities and limitations]. *Kinderkrankenschwester* 26(8), 315–7.

Barnett-Page, E., & Thomas, J. (2009). *Methods for the Synthesis of Qualitative Research: A Critical Review*. Economic and Social Research Council.

Chamberlain, B. (2007). The differences between meta-analysis and meta-study: part I. *Clinical Nurse Specialist* 21(5), 229–30.

Crowther, M., Lim, W., & Crowther, M. A. (2010). Systematic review and meta-analysis methodology. *Blood* 116(17), 3140–6.

Cullum, N. (2000). Users' guides to the nursing literature: An introduction. *Evidence Based Nursing* 3(3), 71–2.

Cullum, N., Ciliska, D., Haynes, B., & Marks, S. (2008). *Evidence-Based Nursing: An Introduction*. Oxford: Blackwell Publishing.

Davies, K. (2007). The information-seeking behaviour of doctors: A review of the evidence. *Health Information & Libraries Journal* 24(2), 78–94.

Downe, S. (2008). Metasynthesis: A guide to knitting smoke. *Evidence Based Midwifery* 6(1), 4–8.

Egger, M., Smith, G., & Altman, D. (2001). *Systematic Reviews in Health Care: Meta-analysis in Context*, 2nd edn. Singapore: BMJ.

Evans, D. (2002). Systematic reviews of interpretive research: Interpretive data synthesis of processed data. *Australian Journal of Advanced Nursing* 20(2), 22–6.

Fernandez, R., & Griffiths, R. (2008). *Water for Wound Cleansing*. Cochrane Database of Systematic Reviews (1) CD003861.

Fernandez, R., & Tran, D. (2009). The meta-analysis graph. Clearing the haze. *Clinical Nurse Specialist*, 23(2), 57–60.

Fineout-Overholt, E., Levin, R. F., & Melnyk, B. M. (2004). Strategies for advancing evidence-based practice in clinical settings. *Journal of the New York State Nurses' Association* 35(2), 28–32.

Fineout-Overholt, E., O'Mathúna, D. P., & Kent, B. (2008). How systematic reviews can foster evidence-based clinical decisions. *Worldviews on Evidence-Based Nursing* 5(1), 45–8.

Flemming, K. (2007). The synthesis of qualitative research and evidence-based nursing. *Evidence Based Nursing* 10(3), 68–71.

Gøtzsche, P. C., Hrobjartsson, A., Maric, K., & Tendal, B. (2007). Data extraction errors in meta-analyses that use standardized mean differences. *JAMA* 298(4), 430–7.

Halcomb, E. J., Fernandez, R., Griffiths, R., Newton, P. J., & Hickman, L. (2008). The infection control management of MRSA in acute care. *International Journal of Evidence-Based Healthcare* 6(4), 440–67.

Higgins, J., & Green, S. (2008). *Cochrane Handbook for Systematic Reviews of Interventions* (Vol. Version 5.0.0): The Cochrane Collaboration.

Higgins, J. P., Thompson, S. G., Deeks, J. J., & Altman, D. G. (2003). Measuring inconsistency in meta-analyses. *British Medical Journal* 327(7414), 557–60.

Hopewell, S., Clarke, M., Lefebvre, C., & Scherer, R. (2007). *Handsearching Versus Electronic Searching to Identify Reports of Randomized Trials*. Cochrane Database of Systematic Reviews (2), MR000001.

Hopewell, S., McDonald, S., Clarke, M., & Egger, M. (2007). *Grey Literature in Meta-Analyses of Randomized Trials of Health Care Interventions*. Cochrane Database of Systematic Reviews(2), MR000010.

Ioannidis, J. P., Patsopoulos, N. A., & Rothstein, H. R. (2008). Reasons or excuses for avoiding meta-analysis in forest plots. *British Medical Journal* 336(7658), 1413–5.

Jadad, A., & Enkin, M. (2007). *Randomized Controlled Trials: Questions, Answers and Musings*, 2nd edn. Singapore: Blackwell BMJ Books.

Jones, A. P., Remmington, T., Williamson, P. R., Ashby, D., & Smyth, R. L. (2005). High prevalence but low impact of data extraction and reporting errors were found in Cochrane systematic reviews. *Journal of Clinical Epidemiology* 58(7), 741–2.

Leong, S. T. (2007). Systematic review made simple for nurses. *Nursing* 16(2), 104–10.

Littell, J., Corcoran, J., & Pillai, V. (2008). *Systematic Reviews and Meta-Analysis*. Oxford and New York: Oxford University Press.

Melnyk, B. M., & Fineout-Overholt, E. (2006). Consumer preferences and values as an integral key to evidence-based practice. *Nursing Administration Quarterly* 30(2), 123–7.

Melnyk, B. M., Fineout-Overholt, E., Fischbeck Feinstein, N., Li, H., Small, L., Wilcox, L., & Kraus, R. (2004). Nurses' perceived knowledge, beliefs, skills, and needs regarding evidence-based practice: Implications for accelerating the paradigm shift. *Worldviews on Evidence-Based Nursing* 1(3), 185–93.

Moher, D., Jadad, A. R., Nichol, G., Penman, M., Tugwell, P., & Walsh, S. (1995). Assessing the quality of randomized controlled trials: An annotated bibliography of scales and checklists. *Control Clinical Trials* 16(1), 62–73.

Montori, V. M., Wilczynski, N. L., Morgan, D., & Haynes, R. B. (2005). Optimal search strategies for retrieving systematic reviews from Medline: Analytical survey. *British Medical Journal* 330(7482), 68.

Nasseri-Moghaddam, S., & Malekzadeh, R. (2006). 'Systematic review': Is it different from the 'traditional review'? *Archives of Iranian Medicine* 9(3), 196–9.

NHMRC (National Health and Medical Research Council) (2009). NHMRC levels of evidence and grades for recommendations for developers of guidelines. Retrieved 9 October 2010, from <http://www.nhmrc.gov.au/_files_nhmrc/file/guidelines/evidence_statement_form.pdf>

Patrick, T. B., Demiris, G., Folk, L. C., Moxley, D. E., Mitchell, J. A., & Tao, D. (2004). Evidence-based retrieval in evidence-based medicine. *Journal of the Medical Library Association* 92(2), 196–9.

Pearson, A., Field, J., & Jordan, Z. (2007). *Evidence-Based Clinical Practice in Nursing and Healthcare: Assimilating Research, Experience and Expertise*. Adelaide: Blackwell Publishing.

Pearson, A., Porritt, K. A., Doran, D., Vincent, L., Craig, D., Tucker, D., et al. (2006). A comprehensive systematic review of evidence on the structure, process, characteristics and composition of a nursing team that fosters a healthy work environment. *International Journal of Evidence-Based Healthcare* 4(2), 118–59.

Perera, R., & Heneghan, C. (2008). Interpreting meta-analysis in systematic reviews. *Evidence Based Medicine* 13(3), 67–9.

Polit, D., & Beck, C. (2008). *Nursing Research: Generating and Assessing Evidence for Nursing Practice*. New York: J. B. Lippincott.

Richardson, W. S., Wilson, M. C., Nishikawa, J., & Hayward, R. S. (1995). The well-built clinical question: A key to evidence-based decisions. *ACP Journal Club* 123(3), A12–13.

Weller, A. C. (2004). Mounting evidence that librarians are essential for comprehensive literature searches for meta-analyses and Cochrane reports. *Journal of the Medical Library Association* 92(2), 163–4.

Yoshii, A., Plaut, D. A., McGraw, K. A., Anderson, M. J., & Wellik, K. E. (2009). Analysis of the reporting of search strategies in Cochrane systematic reviews. *Journal of the Medical Library Association* 97(1), 21–9.

Zeitz, K., & McCutcheon, H. (2005). Tradition, rituals, and standards, in a realm of evidenced based nursing care. *Contemporary Nurse* 18(3), 300–8.

Zhang, L., Ajiferuke, I., & Sampson, M. (2006). Optimizing search strategies to identify randomized controlled trials in MEDLINE. *BMC Medical Research Methodology* 6, 23.

CHAPTER 15

Disseminating Research

Penny Paliadelis, Glenda Parmenter and Jackie Lea

Chapter learning outcomes

By the end of this chapter you will be able to:

▶ understand research dissemination as an essential part of the research process

▶ recognise the importance of sharing research that contributes to the body of nursing and midwifery knowledge

▶ identify the core why, how and where components of preparing research findings for dissemination

▶ recall the different avenues available to share research findings

▶ identify barriers to the dissemination of nursing and midwifery research and related strategies for overcoming them

▶ explain how to access relevant guidelines for abstract and manuscript submissions.

KEY TERMS

Abstract
Collaboration
Conference
Dissemination
Peer review
Publish
Scholarship
Target audience

Introduction

The aim of this chapter is to demystify the process of disseminating nursing and midwifery knowledge. It will present a discussion of writing for publication focusing on developing your understanding of how and where to publicise research findings and professional knowledge. The importance of disseminating research findings will be discussed. The barriers to publishing will be identified and strategies for overcoming them will be provided. Some approaches will be presented that will assist in maximising opportunities to publish or present research findings by targeting the right journal or conference. In addition, strategies for developing and preparing conference presentations, journal manuscripts and project reports will also be outlined. Case study examples of Australian conference papers and journal articles will be used to demonstrate the process of turning research outcomes and/ or clinical innovations into publications, reports, media releases and conference papers.

Avenues for research dissemination and how to target the right one

The importance of disseminating research has been discussed; now we move on to the how and where of dissemination. The most common vehicles for disseminating research are conference and poster presentations, journal articles, books and book chapters, policies, guidelines, reports and media releases. This section will give you practical advice and tips on how to prepare each of these successfully. The first and most important step is to target the most appropriate means of dissemination for your particular project.

Conference papers and posters

It is important to be aware of up-and-coming conferences and seminars and when the calls for abstracts are being made, as this will give you the opportunity to put your work forward. Most national and international conferences call for abstracts up to 12 months before the conference. This allows plenty of time for the abstracts to be peer-reviewed and the results communicated to the author(s). Once your abstract is accepted for a presentation or poster, you need to confirm your attendance and pay conference registration fees and book travel and accommodation, if required.

However, before you can submit your abstract for consideration you must first know how to find calls for conference abstracts. One strategy for becoming aware of such calls is to look for preliminary conference notices in Australian and international nursing publications, such as the *Nursing Review*, the *Australian Journal of Nursing*, or the *Journal of Nursing Scholarship*. In addition, belonging to professional nursing bodies such as the Royal College of Nursing Australia or an interest group such as Palliative Care Australia will assist in identifying appropriate conferences to showcase your work. Membership of professional groups will provide you with information about upcoming conferences, and national and international organisations such as the International Council of Nurses have conference alerts on their website.

A further strategy for finding calls for conference papers is to use a popular search engine like Google and be specific about what you are looking for. For example, if you have completed a research project that explored more effective pain assessment tools for elderly post-operative patients, you may want to search for 'pain management conferences 2011'. This strategy will give you a list of conferences both in Australia and internationally. However, if you only want to present your work locally then you may need to change your search term to something more specific such as 'nursing conferences in Queensland 2011'. Another suggestion for finding calls for conference papers is to search for conferences that target specific research methodologies. For example, there is an annual International Qualitative Health Research Conference, which is entirely devoted to the presentation and discussion of a range of qualitative methodological approaches.

Once you have identified a conference that is relevant to your research, you need to consider the conference themes, abstract instructions and deadlines. Each conference will have different requirements and you need to tailor your abstract to fit the guidelines (see Research in practice 15.4 for examples of abstracts). If you have not attended many conferences and you are a little nervous about public speaking then maybe you should rehearse your presentation with colleagues and friends. Feedback on the timing of your slides, the information on them and the pace of your presentation is valuable. Another option is submitting an abstract for a poster presentation. Information about how to present your research as a conference paper or poster is outlined in many articles. For example, Taggart and Arslanian (2000) and Keely (2004) outline the steps to the construction and formatting of a poster that will assist you in presenting an easy-to-read, informative and well-designed poster.

▶▶▶ TERMS, TIPS AND SKILLS

Before presenting at a conference or seminar, practise delivering your oral presentation in front of fellow students or offer to deliver it as an informal in-service to clinical colleagues.

The example of a poster presentation in Figure 15.1 demonstrates that a poster can be used as a powerful vehicle for dissemination. In this case the focus of the poster is not on a research study, rather it is a reflection on caring for a patient admitted to hospital with a cardiac dysfunction in both a rural and metropolitan setting. (This poster was presented at a Cardiac Conference in NSW in 2004 and won the award for Best Poster.)

Another matter that needs to be considered when submitting a conference abstract concerns the dates and location of the conference. While it might be flattering to have an abstract accepted for an international health promotion conference in Helsinki, it is important to consider whether you can find the funding to cover the costs of attending and presenting your paper or poster. In addition, you will need to discuss leave arrangements with your employer. Remember, the costs of presenting at an international conference can be prohibitive, when you take into account the prices of airfares, accommodation, conference registration, transfers and meals. If you plan ahead, grants to present at international conferences may be available from a number of sources. For example, many employers offer some conference funding. The nursing regulatory body has competitive scholarship rounds, and other nursing organisations, such as the Australian College of Critical Care Nurses, may also have competitive grants available. To secure conference funding you may be required to provide details of the conference, a copy of your accepted abstract and a detailed budget and itinerary.

Figure 15.1 Example of a poster presentation

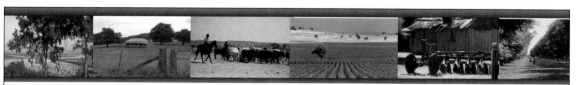

'Going Bush': The challenges for cardiac nurses in rural NSW.
Penny Paliadelis and Helena Sanderson
School of Health, Faculty of Education, Health and Professional Studies, University of New England, Armidale NSW, Australia.

UNE
The University of
NEW ENGLAND

Outinthesticksville Hospital

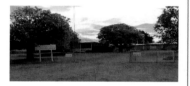

It's 2am, in a rural 22 bed hospital, the Registered Nurse (RN) is looking over the patients notes after settling 18 patients when the A&E bell rings. What is it now? The CCTV screen displays a middle aged man accompanied by a women. The man is clutching his chest. The RN runs to open the A&E door grabbing the EN on her way. It's Bob and Edith Brown who own a property several miles out of town. Bob is pale, diaphoretic and complaining of cental chest pain. Edith says it woke him but she didn't call the ambulance because they live a bit far out of town so they just jumped into the car and drove in.

The EN takes Edith to the waiting room for a cup of tea. The RN administers oxygen, quickly does an ECG while asking Bob about his history. Aspirin 300 mg and anginine are administered and the ECG is assessed.

Bob still has pain, another anginine is administered and the GP 'on call', Dr Letwaitensee is notified. The on call wards-person is contacted at home to get the hospital car ready to drive the bloods to the nearest pathology department. The RN is not accredited to do venipuncture in this hospital. Bob is still in pain, another anginine is given . While waiting for the GP Bob is reassured and the RN gathers what is needed to take bloods, set up a heparin infusion and check the expiry of the Releplase.

It's 2.20 am Bob tells the RN that the pain has eased slightly. The GP arrives, and the wardsperson arrives to take the bloods to another hospital an hour away. The doctor wants another ECG and morphine and thrombolysis administered. Meanwhile the EN informs the RN that one of the patients has fallen out of bed and another is praying at the top of her voice. Finally, the bloods are on their way to the lab and Bob is painfree, thrombolysis has been administered and the ward patients are settled. The GP and the RN discuss the available options and decide to transfer.

Introduction

Providing fast and effective acute cardiac care is challenging in all health facilities. However, in small rural hospitals the challenges are somewhat different to those encountered in metropolitan hospitals. In many rural health services nursing staff are required to care for inpatients as well as be the first line health care professional when patients present to the Accident and Emergency Departments. Services and resources that are taken for granted in metropolitan healthcare may not be readily available in rural hospitals. Foe example, in some rural areas pathology, x-ray and other services are only available in a larger base hospital and interventional cardiology services are non existent in many parts of rural NSW. This poster provides a lighthearted approach to these challenges based on the authors' personal experience.

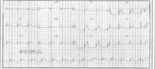

The ECG: Anterior Myocardial Infarction

Conclusion
The challenges for cardiac nurses in the Bush include:

♥ **The tyranny of distance**
♥ **Skills and knowledge**
♥ **Access to specialised facilities**
♥ **Staffing ratios -1 RN :1 EN**
♥ **Access to health facilities**

Bigcitybrightlights Hospital

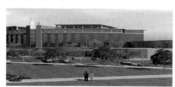

It's 2am, a Registered Nurse is working in the 22 bed A&E department of a 600 bed city hospital. There are people everywhere, when a middle aged man is brought through by the Triage RN. He is pale, diaphoretic and complaining of central chest pain, which he says woke him. A women is with him and the RN sends her to admissions to complete the paper work. The RN takes the client through to the high dependency bay and with the help of an agency nurse quickly connects the patient to a monitor, administers oxygen, takes some bloods and obtains a 12 lead ECG.

An urgent sticker is attached to the bloods and sent to pathology. The RN takes a history and administers 300mg of aspirin and an anginine, while monitoring the vital signs.

The urgent bloods already show slightly elevated Troponin T levels. The RMO looks at the ECG and blood results, agreeing with the diagnosis of an Anterior Myocardial Infarction. The RN administers morphine, starts a GTN infusion, while the RMO checks to see if the cath lab is available within 90 minutes. There is an urgent case in CCU, so Thrombolytic therapy and heparin infusion are administered at 2.45 am. The RN transfers the patient to CCU and moves onto the next patient.

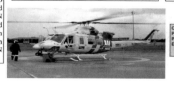

Contacts
Penny Paliadelis   Helena Sanderson
Phone: 02-67733653   Phone :02-67665072
Email: ppaliade@pobox.une.edu.au   Email:hsanders@pobox.une.edu.au

Preparing manuscripts for scholarly journals

If you are searching for an appropriate journal in which to publish an article about your project, one obvious place to start is your own reference list. For example, if you found that you drew on a number of articles from the *Journal of Nursing Management* to inform your project, this may be the right journal to target when writing your manuscript. Always have a look at the types of articles that the journal publishes, look at the focus, the content, the style and the length of published articles and consider whether you can write about your project in a similar style (McIntyre et al. 2007; Saver 2006b). University or hospital librarians can also help with finding the right journal for your manuscript. Having identified a journal that is relevant to your project and/or your target audience, the next step is to go to the journal website and review the author guidelines. The information provided is vital, as in order for your submission to be considered for publication you must comply with the stated word limit, formatting and referencing style, so that the editor will consider your manuscript appropriate for peer review. Reputable scholarly journals send manuscripts out to at least two reviewers in a double-blind process. This means that the reviewers do not know who the authors are, and the authors do not know who the reviewers are. Reviewers of manuscripts for publication are usually asked to comment on style, structure, originality, significance, interest and scientific and technical soundness. The editor then makes the decision to accept the manuscript for publication, accept with changes, or reject the manuscript as not suitable for publication. In most cases the reviewers' feedback is sent to the authors along with the editor's decision.

RESEARCH IN PRACTICE 15.1

15.1

PEER REVIEW

Below is an extract of feedback provided by three peer-reviewers that was sent to the authors of a literature review submitted to an international nursing journal. Please take note of the constructive tone of the comments. This article was later revised, based on the feedback provided, and following a further peer review it was accepted for publication.

Reviewer: 1

Comments to the Author

With some minor changes I think this article will make a contribution to nursing knowledge. I would like to see the title of the article changed to more clearly identify that this is a literature review. The introductory section is a little confusing, as there are multiple subheadings that are not really needed. I can see no need for the 'Literature Review Methodology', nor is there any discussion or evidence provided regarding how a narrative approach was utilised. I think the whole idea of a methodology for a literature review is redundant.

Reviewer: 2

Comments to the Author

Although a very important and potentially interesting topic, the manuscript contains several major weaknesses which in my view need to be addressed prior to considering the paper for publication. These weaknesses are outlined below:

The methodology used in the literature review needs much stronger justification as to why a narrative approach has been adopted and how this differs from such approaches as an integrative review. Indeed, it is unclear from the manuscript how the adopted approach to the literature review contributes to knowledge about cardiovascular disease risk reduction.

Several concepts seemed to have been identified to provide a framework for the literature review but there seems little analysis of these concepts or how they might inform the review. The author also includes the concept of adherence and provides a rather simplistic definition before going on to include literature on adherence as part of the literature search. Once again there is no justification for focusing on adherence in a literature review about risk reduction.

The framework for organising the literature appears unclear. It appears to be based on the methodology of the studies rather than a conceptual framework, which might be a more appropriate approach to contribute to an understanding of risk reduction.

The style of the paper would also benefit from some revision as the authors are inclined to make inappropriate generalisations and assumptions that are not supported with evidence.

Reviewer: 3

Comments to the Author

Methods section was rather weak and did not provide sufficient background to assess the rigour of the review process. I'm not convinced this paper provides significant new information or innovation in assessing this area of scholarship.

The review process for most major nursing journals can take many months, and it is quite common for the reviewers' feedback to indicate that some changes are required before the paper is suitable for publication. For novice authors, this can be a long and daunting process. But it is important not to become disheartened, as all authors have had manuscripts sent back to them requiring substantial changes, while some may have had manuscripts rejected. Sometimes the journal is not the right one in which to publish your work, or maybe you do not make the significance of your project clear (Saver 2006c). Most journals now manage the entire process of submission and review online. Figure 15.2 illustrates the stages in the online submission process. Always read the reviewers' feedback carefully, use their suggestions to polish your manuscript, and most importantly remember that this is a learning process—all successful authors were once novices!

Another important thing to consider when preparing a manuscript for publication is that journals have very strict requirements about the originality of the work under

Figure 15.2   Stages of online manuscript submission

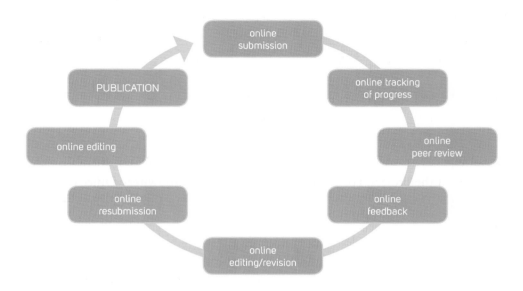

consideration. Upon submission of your manuscript, you will be asked to sign a declaration that the work has not been previously published, nor is it under consideration for publication elsewhere. This precludes you from submitting the same manuscript to several journals at once (Saver 2006c).

Books and book chapters

If you believe that you have a new project, idea or information that may be suitable to be published as a nursing or midwifery textbook then usually the first strategy is to approach a publisher to ask how you go about submitting a book proposal. Many publishers have instructions for potential authors on their websites. Most publishing houses ask for the potential author(s) to produce a clear and compelling case for publication. This will usually include one or more sample chapters and your review of whether similar texts are available and how your text will differ. Once the publisher considers the proposal, they may conduct market research. This means that they send your proposal and sample chapter(s) to experts in the field, and based on the feedback, they may decline your proposal or agree to publish. If your proposal is accepted you will receive a book contract. You will then have to agree on a timeline for submission of chapters or the entire manuscript and a proposed publication date. A similar process occurs with book chapters. However, it is common for editors of the book, or those who submitted the initial proposal, to invite contributors to write specific chapters (Happell 2008). Royalty payments will be negotiated and may vary from one publisher to another.

Policies, guidelines and reports

The requirements for writing up and disseminating research or quality projects as policies, guidelines or formal reports will vary depending on the end-user of these documents and the nature of the publication. While it is important that all policy documents are clear and well written and disseminated to all relevant stakeholders, if it is not a publicly available document, the audience for such a report may be limited. However, this type of dissemination does not generally preclude the authors producing a manuscript about the project for publication in a relevant journal or as a conference presentation or poster.

If you have completed a funded research project, you will probably need to compile a formal report that may be published on a website or as a publicly available record of the outcomes of the project. For example, the Nursing and Midwifery Office of NSW Health has links to reports of research projects that have been funded by this department over the past few years. Larger research projects that have attracted significant public funding may be written up as published reports, which may then be used to inform new statewide or national health policy. Many funding bodies have strict guidelines about how such reports are presented; similarly, public and private health organisations have policy templates and may even have departments dedicated to researching and writing new policies.

15.1 **RESEARCH AND EVIDENCE-BASED PRACTICE 15.1**

DISSEMINATION OF QUALITY STUDY ON A BUSY MEDICAL WARD

Nurses on a busy medical ward conducted a quality project that explored the number of injuries caused by pre-packaged metal closure clips that are included with many brands of bandages. The results of this study were disseminated as an internal policy document that required staff to cease using these devices and dispose of them in a sharps container. The number of injuries resulting from the use of these clips was dramatically reduced. Do you think that an article about this study would be useful if it was disseminated more widely?

▶▶▶   TERMS, TIPS AND SKILLS

If you are or have been involved in any projects, think about how the findings of the project could best be disseminated.

Media releases

In some situations your funding or employing organisation may ask you to prepare a media release about a project that is controversial or has popular appeal. Alternatively, a newspaper or television station may contact you for your comments on a current issue relating to your organisation or area of expertise. For example, if you have completed a project that identifies effective strategies for recruiting and retaining health professionals in rural areas, local media may wish to interview you, as this topic is of national and even global concern. The dissemination of information via media releases and reports is quite different from other forms of dissemination, as newspaper articles, news reports and radio interviews are usually short and only cover the key points. Another useful tip is to have a look at the press releases of nursing organisations, such as the Australian Nursing and Midwifery Council, as this will give you some ideas about how to write a media release. You will also need to make yourself aware of your employer's guidelines regarding media releases before you proceed. If the research project is funded it is important to review the contract to ensure that media releases are permitted. There are a number of websites listed in Weblinks below that provide valuable information about how to prepare a press release and talk to the media.

▶▶▶   TERMS, TIPS AND SKILLS

Access some recent media releases from professional bodies such as the Australian Nursing and Midwifery Council or the new Nursing and Midwifery Board of Australia and note the key elements/information included in the media release.

Barriers to publishing and strategies for overcoming them

There are many avenues for disseminating and publishing research findings and these can take the form of theses, books, project reports, journal articles, conference papers and posters, policy documents, procedure manuals and media releases. However, too few nurses and midwives share their work through publication and many find the writing part of the research process daunting (Wills 2000; Woodward et al. 2007). This is particularly evident within the clinical context where few nurses write and publish about their daily practice (Beal et al. 2008). The reason for this is that nurses and midwives encounter a number of barriers to writing and presenting their writing for publication. These barriers take four broad forms: cultural, knowledge, resource and personal barriers, and the following is a discussion of these four barriers together with some suggestions for overcoming them.

Strategies for overcoming cultural barriers

A significant barrier to writing for publication is the culture of nursing itself. This culture has a strong tradition of favouring verbal communication over the written form (Miracle 2003). A great deal of nursing knowledge is passed on through conversations held in tearooms and at handover, and in more formal settings such as nursing conferences and seminars. In addition, there is a tendency among nurses to undervalue the role of nurse researchers and their contribution to the profession and to health care in general (Bragadottir 1998). Culture change happens slowly, but this change is rapidly gathering pace in nursing, with many more clinicians now becoming interested and participating in the dissemination of their clinical innovations and research findings (Happell 2008). A significant influence on culture change is the growing number of nurses who consult the nursing literature to inform their practice. In addition, health service initiatives such as quality improvement and clinical practice development projects are creating opportunities for clinical staff to undertake local projects that are supported by health management. Such initiatives are just one way in which the culture of nursing is being transformed to become a more research-based and evidence-based one (NSW Health Nursing & Midwifery Office 2009).

▶▶▶ TERMS, TIPS AND SKILLS

Before commencing writing make sure you have a suitable workspace, some quiet time and access to relevant resources.

Strategies for overcoming knowledge barriers

A second barrier to publishing nursing research is a lack of knowledge about the types of papers that are suitable for publication. Many nurses believe that research and publication are the domain of academics and that the work of clinicians is not suitable for dissemination. While the research and publication work of academics is important, it is vital that clinically based nurses make local research outcomes, and the experiences that arise from them, widely known (Beal et al. 2008). These publications may take the form of research, quality assurance projects, case studies, clinical innovations or experiences, reflections on practice, or an opinion or comment on a nursing topic.

Writing can be a challenging task and not knowing where or how to begin is a powerful deterrent. Nurses often require support to enhance their writing skills and strengthen their approaches to the task of writing. However, there is usually very little in the way of support for novice writers, and finding mentors within the clinical setting can be difficult (Reid & Fuller 2005). Nurses may also be unaware of the writing and publication process and confused about the most appropriate journal in which to present their work.

A first step to becoming a published author is to read and familiarise yourself with the range of nursing publications that are available. This will give you an insight into the journals that might be appropriate for your area of expertise or interest and the types of papers that you might develop for publication. It will also help you to prepare your own manuscript. While reading, you can note aspects of style, expression and presentation that you found particularly relevant and that give you ideas for developing your own paper. Later in this chapter some tips on how to identify appropriate journals for publication of your own papers will be provided.

Attendance and presentation at conferences, seminars and workshops is another opportunity for sharing your professional knowledge. It also raises your profile among your colleagues and allows you the opportunity to set up collaborative projects. While successful conference presentation does not require complex skills, the trick is to make your presentation interesting, engaging and succinct. Many nurses who attend conferences realise that they could have presented a paper themselves (Billings & Kowalski 2009b). So while attending presentations, think critically about aspects of the presentation as this will help you in preparing your own.

A lack of knowledge about how to approach the task of writing can be overcome in a number of ways. The first is to be aware of the steps in the writing process. These steps are set out by Hislop and associates (2008): target a journal; draft an abstract; get pre-peer review; develop a detailed outline of the paper; write drafts of all sections of the paper; and revise the draft using a revision-feedback-revision cycle. An important aspect of this approach is that it breaks the larger task into a number of smaller, more doable ones. There is a tendency for novice writers to see writing as one large and overwhelming task, the prospect of which puts them off even beginning the process.

A further way to add to your writing and publishing knowledge and skills is to do a writing course, or to join or initiate a writers' support group (Bakas et al. 2006). This brings together a group of like-minded people who are able to give each other the necessary support and encouragement in gaining skills in writing and publishing. Such groups also provide structure in the form of agreed timelines with collaborators and an expectation that you will continue to work on your project. This helps to sustain motivation and also provides feedback on your progress from your peers and from the more experienced members of the group (Drotar 2000).

▶▶▶ TERMS, TIPS AND SKILLS

If you are a novice writer seek out an experienced author who can mentor you in the writing process.

One strategy for gaining support and encouragement from others is to collaborate with one or more colleagues on a joint paper. This is an excellent way to share the load of writing for publication as it gives you a smaller workload and the support and encouragement of other team members. You can bounce ideas off each other and review each other's work. If possible, it is useful to have at least one member of the writing team who has experience in writing and publishing. This might be achieved by approaching a nurse academic who has an interest in your work to join the writing team as a mentor. If you do decide to collaborate on a joint paper, it is wise to discuss authorship at the outset and how and in what order authors' names will appear on the finished paper. In general, those authors have right of authorship who have contributed significantly to the conception and design of the project, the analysis and interpretation of research data, and/or drafting significant parts of the work or critically revising it so as to contribute to the interpretation (Campanelli et al. 2007; NHMRC 2007).

RESEARCH IN PRACTICE 15.2

15.2 DISSEMINATION OF RESEARCH FINDINGS

A small research team made up of novice and experienced researchers wanted to explore the factors that attract final-year nursing students to seek employment in rural areas. Members of the team worked together to plan the research methodology and conduct the data collection and analysis. Once the study was complete a meeting was held to discuss how the research findings would be disseminated. Tasks were shared among team members, pairing more experienced writers and presenters with novices. One researcher prepared abstracts for submission to an international evidence-based practice conference and a national nursing education conference. These abstracts were proofread for accuracy and clarity by experienced team members prior to submission. Both abstracts were accepted and conference papers were prepared. Again, more experienced team members provided critical review, support and guidance. The team then jointly submitted a manuscript for consideration to the journal *The Collegian*, and following feedback and revision, the paper was published in 2008. The article is listed in References (Lea et al. 2008).

Strategies for addressing a lack of time and resources

A third barrier to writing and publishing for nurses and midwives is a lack of time and resources. Most clinically based staff are shift workers who are often very tired, so the energy and motivation to write may be lacking. In addition, many have family responsibilities that make further demands on their time and energy. This makes getting around to the task of writing very difficult, particularly as many nurses view writing or preparing a presentation as an extra commitment on top of their already allocated workload. Nurses may also lack a defined space in which to write and may have to share a computer with work colleagues and/or family members (Pierce 2009).

These barriers can be overcome if you use your organisational skills and assign a portion of your busy life to the task of writing. One strategy for overcoming the pressure of time is to break the writing up into a number of small tasks. It is surprising how much you can achieve in a single hour and if you set it aside regularly this can soon add up to a considerable amount of completed work. Hislop and others (2008) refer to this strategy as 'snack' writing and suggest regular periods of 30 minutes to one hour.

It is useful if you can have a designated workspace with your work materials set out so that you can begin work easily when you have available time. It is also helpful if you have easy access to the internet as this allows you to use a huge range of nursing information that will aid you in your writing endeavours. Obtaining the latest version of a referencing tool, such as EndNote, will also save you a significant amount of time when you come to publish your work and is worth the time it takes to learn how to use the program.

Another strategy in gaining skills in an atmosphere of support is to undertake research as part of a formal course of study at a tertiary institution. This provides you with resources such as a supervision team, access to literature, computer software and sometimes a computer. It also provides a more structured environment in which timelines are set for you to achieve your writing and publishing goals.

Funding to support research, writing and publishing is also available from a number of sources. At present, the NSW Nurses Association offers Edith Cavell Trust Scholarships that fund educational, research and conference attendance activities. The Royal College of Nursing Australia also offers and administers a number of scholarships and grants to support education, training and research. Make yourself aware of what financial support is available to you and apply for it. Some of these funds are easily available and often do not have a large number of applicants, so your chances of success are good. A list of the web addresses of these funding bodies is presented at the end of this chapter.

Strategies for overcoming personal barriers

Underpinning the three preceding barriers are personal barriers, such as negative thoughts and feelings, a lack of confidence in your own writing skills, and unhelpful personal work patterns or habits (Wills 2000). Many nurses lack confidence in their writing skills and this is compounded by a not entirely unfounded fear of rejection. A lack of mentorship and support finds many aspiring writers giving up before they have begun. Despite initial fears about writing, many beginners have overcome their fears to become successful authors. A common problem is that novice authors sit down to write before they are ready and feel frustrated when they can't think of how to start. A wide reading of the relevant literature is the best strategy for addressing this problem as this will confirm some of your knowledge and give you clues to the gaps in the literature that your research might be filling. This will affirm that you are on the right track or give guidance about how to frame your paper.

Novice writers also need to realise that writing skills are not innate but are developed over time and with extensive practice. The more you write the better you will become. It is good practice to have patience with yourself and seek the support and guidance of more experienced mentors to keep on fine-tuning your skills. Also, don't feel that everything you write has to be perfect. It is better to begin with a very rough outline of your work and then fine-tune it in sections. Be aware that all authors write many drafts of their paper before they have produced the finished article.

RESEARCH IN PRACTICE 15.3

15.3

PLANNING A RESEARCH STUDY

You have an idea for an interesting quality project in the nursing home where you work. You would like the staff to have more information about the residents' food likes and dislikes, in an effort to enhance their enjoyment of the meals. You are unsure how to start such a project. Here are some questions to consider that may help you to plan and disseminate this study (see also Chapter 2).

1   What are your initial steps in deciding whether this project is useful and/or viable?
2   What type of methodology would you use and why?
3   Is ethical approval required before undertaking such a study?
4   How would you identify whether there are any colleagues who might collaborate with you on this project?
5   Is there any support, for example, time, expertise or resources, available to you from within your organisation or from your local educational institution?
6   What research and writing skills do you already possess and how might you access support and mentorship in developing these skills?
7   How might you establish a collaborative research and writing group?
8   How might you quarantine a regular period of time in which to work on this project?
9   How would you disseminate the findings of this project?
10   Who would be your target audience?

Summary

This chapter has discussed the importance of having nurses and midwives disseminate their research work and contribute to the evidence base of the profession. It has also presented some strategies for sharing nursing knowledge within the health care context. A great sense of achievement can be derived from seeing your work developed into a published paper or conference presentation. The knowledge that your research and/or clinical innovation is reaching an extensive audience and influencing clinical practice is a source of enormous satisfaction. Publication of your work also has the potential to enhance your career progression. To add these dimensions to your practice, consider the tips that have been presented in this chapter and remember that all accomplished presenters and authors were once novices.

IMPLICATIONS FOR EVIDENCE-BASED NURSING AND MIDWIFERY

Since the early 1990s there has been an increasing need for nurses and midwives to support their professional practice with a strong research evidence base (Pierce 2009). Research is meaningless unless an account of the findings can be added to the body of nursing and midwifery knowledge and shared with others. In order to achieve this, the findings of nursing and midwifery research must be disseminated via publications and conference presentations. Publication of research activity and findings serves several functions. First, it shares nursing and midwifery knowledge, skills and experience with the wider population, allowing others to apply, critique or build on them, without unnecessary duplication. Second, it allows nurses to contribute to future nursing practice and theory by challenging traditional views and ensures that we are basing our clinical care on sound, credible and valid evidence (Hodges & Casey 2007; Saver 2006a). This allows nurses to apply the most up-to-date nursing knowledge to their clinical practice, leading to improved outcomes in patient care.

In addition to clinical practice, nurses also have a responsibility to generate and share knowledge and participate in activities of dissemination (Gerrish 2005). This is because the increased demands for efficient and effective health care mean that nurses must be accountable for creating best practice (Billings & Kowalski 2009a, p. 152). Other professions and academic disciplines have long based their knowledge on this concept, but nursing and midwifery, as relatively new academic disciplines, are quickly catching up (Reid & Fuller 2005). Similar to many countries, nursing in Australia has emerged and matured as a profession and we need to document this emergence with a strong body of nursing literature. Therefore, it is important that we are able to gain confidence in the value of our work and of our unique contribution to health care and to put our knowledge into writing so that evidence for practice is available to all (Keen 2007).

Practice exercise 15.1

Identify a journal that is relevant to your area of practice or interest. Go online to access and read the instructions for authors. Ask yourself the following questions:

Are the instructions clear?

What type of referencing style is required and are you familiar with it?

What are the format and word limit requirements for each type of manuscript?

Practice exercise 15.2

Ask colleagues and peers about local or recent clinical innovations or quality projects and discover how or if they have considered disseminating the results of these projects. Then reflect on their responses.

Practice exercise 15.3

If you have recently attended a lecture, workshop, training session or conference, consider the presentation and reflect on it. What worked well for you as an audience member, what was interesting, what parts were boring, irrelevant or unclear? This will assist with planning your own presentation.

Practice exercise 15.4

Below is an example of an abstract submitted for presentation at an Australian Primary Health Care Conference. The conference aimed to explore opportunities for greater integration of primary health care within nursing and broader health services, with an increased focus on interdisciplinary care. Contributions were invited that related to the conference aim with a focus on one of the following streams: Research; Service Delivery; Education or Policy. Abstracts had a 300-word limit.

Based on these guidelines answer the following questions:

- How would you assess the suitability of the following abstract for presentation at this conference?
- Does it contain enough information?
- Which of the conference streams, if any, does it best fit?
- If you were a reviewer for the conference would you accept this paper for an oral presentation, reject it or recommend it for presentation as a poster?

Title: An exploration of the capacity of General Practice Nurses to improve the prevention and management of childhood obesity

Childhood obesity is a worldwide concern that poses a major threat to long-term health by increasing the risk of chronic illnesses. The 2004 NSW Schools Physical Activity and Nutrition Survey has shown that overall, 25% of boys and 23% of girls are either overweight or obese. Given the shortage of General Practitioners, it is beyond their scope to manage this issue and this is particularly so in rural areas. At the same time, the role of General Practice Nurses in Primary Health Care is expanding and has recently been recognised by the allocation of a Provider Item Number by Medicare. However, these nursing roles are relatively new and the specific role that the General Practice Nurse might play in the prevention and management of childhood obesity has not been explored.

This study explored the capacity of rural General Practice Nurses to prevent and manage obesity in children. In particular, this study investigated the existing practices, educational qualifications, organisational expectations and motivation of General Practice Nurses, General Practitioners and General Practice Managers in order to identify the potential for expanding the role of these nurses. This study employed a qualitative methodology and used focus groups conducted with the staff of general practices located in a variety of rural locations within NSW.

This study has identified a number of barriers to such an expanded role as well as strategies that may be employed to assist General Practice Nurses to undertake an active role in the prevention and management of childhood obesity (Paliadelis & Parmenter 2009).

Practice exercise 15.5

List five potential avenues that could be used to disseminate research findings.

Practice exercise 15.6

There are a number of documents generated by reviewing of research systematically and used by clinicians. These documents include clinical guidelines and pathways. Based on your experiences, list specific documents you are aware of.

Answers to practice exercises

15.4

This abstract was accepted as an oral presentation for the Royal College of Nursing, Australia, Primary Health Care Conference, November 2009 under the theme of 'service delivery'.

15.5

Books, journal articles, conference presentations, conference posters, policy and procedure documents, reports and media releases.

15.6

Guideline: Graduate compression stocking for the prevention of post-operative venous thromboembolism.

Pathway: Management of patients with asthma, Management of women who have normal birth.

Further reading

Hislop, J., Murray, R., & Newton, M. (2008). Writing for publication: A case study. *Practice Development in Health Care* 7(3), 156–63.

Keen, A. (2007). Writing for publication: Pressures, barriers and support strategies. *Nurse Education Today* 27, 382–8.

McCleary, L. (2008). Drawing support from a writing group. *Nursing* 38(9), 46–53.

Pierce, L. L. (2009). Writing for publication: You can do it! *Rehabilitation Nursing* 34(1), 3–8.

Saver, C. (2006a). Reap the benefits of writing for publication. *AORN Journal* 83(3), 603–6.

Saver, C. (2006b). Finding and refining an article topic. *AORN Journal* 83(4), 829–32.

Taggart, H., & Arslanian, C. (2000). Creating an effective poster presentation. *Orthopaedic Nursing* 19(3), 47–9.

Weblinks

NSW Health Nursing and Midwifery Scholarship site:

<www.health.nsw.gov.au/nursing/scholarships.asp>

How to Write a Media Release:

<www.flyingsolo.com.au/p239863654_How-to-write-a-media-release.html>

Australian Health Practitioners Regulatory Agency:

<www.ahpra.gov.au>

References

Bakas, T., Farran, C., & Williams, L. (2006). Writing with a collaborative team. *Rehabilitation Nursing* 31(5), 222–4.

Beal, J. A., Riley, J. M., & Lancaster, D. R. (2008). Essential Elements of an Optimal Clinical Practice Environment. *Journal of Nursing Administration* 38(11), 488–93.

Billings, D., & Kowalski, K. (2009a). Lessons learnt when writing a manuscript. *Journal of Continuing Education in Nursing* 40(2), 55–6.

Billings, D., & Kowalski, K. (2009b). Strategies for making oral presentations about clinical issues: Part 1. At the workplace. *Journal of Continuing Education in Nursing* 40(4), 152–3.

Bragadottir, H. (1998). Every nurse can be an author: On writing for publication. *Nursing Forum* 3(14), 29–31.

Campanelli, P. C., Feferman, R., Keane, C., Lieberman, H. J., & Roberon, D. (2007). An advanced practice psychiatric nurse's guide to professional writing. *Perspectives in Psychiatric Care* 43(4), 163–73.

Drotar, D. (2000). Training professional psychologists to write and publish: The utility of a writers' workshop seminar. *Professional Psychology: Research and Practice* 31(4), 453–7.

Gerrish, K. (2005). Getting published: Practicalities, pitfalls and plagiarism. *Journal of Community Nursing* 19(8), 13–15.

Happell, B. (2008). Writing for publication: A practical guide. *Nursing Standard* 22(28), 35–40.

Hislop, J., Murray, R., & Newton, M. (2008). Writing for publication: A case study. *Practice Development in Health Care* 7(3), 156–63.

Hodges, B., & Casey, A. (2007). Writing for publication: A personal view. *Paediatric Nursing* 19(2), 35.

Keely, B. (2004). Planning and creating effective scientific posters. *Journal of Continuing Education in Nursing* 35(4), 182–5.

Keen, A. (2007). Writing for publication: Pressures, barriers and support strategies. *Nurse Education Today* 27, 382–8.

Lea, J., Cruickshank, M., Paliadelis, P., Parmenter, G., Sanderson, H., & Thornberry, P. (2008). The lure of the bush: Do rural placements influence student nurses to seek employment in rural settings? *Collegian* 15(3), 77–82.

Lea, J., Paliadelis, P., Parmenter, G., & Cruickshank, M. (2007). The lure of the bush: Are graduate nurses attracted to rural practice in Australia? *Evidence-Based Practice in Nursing: Paradigms and Dialogues Conference Proceedings*. Hong Kong, The Hong Kong Polytechnic University.

McIntyre, E., Eckermann, S., Keane, M., Magarey, A., & Roeger, L. (2007). Publishing in peer review journals: Criteria for success. *Australian Family Physician* 36(7), 561–2.

Miracle, V. A. (2003). Writing for publication: You can do it! *Dimensions of Critical Care Nursing* 22(1), 31–4.

NHMRC (National Health and Medical Research Council). (2007). *Australian Code for the Responsible Conduct of Research*. Canberra: Australian Government Publishing Service.

NSW Nursing & Midwifery Office 2009 Models of Care. Retrieved 9 October 2010, from <www.health.nsw.gov.au/nursing/practice_development.asp#para_4>

Paliadelis, P., & Parmenter, G. (2009). *An Exploration of the Capacity of General Practice Nurses to Improve the Prevention and Management of Childhood Obesity*. Royal College of Nursing Primary Health Care Conference, November, Adelaide.

Pierce, L. L. (2009). Writing for publication: You can do it! *Rehabilitation Nursing* 34(1), 3–8.

Reid, K., & Fuller, J. (2005). Building a culture of research dissemination in primary health care: The South Australian experience of supporting the novice researcher. *Australian Health Review* 29(1), 6–11.

Saver, C. (2006a). Reap the benefits of writing for publication. *AORN Journal* 8(3), 603–6.

Saver, C. (2006b). Finding and refining an article topic. *AORN Journal* 83(4), 829–32.

Saver, C. (2006c). Legal and ethical aspects of publishing. *AORN Journal* 84(4), 571–5.

Saver, C. (2006d). Tables and figures: Adding vitality to your article. *AORN Journal* 84(6), 945–50.

Taggart, H., & Arslanian, C. (2000). Creating an effective poster presentation. *Orthopaedic Nursing* 19(3), 47–9.

Wills, E. (2000). Strategies for managing barriers to the writing process. *Nursing Forum* 3(4), 5–13.

Woodward, V., Webb, C. & Prowse, M. (2007). The perceptions and experiences of nurses undertaking research in the clinical setting. *Journal of Research in Nursing* 12, 227–44.

Glossary

Abstract

A brief synopsis outlining the focus of a conference paper, article, report or poster and usually submitted for peer review.

Action research

A method of enquiry in which an individual or group actively engage as researchers in a process of change to address actual or emergent problems in their specific area of practice.

Alpha error

This implies that one falsely assumes a significant difference between groups, when in reality there is none.

Anonymity

Lack of personal identifiable information or no name.

Attribute

A quality or characteristic ascribed to a person or thing.

Audit

A process of observing and recording events or scrutinising pre-existing records for subsequent comparison to standards.

Autoethnography

The study of oneself within the context of the culture in which one lives.

Beneficence

This is the term used to mean 'doing good'.

Beta error

This implies that one fails to detect an existing difference as significant.

Bias

Any influence that produces distortion in the results of the study.

Bricolage

A research method that creatively amalgamates or synthesises a range of methodologies and strategies deemed appropriate by the researcher as the study unfolds in pursuit of the most robust and accurate explication of findings.

Case control study

A study that compares a group of well individuals with a group of individuals who have the illness or health condition of interest. The two groups are compared with respect to past exposure to risk factors.

Causality

A relationship of cause and effect. It has a minimum of three conditions: a strong relationship between the proposed cause and effect; the proposed cause must precede the effect in time; and the proposed cause must be present whenever the effect occurs.

Clarifying question

Simple questions of fact used to clarify the dilemma.

Closed-ended question

A question that limits responses to predetermined categories. A closed-ended question will normally be answered using a simple "yes/no", or "strongly agreed/agreed/strongly not agreed/not agreed".

Cluster sampling

A method where a random selection of a subset of usually geographically dispersed components of the population (hospitals) is made and forms the sample.

Code

A name given to data that has been broken into component parts.

Cohort study

A study in which a group free of illness is observed for exposure to risk factors that are hypothesised to increase or decrease the chance of getting the illness. The study group will be followed up through time in order to compare the frequency of the illness of groups who have different levels of exposure.

Collaboration

A creative process where two or more people or organisations work together to achieve a common goal.

Concept

A mental idea based on observations of behaviours or characteristics, for example pain and stress.

Concurrent mixed methods design

A design where the quantitative and qualitative data collection and data analysis are carried out in the same timeframe.

Conference

A meeting or gathering for discussion and sharing of ideas.

Confidence interval

A statement about the target population based on values derived from a sample. It tells us where the true value from the target population is likely to be.

Confidentiality

This is when the researcher promises to protect the identity of the participant either by allocating a code number or pseudonym to the participant.

Confounding

Confounding occurs when extraneous variables that are correlated to both the study factor and the outcome distort the bivariate association between study factor and outcome.

Confounding variable

An independent variable that varies systematically with the hypothetical causal variable under study. When uncontrolled, the effects of a confounding variable cannot be distinguished from those of the study variable.

Constant comparison

The process whereby the data and the concepts created from analysis are compared to ensure that they are a good fit and re-evaluated if they are not.

Construct

A construct (with the accent on the first syllable) is an object of perception used frequently in mental health research.

Construct validity

The extent to which a scale measures the underlying construct.

Content validity

The extent to which items on a scale reflect the concept being measured.

Convenience sampling

An approach where a researcher locates a sample that is 'convenient' or easily accessed.

Correlation study

A study that explores the interrelationship among study variables without any active intervention introduced by researchers.

Criterion validity

Used to evaluate whether or not a scale measures what it is supposed to measure by comparing it with another measure known to be valid.

Critical appraisal

A term used to assess the outcomes for evidence of a research study's effectiveness.

Critical social theory

A theory or an intellectual form that has criticism at the centre of its knowledge production. Broad range of ideas and frameworks are used to help people question, deconstruct, and then reconstruct knowledge.

Critical theory

A philosophical belief system and research method aimed at identifying unrecognised social structures and processes that lead to human oppression, preventing individual and group empowerment and emancipation.

Critique

To critique is to read and examine the strengths and limitations of a published study.

Crossover study

A study that administers more than one treatment sequentially to each participant so that comparison can be made of the effects of different treatments on a dependent variable for the same participant.

Cross-sectional study

A study based on observation of a phenomenon at a single time for the purpose of inferring trends over time.

Data extraction

A term used to describe the process of extracting the methods and results from existing research studies for further meta-analysis or presentation in summary tables within a systematic review.

Deductive approach

A method of moving from the general to the specific: from the macro to the micro.

Deductive hypothesis

A hypothesis that begins with theories as a starting point, which then are applied to particular situations.

Dependent variable

The outcome variable hypothesised to depend on or be caused by other independent variables.

Descriptive study

This aims to accurately describe characteristics of persons, places, situations or groups, and the frequency with which certain phenomena occur.

Dissemination

The circulation of your research, which means publishing it or presenting it as a conference paper.

Emphasis dimensions

These consider the status of the qualitative and quantitative element in the study.

Epidemiology

A discipline that describes, quantifies and postulates casual mechanisms for health phenomena in populations.

Epistemology

A philosophical discipline concerned with the ways in which people acquire knowledge about the world in which they live.

Equivalence or interrater reliability

This means comparing the degree to which two raters measuring the same event obtain the same results.

Ethnography

A qualitative research method designed to explore cultural patterns of behaviour—social interactions and associated meanings—for individuals, groups and communities.

Ethnomethodology

A research method designed to explore everyday routine activities or ways by which a group of people within a particular context make sense of their situation.

Ethnonursing

A research method used to explore and describe care patterns in cultures.

Evidence-based practice

A process that requires the practitioner to identify knowledge gaps, find research evidence to address knowledge gaps, and determine the relevance of the evidence to a particular client's situation.

Experimental research

Research in which researchers control and manipulate an independent variable in order to evaluate the resulting change of a dependent variable, and the researchers randomly assign participants to different conditions.

Extraneous variable

A variable that confounds the relationship between the independent and the dependent variables and that needs to be controlled either in the research design or through statistical procedures.

Familiarisation

The process of becoming familiar with the data. The process often begins by transcribing the data, reading and rereading the transcript and continuing on through the process of analysis.

Feminism

Feminism refers to a range of feminist thought and approaches to enquiry concerned with the social structures and processes that lead to gender inequality and oppression with the aim of achieving emancipation and equality.

Focus group

A focus group is a form of qualitative research in which a group of people are asked about their perceptions, opinions, beliefs and attitudes towards a study topic or question. Questions are asked in an interactive group setting where participants are free to talk with other group members.

Grey literature

Unpublished literature in the form of theses, government reports or conference proceedings.

Grounded theory

A systematic process of enquiry in which the researcher engages in a process of constant comparative analysis of data at each stage of the research process in order to generate theories about a particular phenomenon of concern.

Hermeneutics

The interpretation of information or data.

Heuristics

A process of internal search with the aim of exploring and discovering personal insights and understanding of a phenomenon of intense interest to the researcher.

Homogeneity or internal consistency

The extent (strength of association) to which all items in the scale measure the same concept or construct. The most commonly used test of consistency is the Cronbach's alpha coefficient.

Human research ethics committees (HRECs)

HRECs are established to approve human research ethics applications.

Human rights

In research this applies to the participant being fully informed about the research as well as being able to withdraw from participating at any stage.

Hypothesis

A hypothesis is a statement about the relationship between two variables (factors or characteristics in a study).

Impact factor

Calculated for each journal based on citation of articles across a year. The higher the impact factor the more widely read the journal is.

IMRaD

An acronym for Introduction, Method, Results and Discussion used when writing a research paper.

Independent variable

The variable expected to cause or influence the dependent variable. In an experimental study, researchers manipulate this independent variable.

Inductive approach

A method of moving from the specific to the general—from empirical data to theory generation.

Inductive hypothesis

A generalisation based on observed relationships.

Likert scale

Used to measure attitudes and beliefs. The degree of agreement or disagreement to a statement of a question is assigned a numerical value.

Measures of central tendency

These describe where the main part of the distribution of numerical data is. Measures of dispersion describe its variability.

Meta-analysis

A statistical method used to combine the results of several studies that address a set of related research hypotheses.

Meta-synthesis

A qualitative approach for drawing inferences from similar or related studies, identifying key features, and presenting findings representative of all data.

Method

The prescribed systematic procedures and protocols involved in carrying out a research project.

Methodology

The theoretical or philosophical framework that underpins and guides the research process throughout the study; the principles that embody a research approach and guide the researcher in the application of methods. The longer word is often used to mean just 'method', and the student needs to be aware of possible confusion here.

Mixed methods research

Research which systematically combines the collection and analysis of qualitative and quantitative data.

Model

A structure or framework designed to symbolise a concept or phenomenon.

Moral concerns

In carrying out our research with vulnerable people, researchers need to be more morally responsible for their lives and well-being in such a way that they are not making them even more vulnerable.

Multivariable procedures

Methods, most widely used in the health sciences, that enable the simultaneous assessment of the effects of several study factors on the outcome as well as adjustment for confounding.

Naturalist

One who is concerned with exploring phenomena as they occur in their natural setting.

Non-experimental research

Research in which researchers collect data without introducing any manipulation or change.

Non-maleficence

This is the term used to mean 'doing no harm'.

Non-participant observation (covert)

Observations of participants where they are not aware of being observed.

Non-participant observation (overt)

Observation of participants (with their full knowledge) by a researcher who does not take an active part in the situation.

Ontology

A philosophical discipline concerned with the beliefs people hold about the nature of reality and human existence.

Open-ended question

A form of question that requires the participant to answer in his or her own words. It allows a spontaneous, unstructured response and sometime called subjective question.

Paradigm

A worldview underpinned by philosophical assumptions and beliefs.

Parameter

The number or data that describe a population.

Participant observation

A method of qualitative research in which the researcher understands the contextual meanings of an event or events through participating and observing as a subject in the research. The degree of sharing in activities between the researcher and the participant ranges from full participation to onlooker.

Peer review

The process of subjecting scholarly work, research or ideas to the scrutiny of others who are peers in the same field or discipline area.

Peer-reviewed journal

A journal that publishes a paper that has been submitted to an editorial committee and passed by a process of blinded peer review before it is accepted for publication.

Phenomenology

A philosophical movement and a mode of enquiry that aims to understand the essential structures or essence of phenomena of individuals' everyday experiences.

Phenomenon

Any observable thing or occurrence that is worth noting; plural, phenomena.

Placebo effect

The reported response or change in the dependent variable by an individual who does not receive an intervention or receives an inert intervention.

Population

A complete set of persons or objects that possess some common characteristic of interest to a researcher.

Positivist

Someone who believes in the concepts of an objective reality and the notion of determinism.

Probability sampling

A method where each case has a similar opportunity of being selected.

Probing question

Question aimed to help the participant think more deeply about the study issue. It is used to search in-depth information or to examine thoroughly about the study topic.

Problem statement

A problem statement describes what the situation is that requires changing or understanding and how the study will address this situation or problem.

Program evaluation

A study that assesses how well a program is working. The evaluation can be a process or an outcome evaluation.

Psychometric scale

A set of written questions or statements designed to measure a particular concept such as anxiety or stress.

Publish

To disseminate literature or information to others, generally in a printed format.

Purposive sampling

Used where the researcher recruits participants to the study based on some attribute that the researcher feels is appropriate.

P-value

The p-value gives the probability that an observed difference (or an even larger difference) is attributable to chance alone. The p-value is the result of a statistical test. When a p-value is small (usually < 0.05) then the result is called statistically significant.

Qualitative research approach

A systematic and rigorous approach to the study of phenomena present in the social and relational world of human beings. It emphasises words rather than numbers in the process of data collection and analysis. The focus of qualitative research is on the generation of theories.

Qualitative research methods

Inductive research methods such as grounded theory, ethnography or phenomenology, which explore and emancipate human experience.

Quantitative data

These can be either categorical or numerical; statistical methods are directly linked to the type of data investigated.

Quantitative research

A systematic investigation with a rigorous and controlled design, using precise measurements and obtaining quantifiable information to answer a research question.

Quantitative research methods

Deductive research methods such as randomised control trials, quasi-experimental studies, cohort studies, observational, descriptive or exploratory designs. These methods test for cause and effect, explore relationships between variables and control variables.

Quasi-experimental research

Research in which the researchers manipulate an independent variable in order to evaluate the change of a dependent variable. However, not all of the following conditions are met in such a study: random allocation of treatment condition to participants, and a comparison group of participants to those who receive the manipulation. There is some control to increase the internal validity of the results.

Random selection

A sampling method in which every case has the same opportunity to be selected for the study.

Reliability

The degree of consistency or dependability with which an instrument measures the attribute it is intended to measure.

Research design

The overall plan for answering a research question, including an appropriate detailed plan for enhancing the integrity of the study.

Research hypothesis

A quantitatively stated and falsifiable scientific question which a study is designed to answer with statistical confidence.

Research proposal plan/protocol

A research proposal plan or protocol is the initial plan developed by the researcher to explain the research process to be undertaken.

Research question

A research question(s) represent(s) the question being asked by the research—the issue it sets out to explore.

Review protocol for systematic review

A well-defined document that provides explicit strategies to undertake a systematic review so that bias is reduced.

Risk

Risk refers to the level of either emotional or physical discomfort a potential participant may experience when being involved in research.

Sample

A subset of cases with the same characteristics as the original population.

Scholarship

The conduct of scholarly pursuits, usually within the academic world.

Searching the literature for a systematic review

A defined scope of literature with prior specification of eligibility criteria such as inclusion and exclusion criteria for a selected article.

Semantic differential scales

Scales designed to ask respondents their position or attitude to a concept using two adjectives at opposite ends of a continuum.

Semistructured interview

A flexible set of questions which allow new questions to be brought up during the interview as a result of what the participant says. The interviewer in a semi-structured interview generally has a framework of research topic to be explored.

Sequential mixed methods design

A design where the quantitative and qualitative data collection are in separate timeframes.

Stability or test-retest reliability

The ability of a scale to produce the same or similar results with the same group of participants on two (or more) occasions.

Statistic

The number or data that describe a sample.

Statistical hypothesis tests for difference

Procedures that allow the calculation of the likelihood of an observed difference between two or more groups that are compared.

Statistical inference

The ability of statistics to use information from a sample and transfer the results to a wider target population.

Stratified random selection

A sampling method where a similar proportion of cases to the population are selected in each stratum.

Structured interview

A formalised set of questions used to collect quantitative research data when the order in which questions are asked of survey respondents is standardised. It is also known as a standardised interview or a researcher-administered survey.

Systematic review

A method used to review the existing literature on a particular question, by identifying, appraising, selecting and synthesing all high-quality research evidence relevant to that question.

Systematic sampling

A method where every n th case (set interval) is selected from the population.

Target audience

The primary group of people who are most interested in the content of a conference paper or journal article.

Theme

A theme is generated when similar ideas from participants expressed in the data are brought together. The theme may be labelled using a word or expression taken directly from the data or else named by the researcher to best characterise the collection of data.

Theoretical sampling

A process where findings from a small number of cases determine theoretically important aspects that direct subsequent sample or case selection.

Theoretical saturation

The point at which no further data collection or coding is required because no new instances are to be found in the data.

Theory

A set of interrelated assumptions put forward to describe or explain a given phenomenon.

Time dimensions

These relate to when the phases of the mixed methods study are carried out.

Trianglulation

The process of integrating the results from multiple sources of data or research methods in the same study. The word is a metaphor from engineering surveying, where readings are taken from several viewpoints.

Type I error

An error where the null hypothesis is rejected when it is in fact true.

Type II error

The failure to reject the null hypothesis when the null hypothesis is false.

Unstructured interview

It is a method of interview where questions can be changed or adapted to meet the participant's understanding or belief. Questions can be influenced by each individual person's responses.

Validity

The degree to which a measurement instrument measures what it is intended to measure.

Variable

A characteristic or factor that will vary within a study (e.g. age, blood pressure, depression scores).

Visual Analogue Scale (VAS)

A straight line, 100 mm in length, with anchors representing the extremes of the particular concept being measured.

Vulnerable people

Individuals who are marginalised and discriminated against in society because of their social situation—class, ethnicity, gender, age, illness, disability, and sexual preferences. They are often difficult to reach and require special considerations when they are involved in research. The term is also used to refer to people who are difficult to access in societies.

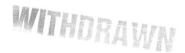

Index

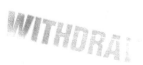